AMINO ACIDS: BIOCHEMISTRY AND NUTRITION

Edited by
Kristy June

ArclerPress

Amino Acids: Biochemistry and Nutrition

Edited by Kristy June

Edition 2018

Published by
Arcler Press LLC
708 3rd Avenue, 6th Floor
New York
NY 10017
United States of America
www.arclerpress.com

ISBN: 978-1-68094-521-8 (Hardback)

Printed in United States of America

Library of Congress Control Number: 2017933227

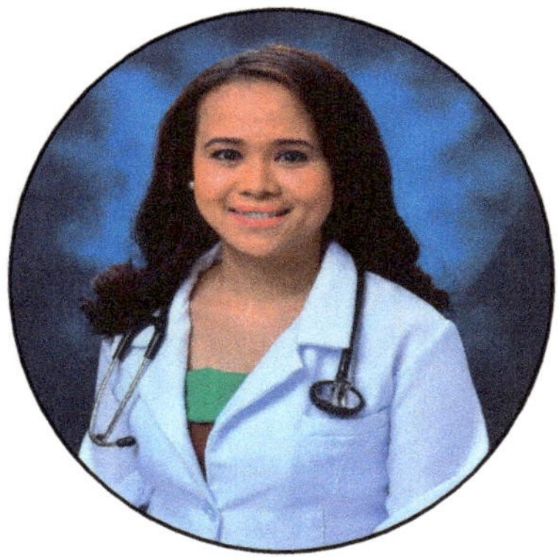

About the Editor

Kristy June

Kristy June is a Doctor of Medicine who also masters copyediting and proofreading scientific and academic research papers. She finished Bachelor of Science in Biology Major in Ecology and Entomology in the University of the Philippines Mindanao as her undergraduate degree where she started engaging herself into writing, editing and proofreading articles and books for publications. She is currently working as both a Medical Doctor and an Editor

Table of Contents

2 PEPTIDES: CLASSES AND SYNTHESIS

3 PROTEINOGENIC AMINO ACIDS

4 NON-PROTEINOGENIC AMINO ACIDS

5 PROTEIN CATABOLISM

6 GENETIC CODE

7 PEPTIDE SYNTHESIS

8 ESSENTIAL OF HUMAN NUTRITION/AMINO ACIDS

9 KETOGENIC AMINO ACID

List of Abbreviations

ALA	Alpha-Linolenic Acid
ATP	Adenosine Triphosphate
BV	Biological Value
BCAA	Branched-Chain Amino Acid
CSF	Cerebrospinal Fluid
CLIP	Corticotropin-Like Intermediate Peptide
DCC	Dicyclohexylcarbodiimide
DRI	Dietary Reference Intake
DIC	Diisopropylcarbodiimide
DMF	Dimethylformamide
DHA	Docosahexaenoic Acid
EPA	Eicosapentaenoic Acid
EMS	Eosinophilia-Myalgia Syndrome
FAO	Food and Agriculture Organization of the United Nations
FDA	Food and Drug Administration
GABA	Gamma-Amino-Butyric Acid
NIR	Near-Infrared Reflectance
PP	Pancreatic Polypeptide
PKU	Phenylketonuria
PEG	Polyethylene Glycol
PTM	Post-Translational Modification
PXR	Pregnane X receptors
POMC	Pro-Opiomelanocortin

PER	Protein Efficiency Ratio
SPPS	Solid-Phase Peptide Synthesis
SIP	Structure-Inducing Probes
tRNA	Transfer RNA
TFA	Trifluoroacetic Acid
TIPS	Triisopropylsilane

Preface

Proteins are large, complex molecules essential for the normal function of the human body, specifically in the structure, function and regulation of tissues and organs. They are made up of hundreds of smaller units called amino acids that are attached to one another by peptide bonds, forming a long chain. Amino acids form polymers through a nucleophilic attack by the amino group of an amino acid at the electrophilic carbonyl carbon of the carboxyl group of another amino acid. The carboxyl group of amino acid must first be activated to provide a better leaving group than OH-. The resulting link between amino acids is an amide link, which biochemists call a peptide bond. In this reaction, water is released. In reverse reaction, the peptide bond can be cleaved by water (hydrolysis). When two amino acids link together to form an amide link, the resulting structure is called a dipeptide. Likewise, we can have tripeptides, tetrapeptides, and other polypeptides. At some point, when the structure is long enough, it is called protein. There are many different ways to represent the structure of a polypeptide or protein, each showing different amount of information.

The key elements of an amino acid are carbon, hydrogen, oxygen, and nitrogen, though other elements are found in the side-chains of certain amino acids. They can be classified according to the core structural functional groups' locations as alpha- (α-), beta- (β-), gamma- (γ-) or delta- (δ-) amino acids; other categories relate to polarity, pH level, and side-chain group type (aliphatic, acyclic, aromatic, containing hydroxyl or sulfur, etc.). In different forms of proteins, amino acids comprise the second largest component (water is the largest) of human muscles, cells and other tissues. Outside proteins, amino acids perform critical roles in processes, such as neurotransmitter transport and biosynthesis.

In biochemistry, amino acids having both the amine and the carboxylic acid groups attached to the first (alpha-) carbon atom have particular importance. They are known as 2-, alpha-, or α-amino acids (generic formula H2NCHRCOOH in most cases, where R is an organic substituent known as a "side-chain"); often the term "amino acid" is used to refer specifically to these. Many important proteinogenic and non-proteinogenic amino acids also play a critical non-protein roles within the body. Because of their biological significance, amino acids are important in nutrition and are commonly used in nutritional supplements, fertilizers, and food technology. Industrial uses include the production of drugs, biodegradable plastics, and chiral catalysts.

Content Coverage

Chapter One introduces the general study of history and importance of amino acids. Because of their biological significance, amino acids are important in nutrition and are commonly used in nutritional supplements, fertilizers, and food technology. Industrial uses include the production of drugs, biodegradable plastics, and chiral catalysts.

Chapter Two presents an emphasis on peptides that are distinguished from proteins on the basis of size, and as an arbitrary benchmark can be understood to contain approximately 50 or fewer amino acids.

Chapters Three and *Four* discuss about the proteinogenic and non-proteinogenic amino acids, respectively. Throughout known life, there are 23 proteinogenic amino acids, 20 in the standard genetic code and an additional 3 that can be incorporated by special translation mechanisms, while non-proteinogenic, or "unnatural" amino acids are those not naturally encoded or found in the genetic code of any organisms.

Chapter Five presents a comprehensive study of protein metabolism that cause both the building, or synthesis, of amino acids into proteins and the breakdown, or catabolism, of proteins into amino acids.

Chapters Six and *Seven* are genetic code and peptide synthesis, separately. The genetic code is the set of rules by which information encoded within genetic material (DNA or mRNA sequences) is translated into proteins by living cells. Peptide synthesis is the production of peptides, which are organic compounds in which multiple amino acids are linked via amide bonds, also known as peptide bonds.

Chapters Eight and *Nine* discuss about essential human amino acids and ketogenic amino acid, respectively. The study of nutrition covers the types of food needed to keep an organism thriving and the means by which the organism derives nourishment by the digestive process.

CHAPTER 1

Amino Acid History and Structure

Chapter Contents

- **Introduction**
- **History**
- **General Structure**
- **Occurrence and Functions in Biochemistry**
- **Uses in Industry**
- **Physicochemical Properties of Amino Acids**

A large proportion of human cells, muscles and tissues are made up of Amino acids carry out many important bodily functions, such as providing cell structures. They also play a key role in the transport and storage of nutrients. Amino acids have an influence on the function of organs, glands, tendons and arteries. They are furthermore essential in healing wounds and repairing tissues, especially in the muscles, bones, skin and hair, as well as for the removal of all kinds of waste deposits produced in connection with the metabolism.

INTRODUCTION

Amino acids are biologically important organic compounds containing amine ($-NH_2$) and carboxyl (-COOH) functional groups, along with a side chain (R group) specific to each amino acid. The key elements of an amino acid are carbon, hydrogen, oxygen, and nitrogen, though other elements are found in the side chains of certain amino acids. About 500 amino acids are known (though only 20 appear in the genetic code) and can be classified in many ways. They can be classified according to the core structural functional groups' locations as alpha- (α-), beta- (β-), gamma- (γ-) or delta- (δ-) amino acids; other categories relate to polarity, pH level, and side chain group type (aliphatic, acyclic, aromatic, containing hydroxyl or sulfur, etc.). In the form of proteins, amino acids comprise the second largest component (water is the largest) of human muscles, cells and other tissues. Outside proteins, amino acids perform critical roles in processes, such as neurotransmitter transport and biosynthesis.

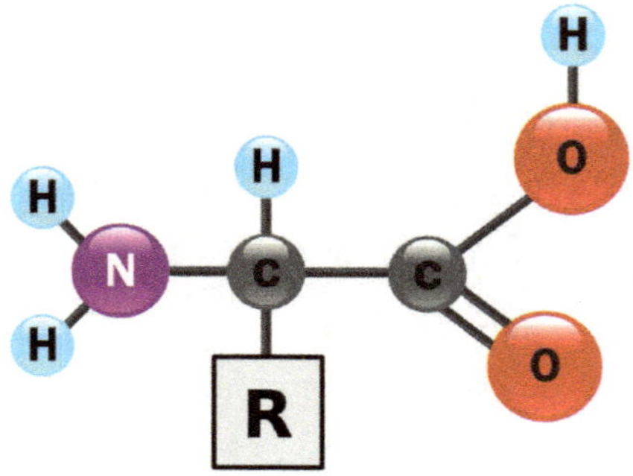

Structure of an Alpha Amino Acid in its Unionized Form

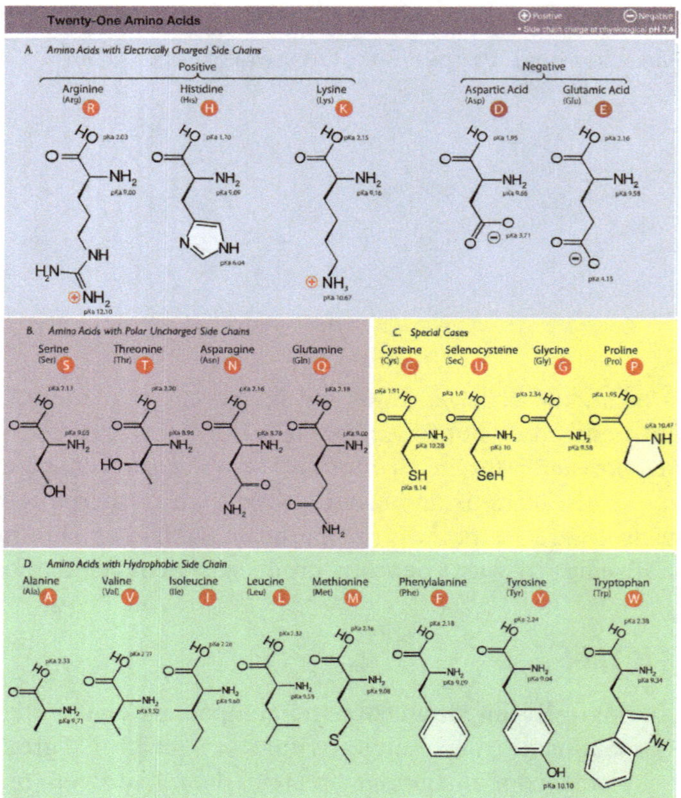

21 proteinogenic α-amino acids found in eukaryotes, grouped according to their side-chains' pK_a values and charges carried at physiological pH 7.4

In biochemistry, amino acids having both the amine and the carboxylic acid groups attached to the first (alpha-) carbon atom have particular importance. They are known as **2-, alpha-,** or **α-amino acids** (generic formula $H_2NCHRCOOH$ in most cases, where R is an organic substituent known as a "side-chain); often the term "amino acid is used to refer specifically to these. They include the 23 proteinogenic ("protein-building") amino acids, which combine into peptide chains ("polypeptides") to form the building blocks of a vast array of proteins. These are all L-stereoisomers ("left-handed isomers), although a few D-amino acids ("right-handed") occur in bacterial envelopes, as neuromodulator (D-serine), and in some antibiotics. Twenty of the proteinogenic amino acids are encoded directly by triplet codons in the genetic code and are known as "standard" amino acids. The other three ("non-standard" or "non-canonical") are selenocysteine (present in many noneukaryotes as well as most eukaryotes, but not coded directly by DNA), pyrrolysine (found only in some archea and one bacterium) and *N*-formylmethionine (which is often the initial amino acid of proteins in bacteria, mitochondria, and chloroplasts). Pyrrolysine and selenocysteine are encoded via variant codons; for example, selenocysteine is encoded by stop codon and SECIS element. Codon–tRNA combinations not found in nature can also be used to expand the genetic code and create novel proteins known as alloproteins incorporating non-proteinogenic amino acids.

Many important proteinogenic and non-proteinogenic amino acids also play critical non-protein roles within the body. For example, in the human brain, glutamate (standard glutamic acid) and gamma-amino-butyric acid ("GABA", non-standard gamma-amino acid) are, respectively, the main excitatory and inhibitory neurotransmitters; hydroxyproline (a major component of the connective tissue collagen) is synthesised from proline; the standard amino acid glycine is used to synthesise porphyrins used in red blood cells; and the non-standard carnitine is used in lipid transport.

Nine proteinogenic amino acids are called "essential for humans because they cannot be created from other compounds by the human body and so must be taken in as food. Others may be conditionally essential for certain ages or medical conditions. Essential amino acids may also differ between species. Because of their biological significance, amino acids are important in nutrition and are commonly used in nutritional supplements, fertilizers, and food technology. Industrial uses include the production of drugs, biodegradable plastics, and chiral catalysts.

HISTORY

The first few amino acids are discovered in the early 19th century. In 1806, French chemists, Louis-Nicolas Vauquelin and Pierre Jean Robiquet isolated, a compound in asparagus that was subsequently named asparagine, the first amino acid discovered. Cystine was discovered in 1810, although its monomer, cysteine, remained undiscovered until 1884. Glycine and leucine were discovered in 1820. The last of the 20 common amino acids to be discovered was threonine in 1935 by William Cumming Rose, who also determined the essential amino acids and established the minimum daily requirements of all amino acids for optimal growth.

Usage of the term *amino acid* in the English language is from 1898. Proteins were found to yield amino acids after enzymatic digestion or acid hydrolysis. In 1902, Emil

Fischer and Franz Hofmeister proposed that proteins are the result of the formation of bonds between the amino group of one amino acid with the carboxyl group of another, in a linear structure that Fischer termed "peptide".

GENERAL STRUCTURE

In the structure shown at the top of the page, **R** represents a side chain specific to each amino acid. The carbon atom next to the carboxyl group (which is therefore numbered 2 in the carbon chain starting from that functional group) is called the α–carbon. Amino acids containing an amino group bonded directly to the alpha carbon are referred to as *alpha amino acids*.These include amino acids such as proline which contain secondary amines, which used to be often referred to as "imino acids".

Isomerism

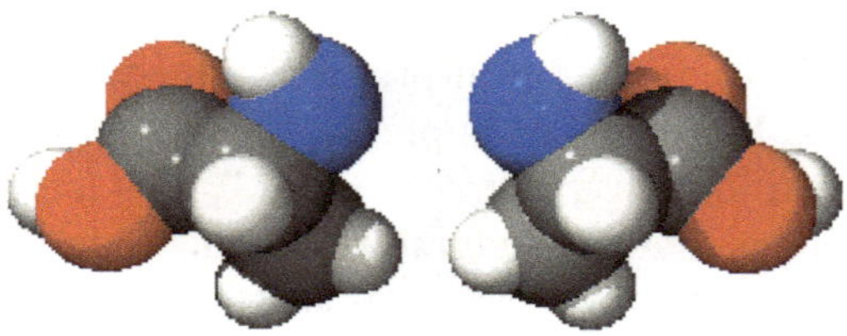

Two enantiomers of alanine, D-alanine and L-alanine.

The alpha amino acids are the most common form found in nature, but only when occurring in the L-isomer. The alpha carbon is a chiral carbon atom, with the exception of glycine which has two indistinguishable hydrogen atoms on the alpha carbon.Therefore, all alpha amino acids but glycine can exist in either of two enantiomers, called L or D amino acids, which are mirror images of each other (*see also Chirality*). While L-amino acids represent all of the amino acids found in proteins during translation in the ribosome, D-amino acids are found in some proteins produced by enzyme posttranslational modifications after translation and translocation to the endoplasmic reticulum, as in exotic sea-dwelling organisms such as cone snails. They are also abundant components of the peptidoglycan cell walls of bacteria, and D-serine may act as a neurotransmitter in the brain. D-amino acids are used in racemic crystallography to create centrosymmetric crystals, which (depending on the protein) may allow for easier and more robust protein structure determination. The L and D convention for amino acid configuration refers not to the optical activity of the amino acid itself but rather to the optical activity of the isomer of glyceraldehyde from which that amino acid can, in theory, be synthesized (D-glyceraldehyde is dextrorotatory; L-glyceraldehyde is levorotatory). In alternative fashion, the *(S)* and *(R)* designators are used to indicate the absolute stereochemistry.

Almost all of the amino acids in proteins are *(S)* at the α carbon, with cysteine being *(R)* and glycine non-chiral. Cysteine has its side chain in the same geometric position as the other amino acids, but the *R/S* terminology is reversed because of the higher atomic number of sulfur compared to the carboxyl oxygen gives the side chain a higher priority, whereas the atoms in most other side chains give them lower priority.

Side Chains

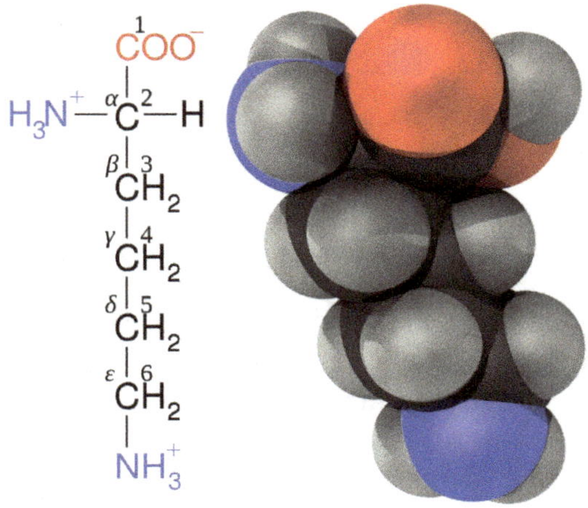

Lysine with carbon atoms

In amino acids that have carbon chain attached to the α–carbon (such as lysine, shown in the right) the carbons are labeled in order as α, β, γ, δ, and so on. In some amino acids, the amine group is attached to the β or γ-carbon, and these are therefore referred to as *beta* or *gamma amino acids*.

Amino acids are usually classified by the properties of their side chain into four groups. The side-chain can make an amino acid a weak acid or a weak base, and a hydrophile if the side-chain is polar or a hydrophobe if it is nonpolar. The chemical structures of the 22 standard amino acids, along with their chemical properties, are described more fully in the article on these proteinogenic amino acids.

The phrase branched-chain amino acids or BCAA refers to the amino acids having aliphatic side-chains that are non-linear; these are leucine, isoleucine, and valine. Proline is the only proteinogenic amino acid whose side-group links to the α-amino group and, thus, is also the only proteinogenic amino acid containing a secondary amine at this position. In chemical terms, proline is, therefore, an imino acid, since it lacks a primary amino group, although it is still classed as an amino acid in the current biochemical nomenclature, and may also be called an N-alkylated alpha-amino acid.

Zwitterions

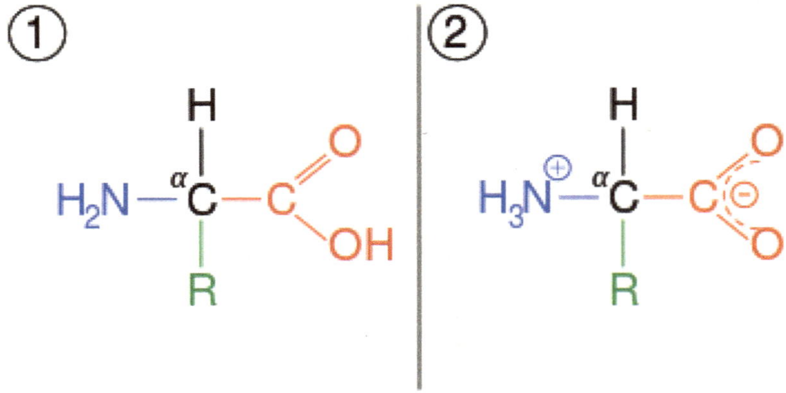

Amino acid in its (1) unionized and (2) zwitterionic forms

The α-carboxylic acid group of amino acids is a weak acid, meaning that it releases a hydron (such as a proton) at moderate pH values. In other words, carboxylic acid groups ($-CO_2H$) can be deprotonated to become negative carboxylates ($-CO_2^-$). The negatively charged carboxylate ion predominates at pH values greater than the pKa of the carboxylic acid group (mean for the 20 common amino acids is about 2.2, see the table of amino acid structures above). In a complementary fashion, the α-amine of amino acids is a weak base, meaning that it accepts a proton at moderate pH values. In other words, α-amino groups (NH_2-) can be protonated to become positive α-ammonium groups ($^+NH_3-$). The positively charged α-ammonium group predominates at pH values less than the pKa of the α-ammonium group (mean for the 20 common α-amino acids is about 9.4).

Because all amino acids contain amine and carboxylic acid functional groups, they share amphiprotic properties. Below pH 2.2, the predominant form will have a neutral carboxylic acid group and a positive α-ammonium ion (net charge +1), and above pH 9.4, a negative carboxylate and neutral α-amino group (net charge −1). But at pH between 2.2 and 9.4, an amino acid usually contains both a negative carboxylate and a positive α-ammonium group, as shown in structure (2) on the right, so has net zero charge. This molecular state is known as a zwitterion, from the German **Zwitter** meaning *hermaphrodite* or *hybrid*.The fully neutral form (structure (1) on the right) is a very minor species in aqueous solution throughout the pH range (less than 1 part in 10^7). Amino acids exist as zwitterions also in the solid phase, and crystallize with salt-like properties unlike typical organic acids or amines.

Isoelectric Point

The variation in titration curves when amino acids are grouped by category can be seen here. With the exception of tyrosine, using titration to differentiate between hydrophobic amino acids is problematic.

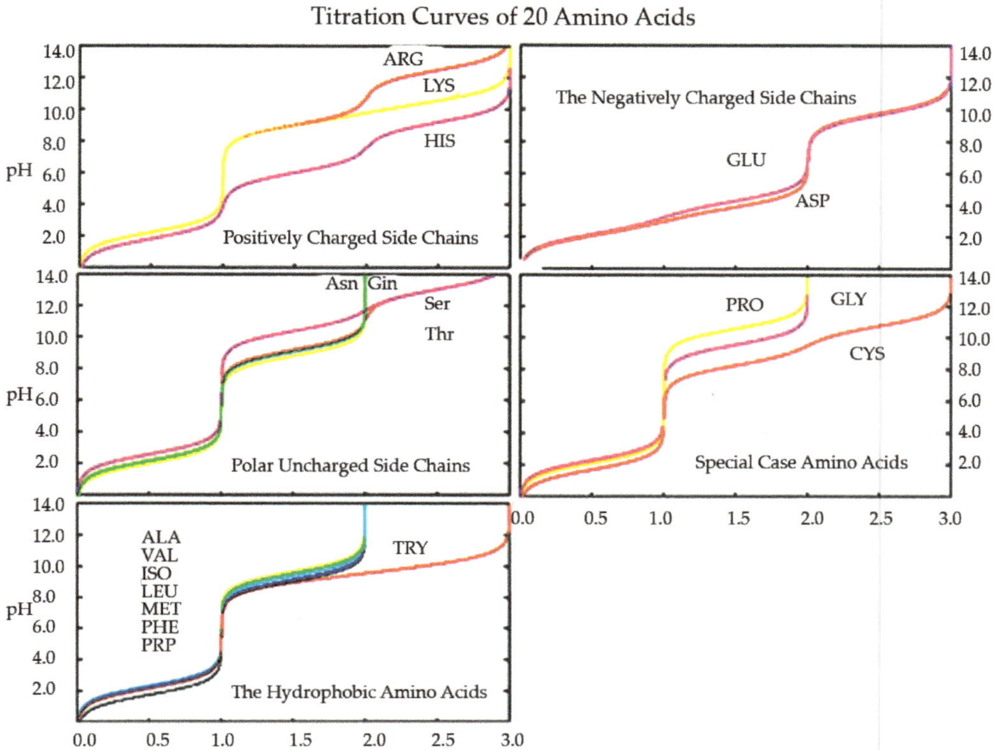

Composite of titration curves of twenty proteinogenic amino acids grouped by side chain category.

At pH values between the two pKa values, the zwitterion predominates, but coexists in dynamic equilibrium with small amounts of net negative and net positive ions. At the exact midpoint between the two pKa values, the trace amount of net negative and trace of net positive ions exactly balance, so that average net charge of all forms present is zero. This pH is known as the isoelectric point pI, so pI = ½(pKa_1 + pKa_2). The individual amino acids all have slightly different pKa values, so have different isoelectric points. For amino acids with charged side chains, the pKa of the side-chain is involved. Thus for Asp, Glu with negative side chains, pI = ½(pKa_1 + pKa_R), where pKa_R is the side chain pKa. Cysteine also has potentially negative side chain with pKa_R = 8.14, so pI should be calculated as for Asp and Glu, even though the side-chain is not significantly charged at neutral pH. For His, Lys, and Arg with positive side chains, pI = ½(pKa_R + pKa_2). Amino acids have zero mobility in electrophoresis at their isoelectric point, although this behaviour is more usually exploited for peptides and proteins than single amino acids. Zwitterions have minimum solubility at their isoelectric point and some amino acids (in particular, with non polar side chains) can be isolated by precipitation from water by adjusting the pH to the required isoelectric point.

OCCURRENCE AND FUNCTIONS IN BIOCHEMISTRY

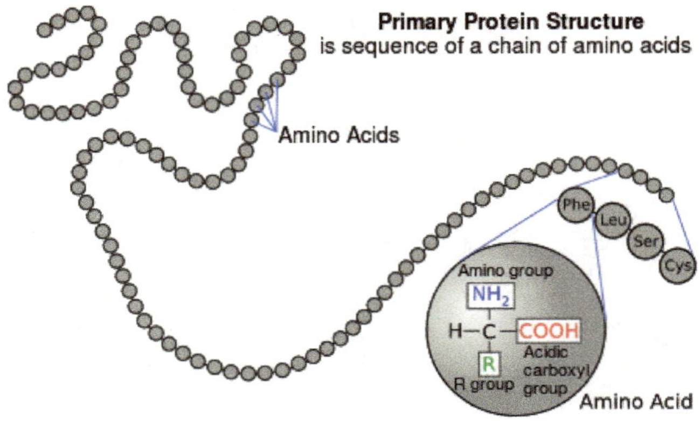

Polypeptide, an unbranched chain amino acid

Proteinogenic Amino Acids

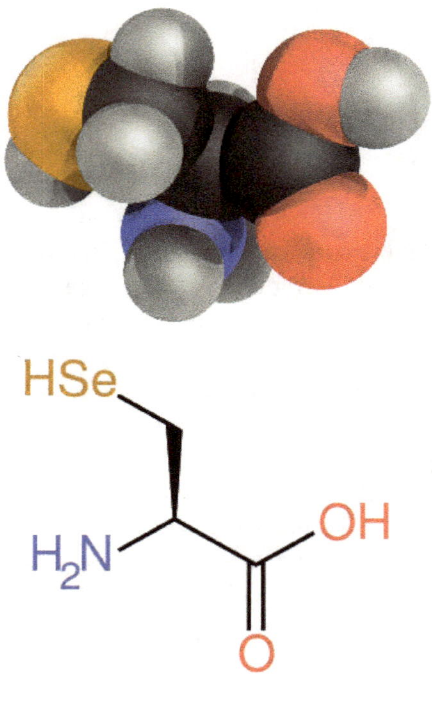

Selenocysteine

Amino acids are the structural units (monomers) that make up proteins. They join together to form short polymer chains called peptides or longer chains called either polypeptides or proteins. These polymers are linear and unbranched, with each amino acid within the chain attached to two neighboring amino acids. The process of making proteins is called *translation* and involves the step-by-step addition of amino acids to a growing protein chain by a ribozyme that is called a ribosome. The order in which the amino acids are added is read through the genetic code from an mRNA template, which is a RNA copy of one of the organism's genes.

Twenty-two amino acids are naturally incorporated into polypeptides and are called proteinogenic or natural amino acids. Of these, 20 are encoded by the universal genetic code. The remaining 2, selenocysteine and pyrrolysine, are incorporated into proteins by unique synthetic mechanisms. Selenocysteine is incorporated when the mRNA being translated includes a SECIS element, which causes the UGA codon to encode selenocysteine instead of a stop codon. Pyrrolysine is used by some methanogenic archaea in enzymes that they use to produce methane. It is coded for with the codon UAG, which is normally a stop codon in other organisms. This UAG codon is followed by a PYLIS downstream sequence.

Non-Proteinogenic Amino Acids

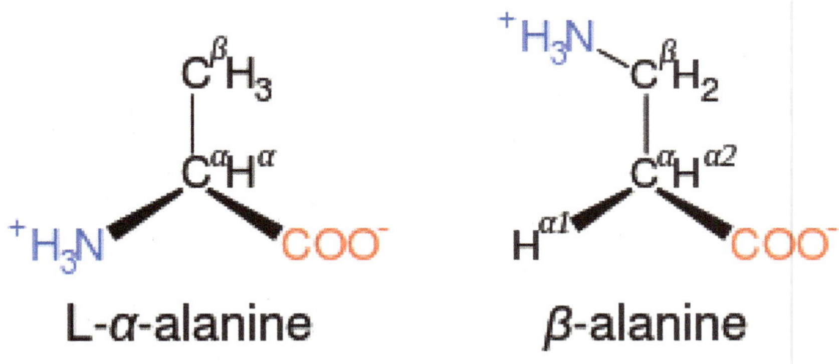

β-alanine and its α-alanine isomer

Aside from the 22 proteinogenic amino acids, there are other amino acids that are called *non-proteinogenic*. Those either are not found in proteins (for example, carnitine, GABA) or are not produced directly and in isolation by standard cellular machinery (for example, hydroxyproline and selenomethionine).

Non-proteinogenic amino acids that are found in proteins are formed by post-translational modification, which is modification after translation during protein synthesis.

These modifications are often essential for the function or regulation of a protein; for example, the carboxylation of glutamate allows for better binding of calcium cations, and the hydroxylation of proline is critical for maintaining connective tissues. Another example is the formation of hypusine in the translation initiation factor EIF5A, through modification of a lysine residue. Such modifications can also determine the localization of the protein, e.g., the addition of long hydrophobic groups can cause a protein to bind to a phospholipid membrane.

Some non-proteinogenic amino acids are not found in proteins. Examples include 2-aminoisobutyric acid and the neurotransmitter gamma-aminobutyric acid. Non-proteinogenic amino acids often occur as intermediates in the metabolic pathways for standard amino acids – for example, ornithine and citrulline occur in the urea cycle, part of amino acid catabolism (see below). A rare exception to the dominance of α-amino acids in biology is the β-amino acid beta alanine (3-aminopropanoic acid), which is used in plants and microorganisms in the synthesis of pantothenic acid (vitamin B_5), a component of coenzyme A.

D-Amino Acid Natural Abundance

D-isomers are uncommon in live organisms. For instance, gramicidin is a polypeptide made up from mixture of d- and l-amino acids. Other compounds containing D-amino acid are tyrocidine and valinomycin. These compounds disrupt bacterial cell walls, particularly in Gram-positive bacteria. Only 837 d-amino acids were found in Swiss-Prot database (187 million amino acids analysed).

Non-Standard Amino Acids

The 20 amino acids that are encoded directly by the codons of the universal genetic code are called *standard* or *canonical* amino acids. The others are called *non-standard* or *non-canonical*. Most of the non-standard amino acids are also non-proteinogenic (i.e. they cannot be used to build proteins), but three of them are proteinogenic, as they can be used to build proteins by exploiting information not encoded in the universal genetic code.

The three non-standard proteinogenic amino acids are selenocysteine (present in many non-eukaryotes as well as most eukaryotes, but not coded directly by DNA), pyrrolysine (found only in some archaea and one bacterium), and *N*-formylmethionine (which is often the initial amino acid of proteins in bacteria, mitochondria, and chloroplasts). For example, 25 human proteins include selenocysteine (Sec) in their primary structure, and the structurally characterized enzymes (selenoenzymes) employ Sec as the catalytic moiety in their active sites. Pyrrolysine and selenocysteine are encoded via variant codons. For example, selenocysteine is encoded by stop codon and SECIS element.

In Human Nutrition

When taken up into the human body from the diet, the 20 standard amino acids either are used to synthesize proteins and other biomolecules or are oxidized to urea and carbon dioxide as a source of energy. The oxidation pathway starts with the removal of the amino group by a transaminase; the amino group is then fed into the urea cycle. The other product of transamidation is a keto acid that enters the citric acid cycle. Glucogenic amino acids can also be converted into glucose, through gluconeogenesis. Of the 20 standard amino acids, nine (His, Ile, Leu, Lys, Met, Phe, Thr, Trp and Val), are called essential amino acids because the human body cannot synthesize them from other compounds at the level needed for normal growth, so they must be obtained from food. In addition, cysteine, taurine, tyrosine, and arginine are considered semiessential amino-acids in children (though taurine is not technically an amino acid), because the metabolic pathways that synthesize these amino acids are not fully developed. The amounts required also depend on the age and health of the individual, so it is hard to make general statements about the dietary requirement for some amino acids. Dietary exposure to the non-standard amino acid BMAA has been linked to human neurodegenerative diseases, including ALS.

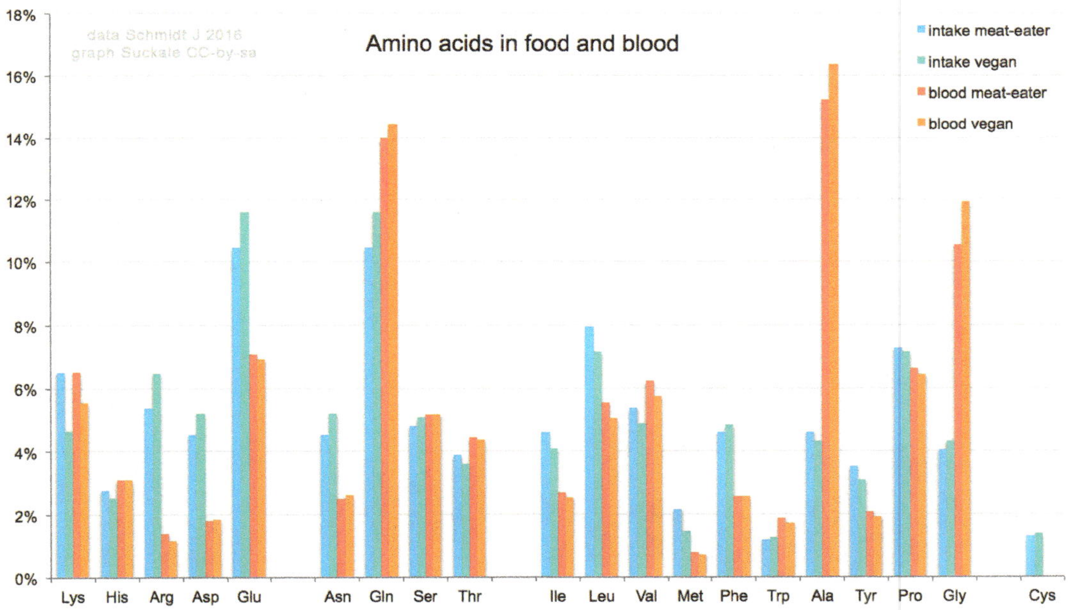

Share of amino acid in different human diets and the resulting mix of amino acids in human blood serum. Glutamate and glutamine are the most frequent in food at over 10%, while alanine, glutamine, and glycine are the most common in blood.

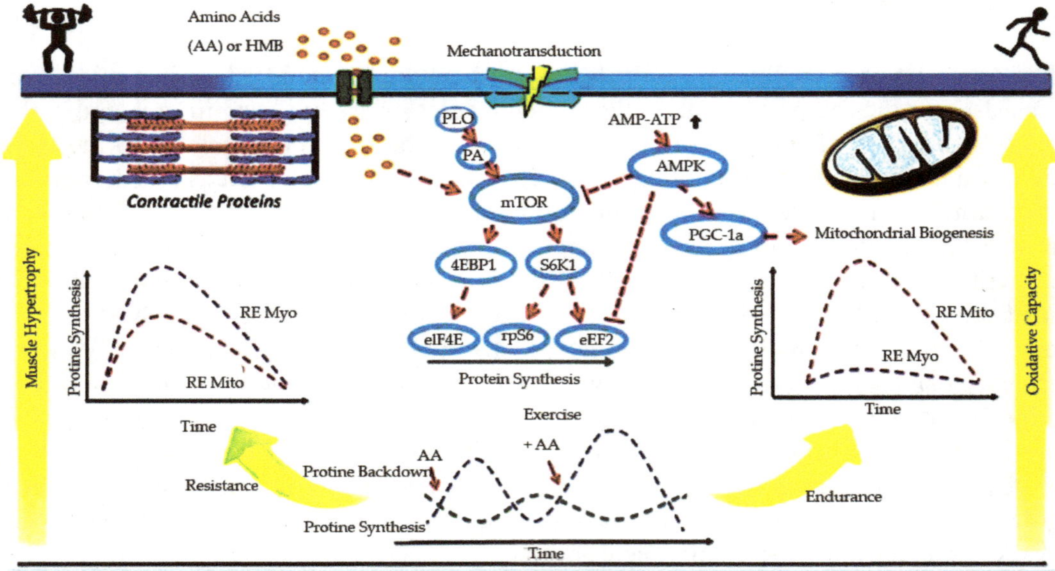

Diagram of the molecular signaling cascades that are involved in myofibrillar muscle protein synthesis and mitochondrial biogenesis in response to physical exercise and specific amino acids or their derivatives. Many amino acids derived from food protein promote the activation of mTORC1 and increase protein synthesis by signaling through Rag GTPases.

Abbreviations and Representations

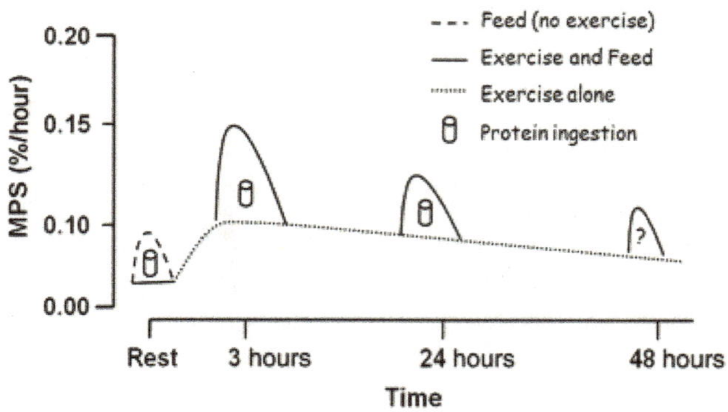

Resistance training stimulates muscle protein synthesis (MPS) for a period of up to 48 hours following exercise (shown by dotted line). Ingestion of a protein-rich meal at any point during this period will augment the exercise-induced increase in muscle protein synthesis (shown by solid lines).

Non-Protein Functions

Biosynthetic Pathways for Catecholamines and Trace Amines in the Human Brain

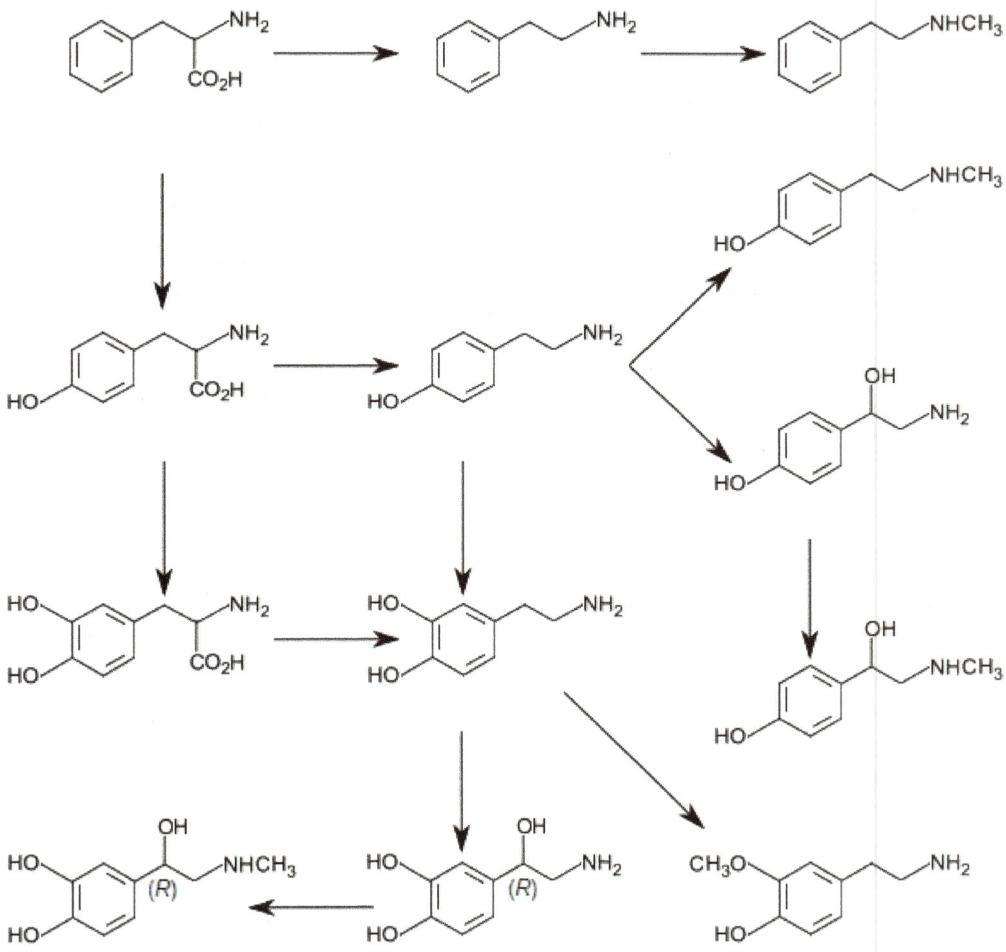

Catecholamines and trace amines are synthesized from phenylalanine and tyrosine in humans.

In humans, non-protein amino acids also have important roles as metabolic intermediates, such as in the biosynthesis of the neurotransmitter gamma-amino-butyric acid (GABA). Many amino acids are used to synthesize other molecules, for example:

- Tryptophan is a precursor of the neurotransmitter serotonin.

- Tyrosine (and its precursor phenylalanine) are precursors of the catecholamineneurotransmittersdopamine, epinephrine and norepinephrine and various trace amines.
- Phenylalanine is a precursor of phenethylamine and tyrosine in humans. In plants, it is a precursor of various phenylpropanoids, which are important in plant metabolism.
- Glycine is a precursor of porphyrins such as heme.
- Arginine is a precursor of nitric oxide.
- Ornithine and S-adenosylmethionine are precursors of polyamines.
- Aspartate, glycine, and glutamine are precursors of nucleotides.

However, not all of the functions of other abundant non-standard amino acids are known.

Some non-standard amino acids are used as defenses against herbivores in plants. For example, canavanine is an analogue of arginine that is found in many legumes, and in particularly large amounts in *Canavalia gladiata* (sword bean). This amino acid protects the plants from predators such as insects and can cause illness in people if some types of legumes are eaten without processing. The non-protein amino acid mimosine is found in other species of legume, in particular *Leucaena leucocephala*. This compound is an analogue of tyrosine and can poison animals that graze on these plants.

USES IN INDUSTRY

Amino acids are used for a variety of applications in industry, but their main use is as additives to animal feed. This is necessary, since many of the bulk components of these feeds, such as soybeans, either have low levels or lack some of the essential amino acids: lysine, methionine, threonine, and tryptophan are most important in the production of these feeds. In this industry, amino acids are also used to chelate metal cations in order to improve the absorption of minerals from supplements, which may be required to improve the health or production of these animals.

The food industry is also a major consumer of amino acids, in particular, glutamic acid, which is used as a flavor enhancer,and aspartame (aspartyl-phenylalanine-1-methyl ester) as a low-calorie artificial sweetener. Similar technology to that used for animal nutrition is employed in the human nutrition industry to alleviate symptoms of mineral deficiencies, such as anemia, by improving mineral absorption and reducing negative side effects from inorganic mineral supplementation.

The chelating ability of amino acids has been used in fertilizers for agriculture to facilitate the delivery of minerals to plants in order to correct mineral deficiencies, such as iron chlorosis. These fertilizers are also used to prevent deficiencies from occurring and improving the overall health of the plants. The remaining production of amino acids is used in the synthesis of drugs and cosmetics.

Similarly, some amino acids derivatives are used in pharmaceutical industry. They include 5-HTP (5-hydroxytryptophan) used for experimental treatment of depression,

L-DOPA (L-dihydroxyphenylalanine) for Parkinson's treatment, and eflornithine drug that inhibits ornithine decarboxylase and used in the treatment of sleeping sickness.

Expanded Genetic Code

Since 2001, 40 non-natural amino acids have been added into protein by creating a unique codon (recoding) and a corresponding transfer-RNA:aminoacyl – tRNA-synthetase pair to encode it with diverse physicochemical and biological properties in order to be used as a tool to exploring protein structure and function or to create novel or enhanced proteins.

Nullomers

Nullomers are codons that in theory code for an amino acid, however in nature there is a selective bias against using this codon in favor of another, for example bacteria prefer to use CGA instead of AGA to code for arginine. This creates some sequences that do not appear in the genome. This characteristic can be taken advantage of and used to create new selective cancer-fighting drugs and to prevent cross-contamination of DNA samples from crime-scene investigations.

Chemical Building Blocks

Amino acids are important as low cost feedstocks. These compounds are used in chiral pool synthesis as enantiomerically pure building blocks.

Amino acids have been investigated as precursors chiral catalysts, e.g., for asymmetric hydrogenation reactions, although no commercial applications exist.

Biodegradable Plastics

Amino acids are under development as components of a range of biodegradable polymers. These materials have applications as environmentally friendly packaging and in medicine in drug delivery and the construction of prosthetic implants. These polymers include polypeptides, polyamides, polyesters, polysulfides, and polyurethanes with amino acids either forming part of their main chains or bonded as side chains. These modifications alter the physical properties and reactivities of the polymers. An interesting example of such materials is polyaspartate, a water-soluble biodegradable polymer that may have applications in disposable diapers and agriculture. Due to its solubility and ability to chelate metal ions, polyaspartate is also being used as a biodegradeable antiscaling agent and a corrosion inhibitor. In addition, the aromatic amino acid tyrosine is being developed as a possible replacement for toxic phenols such as bisphenol A in the manufacture of polycarbonates.

Reactions

As amino acids have both a primary amine group and a primary carboxyl group, these chemicals can undergo most of the reactions associated with these functional groups. These include nucleophilic addition, amide bond formation, and imine formation for the amine group, and esterification, amide bond formation, and decarboxylation for the carboxylic acid group.The combination of these functional groups allow amino acids to be effective polydentate ligands for metal-amino acid chelates. The multiple side-chains of amino acids can also undergo chemical reactions. The types of these reactions are determined by the groups on these sidechains and are, therefore, different between the various types of amino acid.

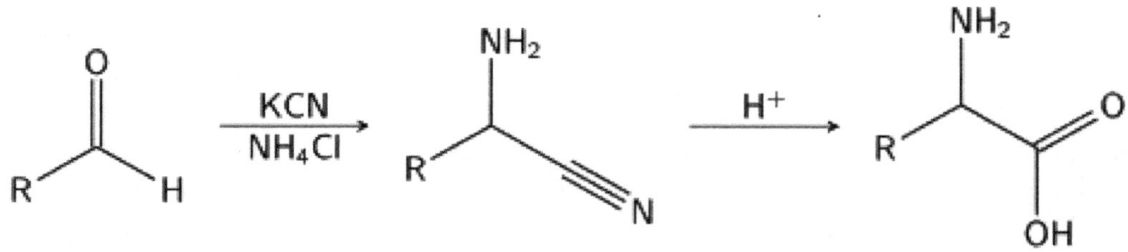

The Strecker amino acid synthesis.

Chemical Synthesis

Several methods exist to synthesize amino acids. One of the oldest methods begins with the bromination at the α-carbon of a carboxylic acid. Nucleophilic substitution with ammonia then converts the alkyl bromide to the amino acid. In alternative fashion, the Strecker amino acid synthesis involves the treatment of an aldehyde with potassium cyanide and ammonia, this produces an α-amino nitrile as an intermediate. Hydrolysis of the nitrile in acid then yields a α-amino acid. Using ammonia or ammonium salts in this reaction gives unsubstituted amino acids, whereas substituting primary and secondary amines will yield substituted amino acids. Likewise, using ketones, instead of aldehydes, gives α,α-disubstituted amino acids. The classical synthesis gives racemic mixtures of α-amino acids as products, but several alternative procedures using asymmetric auxiliaries or asymmetric catalysts have been developed.

At the current time, the most-adopted method is an automated synthesis on a solid support (e.g., polystyrene beads), using protecting groups (e.g., Fmoc and t-Boc) and activating groups (e.g., DCC and DIC).

Peptide Bond Formation

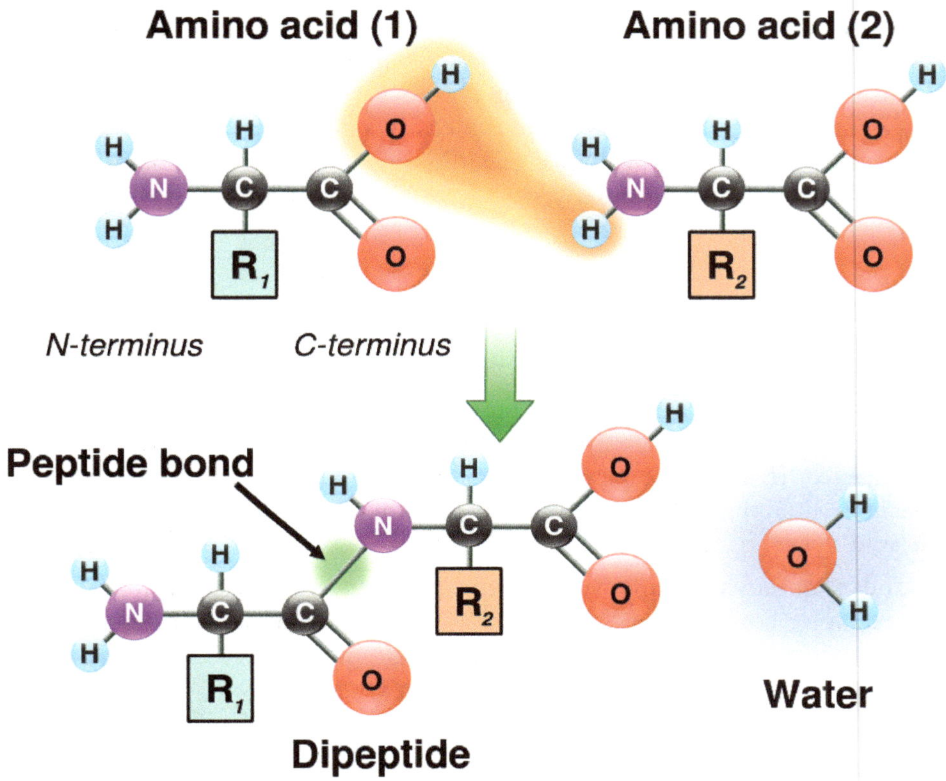

condensation of two amino acids to form a *dipeptide* through a *peptide bond*

As both the amine and carboxylic acid groups of amino acids can react to form amide bonds, one amino acid molecule can react with another and become joined through an amide linkage. This polymerization of amino acids is what creates proteins. This condensation reaction yields the newly formed peptide bond and a molecule of water. In cells, this reaction does not occur directly; instead, the amino acid is first activated by attachment to a transfer RNA molecule through an ester bond. This aminoacyl-tRNA is produced in an ATP-dependent reaction carried out by an aminoacyl tRNA synthetase. This aminoacyl-tRNA is then a substrate for the ribosome, which catalyzes the attack of the amino group of the elongating protein chain on the ester bond. As a result of this mechanism, all proteins made by ribosomes are synthesized starting at their N-terminus and moving toward their C-terminus.

However, not all peptide bonds are formed in this way. In a few cases, peptides are synthesized by specific enzymes. For example, the tripeptide glutathione is an essential part of the defenses of cells against oxidative stress. This peptide is synthesized in two steps from free amino acids. In the first step, gamma-glutamylcysteine synthetase condenses cysteine and glutamic acid through a peptide bond formed between the side-chain carboxyl of the glutamate (the gamma carbon of this side chain) and the amino group of the cysteine. This dipeptide is then condensed with glycine by glutathione synthetase to form glutathione.

In chemistry, peptides are synthesized by a variety of reactions. One of the most-used in solid-phase peptide synthesis uses the aromatic oxime derivatives of amino acids as activated units. These are added in sequence onto the growing peptide chain, which is attached to a solid resin support. The ability to easily synthesize vast numbers of different peptides by varying the types and order of amino acids (using combinatorial chemistry) has made peptide synthesis particularly important in creating libraries of peptides for use in drug discovery through high throughout screening.

Biosynthesis

In plants, nitrogen is first assimilated into organic compounds in the form of glutamate, formed from alpha-ketoglutarate and ammonia in the mitochondrion. In order to form other amino acids, the plant uses transaminases to move the amino group to another alpha-keto carboxylic acid. For example, aspartate aminotransferase converts glutamate and oxaloacetate to alpha-ketoglutarate and aspartate. Other organisms use transaminases for amino acid synthesis, too.

Nonstandard amino acids are usually formed through modifications to standard amino acids. For example, homocysteine is formed through the transsulfuration pathway or by the demethylation of methionine via the intermediate metabolite S-adenosyl methionine, while hydroxyproline is made by a posttranslational modification of proline.

Microorganisms and plants can synthesize many uncommon amino acids. For example, some microbes make 2-aminoisobutyric acid and lanthionine, which is a sulfide-bridged derivative of alanine. Both of these amino acids are found in peptidic lantibiotics such as alamethicin. However, in plants, 1-aminocyclopropane-1-carboxylic acid is a small disubstituted cyclic amino acid that is a key intermediate in the production of the plant hormone ethylene.

Catabolism

Amino acids must first pass out of organelles and cells into blood circulation via amino acid transporters, since the amine and carboxylic acid groups are typically ionized. Degradation of an amino acid, occurring in the liver and kidneys, often involves deamination by moving its amino group to alpha-ketoglutarate, forming glutamate. This process involves transaminases, often the same as those used in amination during synthesis. In many vertebrates, the amino group is then removed through the urea cycle and is excreted in the form of urea. However, amino acid degradation can produce uric acid or ammonia instead. For example, serine dehydratase converts serine to pyruvate and ammonia. After removal of one or more amino groups, the remainder of the molecule can sometimes be used to synthesize new amino acids, or it can be used for energy by entering glycolysis or the citric acid cycle, as detailed in image at right.

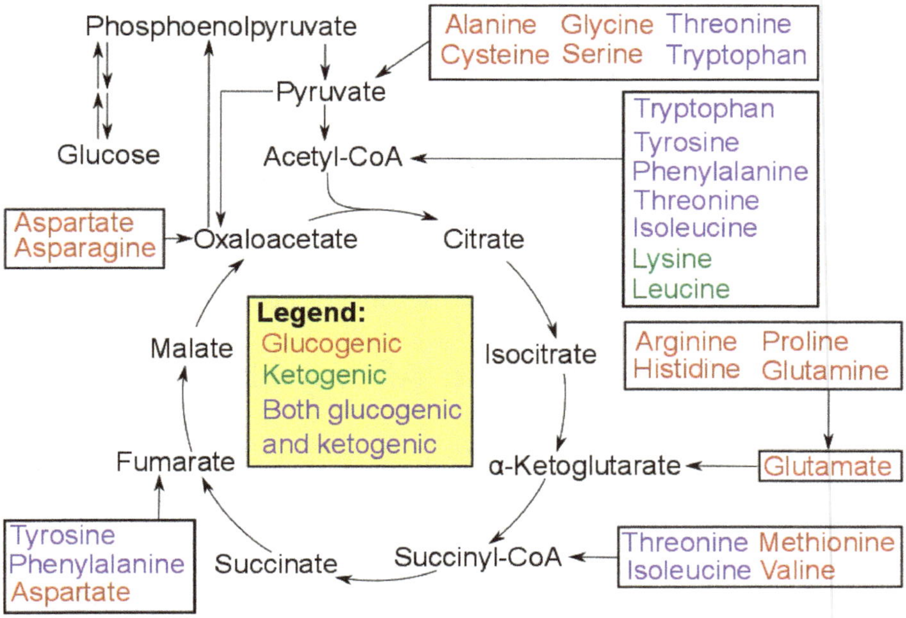

Catabolism of proteinogenic amino acids. Amino acids can be classified according to the properties of their main products as either of the following:

* *Glucogenic*, with the products having the ability to form glucose by gluconeogenesis
* *Ketogenic*, with the products not having the ability to form glucose. These products may still be used for ketogenesis or lipid synthesis.
* Amino acids catabolized into both glucogenic and ketogenic products.

PHYSICOCHEMICAL PROPERTIES OF AMINO ACIDS

The 20 amino acids encoded directly by the genetic code can be divided into several groups based on their properties. Important factors are charge, hydrophilicity or hydrophobicity, size, and functional groups. These properties are important for protein structure and protein–protein interactions. The water soluble proteins tend to have their hydrophobic residues (Leu, Ile, Val, Phe, and Trp) buried in the middle of the protein, whereas hydrophilic side-chains are exposed to the aqueous solvent. (Note that in biochemistry, a residue refers to a specific monomer within the polymeric chain of a polysaccharide, protein or nucleic acid.) The integral membrane proteins tend to have outer rings of exposed hydrophobic amino acids that anchor them into the lipid bilayer. In the case part-way between these two extremes, some peripheral membrane proteins have a patch of hydrophobic amino acids on their surface that locks onto the membrane. In similar fashion, proteins that have to bind to positively charged molecules have surfaces rich with negatively charged amino acids like glutamate and aspartate, while proteins binding to negatively charged molecules have surfaces rich with positively charged chains like lysine and arginine. There are different hydrophobicity scales of amino acid residues.

Some amino acids have special properties such as cysteine, that can form covalent disulfide bonds to other cysteine residues, proline that forms a cycle to the polypeptide backbone, and glycine that is more flexible than other amino acids.

Many proteins undergo a range of posttranslational modifications, when additional chemical groups are attached to the amino acids in proteins. Some modifications can produce hydrophobic lipoproteins, or hydrophilic glycoproteins. These type of modification allow the reversible targeting of a protein to a membrane. For example, the addition and removal of the fatty acid palmitic acid to cysteine residues in some signaling proteins causes the proteins to attach and then detach from cell membranes.

Table of Standard Amino acid Abbreviations and Properties

Amino Acid	3-Letter	1-Letter	Side-chain class	Side-chain polarity	Side-chain charge (pH 7.4)	Hydropathy index	Absorbance λ_{max}(nm)	ε at λ_{max} (mM^{-1} cm^{-1})	MW (Weight)	Occurrence in proteins (%)
Alanine	Ala	A	aliphatic	nonpolar	neutral	1.8			89.094	8.76
Arginine	Arg	R	basic	basic polar	positive	−4.5			174.203	5.78
Asparagine	Asn	N	amide	polar	neutral	−3.5			132.119	3.93
Aspartic acid	Asp	D	acid	acidic polar	negative	−3.5			133.104	5.49
Cysteine	Cys	C	sulfur-containing	nonpolar	neutral	2.5	250	0.3	121.154	1.38
Glutamic acid	Glu	E	acid	acidic polar	negative	−3.5			147.131	6.32
Glutamine	Gln	Q	amide	polar	neutral	−3.5			146.146	3.9
Glycine	Gly	G	aliphatic	nonpolar	neutral	−0.4			75.067	7.03
Histidine	His	H	basic aromatic	basic polar	positive(10%) neutral(90%)	−3.2	211	5.9	155.156	2.26
Isoleucine	Ile	I	aliphatic	nonpolar	neutral	4.5			131.175	5.49
Leucine	Leu	L	aliphatic	nonpolar	neutral	3.8			131.175	9.68
Lysine	Lys	K	basic	basic polar	positive	−3.9			146.189	5.19
Methionine	Met	M	sulfur-containing	nonpolar	neutral	1.9			149.208	2.32
Phenylalanine	Phe	F	aromatic	nonpolar	neutral	2.8	257, 206, 188	0.2, 9.3, 60.0	165.192	3.87
Proline	Pro	P	cyclic	nonpolar	neutral	−1.6			115.132	5.02
Serine	Ser	S	hydroxyl-containing	polar	neutral	−0.8			105.093	7.14
Threonine	Thr	T	hydroxyl-containing	polar	neutral	−0.7			119.119	5.53
Tryptophan	Trp	W	aromatic	nonpolar	neutral	−0.9	280, 219	5.6, 47.0	204.228	1.25
Tyrosine	Tyr	Y	aromatic	polar	neutral	−1.3	274, 222, 193	1.4, 8.0, 48.0	181.191	2.91
Valine	Val	V	aliphatic	nonpolar	neutral	4.2			117.148	6.73

Two additional amino acids are in some species coded for by codons that are usually interpreted as stop codons:

21st and 22nd amino acids	3-Letter	1-Letter	MW(Weight)
Selenocysteine	Sec	U	168.064
Pyrrolysine	Pyl	O	255.313

In addition to the specific amino acid codes, placeholders are used in cases where chemical or crystallographic analysis of a peptide or protein cannot conclusively determine the identity of a residue. They are also used to summarise conserved protein sequence motifs. The use of single letters to indicate sets of similar residues is similar to the use of abbreviation codes for degenerate bases.

Ambiguous Amino Acids	3-Letter	1-Letter	
Any / unknown	Xaa	X	All
Asparagine or aspartic acid	Asx	B	D, N
Glutamine or glutamic acid	Glx	Z	E, Q
Leucine or Isoleucine	Xle	J	I, L
Hydrophobic		Φ	V, I, L, F, W, Y, M
Aromatic		Ω	F, W, Y, H
Aliphatic (Non-Aromatic)		Ψ	V, I, L, M
Small		π	P, G, A, S
Hydrophilic		ζ	S, T, H, N, Q, E, D, K, R
Positively charged		+	K, R, H
Negatively charged		−	D, E

Unk is sometimes used instead of **Xaa**, but is less standard.

In addition, many non-standard amino acids have a specific code. For example, several peptide drugs, such as Bortezomib and MG132, are artificially synthesized and retain their protecting groups, which have specific codes. Bortezomib is Pyz-Phe-boroLeu, and MG132 is Z-Leu-Leu-Leu-al. To aid in the analysis of protein structure, photo-reactive amino acid analogs are available. These include photoleucine (**pLeu**) and photomethionine (**pMet**).

REFERENCES

1. A One-Letter Notation for Amino Acid Sequences. European Journal of Biochemistry. 5 (2): 151–153. 1 July 1968. doi:10.1111/j.1432-1033.1968.tb00350.x.
2. Alpha amino acid – Medical definition. Merriam-Webster dictionary.
3. amino acid. Cambridge Dictionaries Online. Cambridge University Press. 2015. Retrieved 3 July 2015.
4. Amino. Dictionary.com. 2015. Retrieved 3 July 2015.
5. amino. FreeDictionary.com. Farlex. 2015. Retrieved 3 July 2015.
6. Chapter 1: Proteins are the Body›s Worker Molecules. The Structures of Life. National Institute of General Medical Sciences. 27 October 2011. Retrieved 20 May 2008.

7. etymonline.com entry for amino. www.etymonline.com. Retrieved 19 July 2010.
8. Lethal DNA tags could keep innocent people out of jail. New Scientist. 2 May 2013.
9. Nomenclature and Symbolism for Amino Acids and Peptides. IUPAC-IUB Joint Commission on Biochemical Nomenclature. 1983. Archived from the original on 9 October 2008. Retrieved 17 November 2008.
10. Anfinsen CB, Edsall JT, Richards FM (1972). Advances in Protein Chemistry. New York: Academic Press. pp. 99, 103. ISBN 978-0-12-034226-6.
11. Brook MS, Wilkinson DJ, Phillips BE, Perez-Schindler J, Philp A, Smith K, Atherton PJ (January 2016).Skeletal muscle homeostasis and plasticity in youth and ageing: impact of nutrition and exercise. Acta Physiologica. 216 (1): 15–41. doi:10.1111/apha.12532. PMC 4843955. PMID 26010896.
12. Creighton, Thomas H. (1993).Chapter 1. Proteins: structures and molecular properties. San Francisco: W. H. Freeman. ISBN 978-0-7167-7030-5.
13. Hausman, Robert E.; Cooper, Geoffrey M. (2004). The cell: a molecular approach. Washington, D.C: ASM Press. p. 51. ISBN 0-87893-214-3.
14. Elzanowski A, Ostell J (7 April 2008).The Genetic Codes. National Center for Biotechnology Information (NCBI). Retrieved 10 March 2010.
15. Freifelder, D. (1983). Physical Biochemistry (2nd ed.). W. H. Freeman and Company. ISBN 0-7167-1315-2.[page needed]
16. Frontiers in Drug Design and Discovery ed. Atta-Ur-Rahman & others, p.299
17. Leuchtenberger W, Huthmacher K, Drauz K (November 2005).Biotechnological production of amino acids and derivatives: current status and prospects. Applied Microbiology and Biotechnology. 69 (1): 1–8. doi:10.1007/s00253-005-0155-y. PMID 16195792.
18. Modeling Electrostatic Contributions to Protein Folding and Binding – Tjong, p.1 footnote
19. Phillips SM (May 2014).A brief review of critical processes in exercise-induced muscular hypertrophy. Sports Med. 44 Suppl 1: S71–S77. doi:10.1007/s40279-014-0152-3. PMC 4008813. PMID 24791918.
20. Wang Q, Parrish AR, Wang L (March 2009).Expanding the genetic code for biological studies. Chem. Biol. 16 (3): 323–36. doi:10.1016/j.chembiol.2009.03.001. PMC 2696486. PMID 19318213.
21. Xie J, Schultz PG (December 2005).Adding amino acids to the genetic repertoire. Current Opinion in Chemical Biology. 9 (6): 548–54. doi:10.1016/j.cbpa.2005.10.011. PMID 16260173.
22. Aasland, Rein; Abrams, Charles; Ampe, Christophe; Ball, Linda J.; Bedford, Mark T.; Cesareni, Gianni; Gimona, Mario; Hurley, James H.; Jarchau, Thomas (20 February 2002).Normalization of nomenclature for peptide motifs as ligands of modular protein domains. FEBS Letters. 513 (1): 141–144. doi:10.1016/S0014-5793(01)03295-1.

23. Albion Laboratories, Inc.Albion Ferrochel Website. Retrieved 12 July 2011.

24. Alexander L, Grierson D (October 2002).Ethylene biosynthesis and action in tomato: a model for climacteric fruit ripening. Journal of Experimental Botany. 53 (377): 2039–55. doi:10.1093/jxb/erf072. PMID 12324528.

25. Ashmead, H. DeWayne (1986). Foliar Feeding of Plants with Amino Acid Chelates. Park Ridge: Noyes Publications.

26. Ashmead, H. DeWayne (1993). The Role of Amino Acid Chelates in Animal Nutrition. Westwood: Noyes Publications.

27. Baumann E (1884).Über cystin und cystein. Z Physiol Chem. 8 (4): 299–305. Archived from the original on 14 March 2011. Retrieved 28 March 2011.

28. Bhattacharjee A, Bansal M (March 2005).Collagen structure: the Madras triple helix and the current scenario. IUBMB Life. 57 (3): 161–72. doi:10.1080/15216540500090710. PMID 16036578.

29. Blaser, Hans Ulrich (1992).The chiral pool as a source of enantioselective catalysts and auxiliaries. Chemical Reviews. 92 (5): 935–52. doi:10.1021/cr00013a009.

30. Blenis J, Resh MD (December 1993).Subcellular localization specified by protein acylation and phosphorylation. Current Opinion in Cell Biology. 5 (6): 984–9. doi:10.1016/0955-0674(93)90081-Z. PMID 8129952.

31. Bourke SL, Kohn J (2003).Polymers derived from the amino acid l-tyrosine: polycarbonates, polyarylates and copolymers with poly(ethylene glycol). Advanced Drug Delivery Reviews. 55 (4): 447–466. doi:10.1016/S0169-409X(03)00038-3. PMID 12706045.

32. Braconnot HM (1820).Sur la conversion des matières animales en nouvelles substances par le moyen de l›acide sulfurique. Annales de Chimie et de Physique. 2nd Series. 13: 113–25.

33. Broadley KJ (March 2010).The vascular effects of trace amines and amphetamines. Pharmacol. Ther. 125 (3): 363–375. doi:10.1016/j.pharmthera.2009.11.005. PMID 19948186.

34. Brosnan JT (April 2000).Glutamate, at the interface between amino acid and carbohydrate metabolism. The Journal of Nutrition. 130 (4S Suppl): 988S–90S. PMID 10736367.

35. Brosnan JT, Brosnan ME (June 2006).The sulfur-containing amino acids: an overview. The Journal of Nutrition. 136 (6 Suppl): 1636S–1640S. PMID 16702333.

36. Carpino, Louis A. (1992).1-Hydroxy-7-azabenzotriazole. An efficient peptide coupling additive. Journal of the American Chemical Society. 115 (10): 4397–8. doi:10.1021/ja00063a082.

37. Clark, Jim (August 2007).an introduction to amino acids. chemguide. Retrieved 4 July 2015.

38. Coghlan, Andy (225 October 2012).Molecules ‹too dangerous for nature› kill cancer cells. New Scientist.Check date values in: |date= (help)

39. Cox, PA, Davis, DA, Mash, DC, Metcalf, JS, Banack, SA. (2015).Dietary exposure to an environmental toxin triggers neurofibrillary tangles and amyloid deposits in the brain. Proceedings of the Royal Society B. 283 (1823): 20152397. doi:10.1098/rspb.2015.2397. PMC 4795023. PMID 26791617.

40. Coxon KM, Chakauya E, Ottenhof HH, Whitney HM, Blundell TL, Abell C, Smith AG (August 2005).Pantothenate biosynthesis in higher plants. Biochemical Society Transactions. 33 (Pt 4): 743–6. doi:10.1042/BST0330743. PMID 16042590.

41. Cruz-Vera LR, Magos-Castro MA, Zamora-Romo E, Guarneros G (2004). Ribosome stalling and peptidyl-tRNA drop-off during translational delay at AGA codons. Nucleic Acids Research. 32. 18 (15): 4462–8. doi:10.1093/nar/gkh784. PMC 516057. PMID 15317870.

42. Curis E, Nicolis I, Moinard C, Osowska S, Zerrouk N, Bénazeth S, Cynober L (November 2005).Almost all about citrulline in mammals. Amino Acids. 29 (3): 177–205. doi:10.1007/s00726-005-0235-4. PMID 16082501.

43. Davis FA, Reddy RE, Portonovo PS (1994).Asymmetric strecker synthesis using enantiopure sulfinimines: A convenient synthesis of α-amino acids. Tetrahedron Letters. 35 (50): 9351–9354. doi:10.1016/S0040-4039(00)78540-6.

44. Driscoll DM, Copeland PR (2003).Mechanism and regulation of selenoprotein synthesis. Annual Review of Nutrition. 23 (1): 17–40. doi:10.1146/annurev.nutr.23.011702.073318. PMID 12524431.

45. Duthaler, Rudolf O. (1994).Recent developments in the stereoselective synthesis of α-aminoacids. Tetrahedron. 50 (6): 1539–1650. doi:10.1016/S0040-4020(01)80840-1.

46. Ekanayake S, Skog K, Asp NG (May 2007).Canavanine content in sword beans (Canavalia gladiata): analysis and effect of processing. Food and Chemical Toxicology. 45 (5): 797–803. doi:10.1016/j.fct.2006.10.030. PMID 17187914.

47. Elmore, Donald Trevor; Barrett, G. C. (1998). Amino acids and peptides. Cambridge, UK: Cambridge University Press. pp. 48–60. ISBN 0-521-46827-2.

48. Fennema OR. Food Chemistry 3rd Ed. CRC Press. pp. 327–8. ISBN 0-8247-9691-8.

49. For example, ruminants such as cows obtain a number of amino acids via microbes in the first two stomach chambers.

50. Fürst P, Stehle P (June 2004).What are the essential elements needed for the determination of amino acid requirements in humans?. The Journal of Nutrition. 134 (6 Suppl): 1558S–1565S. PMID 15173430.

51. Garattini S (April 2000).Glutamic acid, twenty years later. The Journal of Nutrition. 130 (4S Suppl): 901S–9S. PMID 10736350.

52. Gromer, S., Urig, S., Becker, K. (2004) The Thioredoxin System – From Science to Clinic. Medicinal Research Reviews. 24(1):40–89.

53. Gross RA, Kalra B (2002).Biodegradable Polymers for the Environment. Science. 297 (5582): 803–807. Bibcode:2002Sci...297..803G. doi:10.1126/science.297.5582.803. PMID 12161646.

54. Gutteridge A, Thornton JM (November 2005).Understanding nature›s catalytic toolkit. Trends in Biochemical Sciences. 30 (11): 622–9. doi:10.1016/j.tibs.2005.09.006. PMID 16214343.

55. Hammond AC (May 1995).Leucaena toxicosis and its control in ruminants. Journal of Animal Science. 73 (5): 1487–92. PMID 7665380.

56. Hanessian S (1993).Reflections on the total synthesis of natural products: Art, craft, logic, and the chiron approach. Pure and Applied Chemistry. 65 (6): 1189–204. doi:10.1351/pac199365061189.

57. Hatem, Salama Mohamed Ali (2006).Gas chromatographic determination of Amino Acid Enantiomers in tobacco and bottled wines. University of Giessen. Retrieved 17 November 2008.

58. Heby O, Persson L, Rentala M (August 2007).Targeting the polyamine biosynthetic enzymes: a promising approach to therapy of African sleeping sickness, Chagas› disease, and leishmaniasis. Amino Acids. 33 (2): 359–66. doi:10.1007/s00726-007-0537-9. PMID 17610127.

59. Hertweck C (2011).Biosynthesis and Charging of Pyrrolysine, the 22nd Genetically Encoded Amino Acid. Angewandte Chemie International Edition. 50 (41): 9540–1. doi:10.1002/anie.201103769. PMID 21796749.

60. Holtcamp, W. (2012).The emerging science of BMAA: do cyanobacteria contribute to neurodegenerative disease?. Environmental Health Perspectives. 120 (3): a110–a116. doi:10.1289/ehp.120-a110. PMC 3295368. PMID 22382274.

61. http://opbs.okstate.edu/5753/Amino%20Acids.html

62. Huang J, Corey EJ (2004).A New Chiral Catalyst for the Enantioselective Strecker Synthesis of α-Amino Acids. Orgic Letters. 62 (6): 5027–9. doi:10.1021/ol047698w. PMID 15606127.

63. Hylin, John W. (1969).Toxic peptides and amino acids in foods and feeds. Journal of Agricultural and Food Chemistry. 17 (3): 492–6. doi:10.1021/jf60163a003.

64. Ibba M, Söll D (May 2001).The renaissance of aminoacyl-tRNA synthesis. EMBO Reports. 2 (5): 382–7. doi:10.1093/embo-reports/kve095. PMC 1083889. PMID 11375928.

65. Imura K, Okada A (January 1998).Amino acid metabolism in pediatric patients. Nutrition. 14 (1): 143–8. doi:10.1016/S0899-9007(97)00230-X. PMID 9437700.

66. Ishitani H, Komiyama S, Hasegawa Y, Kobayashi S (2000).Catalytic Asymmetric Strecker Synthesis. Preparation of Enantiomerically Pure α-Amino Acid Derivatives from Aldimines and Tributyltin Cyanide or Achiral Aldehydes, Amines, and Hydrogen Cyanide Using a Chiral Zirconium Catalyst. Journal of the American Chemical Society. 122 (5): 762–6. doi:10.1021/ja9935207.

67. IUPAC, Compendium of Chemical Terminology, 2nd ed. (theGold Book) (1997). Online corrected version: (2006–)Imino acids.

68. Jakubke, Hans-Dieter; Sewald, Norbert (2008).Amino acids. Peptides from A to Z: A Concise Encyclopedia. Germany: Wiley-VCH. p. 20. ISBN 9783527621170 – via Google Books.

69. Jodidi, S. L. (1 March 1926).The Formol Titration of Certain Amino Acids. Journal of the American Chemical Society. 48 (3): 751–753. doi:10.1021/ja01414a033.

70. Jones, Russell Celyn; Buchanan, Bob B.; Gruissem, Wilhelm (2000). Biochemistry & molecular biology of plants. Rockville, Md: American Society of Plant Physiologists. pp. 371–2. ISBN 0-943088-39-9.

71. Joseph S. Fruton (1990).Chapter 5- Emil Fischer and Franz Hofmeister. Contrasts in Scientific Style: Research Groups in the Chemical and Biochemical Sciences,. 191. American Philosophical Society. pp. 163–165. ISBN 0-87169-191-4.

72. Ketchem, Randal R.; Hu, Weidong; Cross, Timothy A. (1993).High-Resolution Conformation of Gramicidin A in a Lipid Bilayer by Solid-State NMR. Science. 261 (5127): 1457–1460. doi:10.1126/science.7690158.

73. Khoury, George A.; Baliban, Richard C.; Floudas, Christodoulos A. (2011). Proteome-Wide Post-Translational Modification Statistics: Frequency Analysis and Curation of the Swiss-Prot Database. Scientific Reports. 1 (90). doi:10.1038/srep00090. PMC 3201773. PMID 22034591.

74. Kivirikko KI, Pihlajaniemi T (1998).Collagen hydroxylases and the protein disulfide isomerase subunit of prolyl 4-hydroxylases. Advances in Enzymology and Related Areas of Molecular Biology. Advances in Enzymology – and Related Areas of Molecular Biology. 72: 325–98. doi:10.1002/9780470123188.ch9. ISBN 9780470123188. PMID 9559057.

75. Konara S, Gagnona K, Clearfield A, Thompson C, Hartle J, Ericson C, Nelson C (2010).Structural determination and characterization of copper and zinc bis-glycinates with X-ray crystallography and mass spectrometry. Journal of Coordination Chemistry. 63 (19): 3335–47. doi:10.1080/00958972.2010.514336.

76. Kostrzewa RM, Nowak P, Kostrzewa JP, Kostrzewa RA, Brus R (March 2005). Peculiarities of L: -DOPA treatment of Parkinson›s disease. Amino Acids. 28 (2): 157–64. doi:10.1007/s00726-005-0162-4. PMID 15750845.

77. Kozlowski, Lukasz P. (2016-10-26).Proteome-pI: proteome isoelectric point database. Nucleic Acids Research: gkw978. doi:10.1093/nar/gkw978. PMID 27789699.

78. Kryukov GV, Castellano S, Novoselov SV, Lobanov AV, Zehtab O, Guigó R, Gladyshev VN (2003).Characterization of mammalian selenoproteomes. Science. 300 (5624): 1439–1443. Bibcode:2003Sci...300.1439K. doi:10.1126/science.1083516. PMID 12775843.

79. Krzycki JA (December 2005).The direct genetic encoding of pyrrolysine. Current Opinion in Microbiology. 8 (6): 706–12. doi:10.1016/j.mib.2005.10.009. PMID 16256420.

80. Kyte J, Doolittle RF (May 1982).A simple method for displaying the hydropathic character of a protein. Journal of Molecular Biology. 157 (1): 105–32. doi:10.1016/0022-2836(82)90515-0. PMID 7108955.

81. Latham, Michael C. (1997).Chapter 8. Body composition, the functions of

food, metabolism and energy. Human nutrition in the developing world. Food and Nutrition Series – No. 29. Rome: Food and Agriculture Organization of the United Nations.

82. Lengyel P, Söll D (June 1969).Mechanism of protein biosynthesis. Bacteriological Reviews. 33 (2): 264–301. PMC 378322. PMID 4896351.

83. Liebecq, Claude, ed. (1992). Biochemical Nomenclature and Related Documents (2nd ed.). Portland Press. pp. 39–69. ISBN 978-1-85578-005-7.

84. Lindemann L, Hoener MC (May 2005).A renaissance in trace amines inspired by a novel GPCR family. Trends Pharmacol. Sci. 26 (5): 274–281. doi:10.1016/j.tips.2005.03.007. PMID 15860375.

85. Lipton JO, Sahin M (October 2014).The neurology of mTOR. Neuron. 84 (2): 275–291. doi:10.1016/j.neuron.2014.09.034. PMC 4223653. PMID 25374355.

86. Figure 2: The mTOR Signaling Pathway

87. Lourenço R, Camilo ME (2002).Taurine: a conditionally essential amino acid in humans? An overview in health and disease. Nutrición Hospitalaria. 17 (6): 262–70. PMID 12514918.

88. Low, K. C.; Wheeler, A. P.; Koskan, L. P. (1996). Commercial poly(aspartic acid) and Its Uses. Advances in Chemistry Series. 248. Washington, D.C.: American Chemical Society.

89. Magee T, Seabra MC (April 2005).Fatty acylation and prenylation of proteins: what›s hot in fat. Current Opinion in Cell Biology. 17 (2): 190–6. doi:10.1016/j.ceb.2005.02.003. PMID 15780596.

90. Marasco D, Perretta G, Sabatella M, Ruvo M (October 2008).Past and future perspectives of synthetic peptide libraries. Current Protein & Peptide Science. 9 (5): 447–67. doi:10.2174/138920308785915209. PMID 18855697.

91. Masumoto S, Usuda H, Suzuki M, Kanai M, Shibasaki M (May 2003).Catalytic enantioselective Strecker reaction of ketoimines. Journal of the American Chemical Society. 125 (19): 5634–5. doi:10.1021/ja034980. PMID 12733893.

92. Matthews BW (2009).Racemic crystallography—easy crystals and easy structures: What›s not to like?. Protein Science. 18 (6): 1135–1138. doi:10.1002/pro.125. PMC 2774423. PMID 19472321.

93. McCoy, R. H.; Meyer, C. E. & Rose, W. C. (1935).Feeding Experiments with Mixtures of Highly Purified Amino Acids. VIII. Isolation and Identification of a New Essential Amino Acid. Journal of Biological Chemistry. 112: 283–302.

94. McMurry, John (1996). Organic chemistry. Pacific Grove, CA, USA: Brooks/Cole. p. 1064. ISBN 0-534-23832-7.

95. Meister A (November 1988).Glutathione metabolism and its selective modification. The Journal of Biological Chemistry. 263 (33): 17205–8. PMID 3053703.

96. Michal, Gerhard; Schomburg, Dietmar, eds. (2012). Biochemical Pathways: An Atlas of Biochemistry and Molecular Biology (2nd ed.). Wiley. p. 5.

97. Park MH (February 2006).The post-translational synthesis of a polyamine-

derived amino acid, hypusine, in the eukaryotic translation initiation factor 5A (eIF5A). Journal of Biochemistry. 139 (2): 161–9. doi:10.1093/jb/mvj034. PMC 2494880. PMID 16452303.

98. Petroff OA (December 2002).GABA and glutamate in the human brain. Neuroscientist. 8 (6): 562–573. doi:10.1177/1073858402238515. PMID 12467378.

99. Pilobello KT, Mahal LK (June 2007).Deciphering the glycocode: the complexity and analytical challenge of glycomics. Current Opinion in Chemical Biology. 11 (3): 300–5. doi:10.1016/j.cbpa.2007.05.002. PMID 17500024.

100. Pisarewicz K, Mora D, Pflueger FC, Fields GB, Marí F (May 2005).Polypeptide chains containing D-gamma-hydroxyvaline. Journal of the American Chemical Society. 127 (17): 6207–15. doi:10.1021/ja050088m. PMID 15853325.

101. Pollegioni, Loredano; Servi, Stefano, eds. (2012). Unnatural Amino Acids: Methods and Protocols. Methods in Molecular Biology – Volume 794. Humana Press. p. v. ISBN 978-1-61779-331-8. OCLC 756512314.

102. Proline at the US National Library of Medicine Medical Subject Headings (MeSH)

103. Proline is an exception to this general formula. It lacks the NH2 group because of the cyclization of the side-chain and is known as an imino acid; it falls under the category of special structured amino acids.

104. Reeds PJ (July 2000).Dispensable and indispensable amino acids for humans. The Journal of Nutrition. 130 (7): 1835S–40S. PMID 10867060.

105. Robert D. Simoni; Robert L. Hill; Martha Vaughan (13 September 2002).The Discovery of the Amino Acid Threonine: the Work of William C. Rose. Journal of Biological Chemistry. 277 (37): 56–58. PMID 12218068.

106. Rodnina MV, Beringer M, Wintermeyer W (January 2007).How ribosomes make peptide bonds. Trends in Biochemical Sciences. 32 (1): 20–6. doi:10.1016/j.tibs.2006.11.007. PMID 17157507.

107. Rodríguez-Caso C, Montañez R, Cascante M, Sánchez-Jiménez F, Medina MA (August 2006).Mathematical modeling of polyamine metabolism in mammals. The Journal of Biological Chemistry. 281 (31): 21799–812. doi:10.1074/jbc.M602756200. PMID 16709566.

108. Rosenthal GA (2001).L-Canavanine: a higher plant insecticidal allelochemical. Amino Acids. 21 (3): 319–30. doi:10.1007/s007260170017. PMID 11764412.

109. Sakami W, Harrington H (1963).Amino acid metabolism. Annual Review of Biochemistry. 32 (1): 355–98. doi:10.1146/annurev.bi.32.070163.002035. PMID 14144484.

110. Sanda F, Endo T (1999).Syntheses and functions of polymers based on amino acids. Macromolecular Chemistry and Physics. 200 (12): 2651–61. doi:10.1002/(SICI)1521-3935(19991201)200:12<2651::AID-MACP2651>3.0.CO;2-P.

111. Savelieva KV, Zhao S, Pogorelov VM, Rajan I, Yang Q, Cullinan E, Lanthorn TH (2008). Bartolomucci A, ed.Genetic disruption of both tryptophan hydroxylase genes dramatically reduces serotonin and affects behavior in models sensitive

to antidepressants. PLoS ONE. 3 (10): e3301. Bibcode:2008PLoSO...3.3301S. doi:10.1371/journal.pone.0003301. PMC 2565062. PMID 18923670.

112. Shemin D, Rittenberg D (1 December 1946).The biological utilization of glycine for the synthesis of the protoporphyrin of hemoglobin. Journal of Biological Chemistry. 166 (2): 621–5. PMID 20276176.

113. Simmons, William J.; Gerhard Meisenberg (2006). Principles of medical biochemistry. Mosby Elsevier. p. 19. ISBN 0-323-02942-6.

114. Simon M (2005). Emergent computation: emphasizing bioinformatics. New York: AIP Press/Springer Science+Business Media. pp. 105–106. ISBN 0-387-22046-1.

115. Smith, Anthony D. (1997). Oxford dictionary of biochemistry and molecular biology. Oxford: Oxford University Press. p. 535. ISBN 978-0-19-854768-6. OCLC 37616711.

116. Smotrys JE, Linder ME (2004).Palmitoylation of intracellular signaling proteins: regulation and function. Annual Review of Biochemistry. 73 (1): 559–87. doi:10.1146/annurev.biochem.73.011303.073954. PMID 15189153.

117. Stegink LD (July 1987).The aspartame story: a model for the clinical testing of a food additive. The American Journal of Clinical Nutrition. 46 (1 Suppl): 204–15. PMID 3300262.

118. Stipanuk, M. H. (2006). Biochemical, physiological, & molecular aspects of human nutrition (2 ed.): Saunders Elsevier.

119. Strecker, Adolph (1850).Ueber die künstliche Bildung der Milchsäure und einen neuen, dem Glycocoll homologen Körper. Justus Liebigs Annalen der Chemie. 75 (1): 27–45. doi:10.1002/jlac.18500750103.

120. Strecker, Adolph (1854).Ueber einen neuen aus Aldehyd – Ammoniak und Blausäure entstehenden Körper. Justus Liebigs Annalen der Chemie. 91 (3): 349–51. doi:10.1002/jlac.18540910309.

121. Stryer, Lubert; Berg, Jeremy Mark; Tymoczko, John L. (2002). Biochemistry. San Francisco: W.H. Freeman. pp. 693–8. ISBN 0-7167-4684-0.

122. Stryer, Lubert; Berg, Jeremy Mark; Tymoczko, John L. (2002). Biochemistry. San Francisco: W.H. Freeman. pp. 639–49. ISBN 0-7167-4684-0.

123. Suchanek M, Radzikowska A, Thiele C (April 2005).Photo-leucine and photo-methionine allow identification of protein-protein interactions in living cells. Nature Methods. 2 (4): 261–7. doi:10.1038/nmeth752. PMID 15782218.

124. Tejero J, Biswas A, Wang ZQ, Page RC, Haque MM, Hemann C, Zweier JL, Misra S, Stuehr DJ (November 2008).Stabilization and characterization of a heme-oxy reaction intermediate in inducible nitric-oxide synthase. The Journal of Biological Chemistry. 283 (48): 33498–507. doi:10.1074/jbc.M806122200. PMC 2586280. PMID 18815130.

125. Théobald-Dietrich A, Giegé R, Rudinger-Thirion J (2005).Evidence for the existence in mRNAs of a hairpin element responsible for ribosome dependent pyrrolysine insertion into proteins. Biochimie. 87 (9–10): 813–7. doi:10.1016/j.biochi.2005.03.006. PMID 16164991.

126. Thombre SM, Sarwade BD (2005).Synthesis and Biodegradability of Polyaspartic Acid: A Critical Review. Journal of Macromolecular Science, Part A. 42 (9): 1299–1315. doi:10.1080/10601320500189604.

127. Turner BL, Harborne JB (1967).Distribution of canavanine in the plant kingdom. Phytochemistry. 6 (6): 863–66. doi:10.1016/S0031-9422(00)86033-1.

128. Turner EH, Loftis JM, Blackwell AD (March 2006).Serotonin a la carte: supplementation with the serotonin precursor 5-hydroxytryptophan. Pharmacology & Therapeutics. 109 (3): 325–38. doi:10.1016/j.pharmthera.2005.06.004. PMID 16023217.

129. Urry DW (2004).The change in Gibbs free energy for hydrophobic association: Derivation and evaluation by means of inverse temperature transitions. Chemical Physics Letters. 399 (1–3): 177–83. doi:10.1016/S0009-2614(04)01565-9.

130. van Heijenoort J (March 2001).Formation of the glycan chains in the synthesis of bacterial peptidoglycan. Glycobiology. 11 (3): 25R–36R. doi:10.1093/glycob/11.3.25R. PMID 11320055.

131. Vauquelin LN, Robiquet PJ (1806).The discovery of a new plant principle in Asparagus sativus. Annales de Chimie. 57: 88–93.

132. Vermeer C (March 1990).Gamma-carboxyglutamate-containing proteins and the vitamin K-dependent carboxylase. The Biochemical Journal. 266 (3): 625–36. doi:10.1042/bj2660625. PMC 1131186. PMID 2183788.

133. Wagner I, Musso H (November 1983).New Naturally Occurring Amino Acids. Angewandte Chemie International Edition in English. 22 (11): 816–28. doi:10.1002/anie.198308161.

134. Wang X, Li J, Dong G, Yue J (February 2014).The endogenous substrates of brain CYP2D. Eur. J. Pharmacol. 724: 211–218. doi:10.1016/j.ejphar.2013.12.025. PMID 24374199. The highest level of brain CYP2D activity was found in the substantia nigra ... The in vitro and in vivo studies have shown the contribution of the alternative CYP2D-mediated dopamine synthesis to the concentration of this neurotransmitter although the classic biosynthetic route to dopamine from tyrosine is active. ... Tyramine levels are especially high in the basal ganglia and limbic system, which are thought to be related to individual behavior and emotion (Yu et al., 2003c). ... Rat CYP2D isoforms (2D2/2D4/2D18) are less efficient than human CYP2D6 for the generation of dopamine from p-tyramine. The Km values of the CYP2D isoforms are as follows: CYP2D6 (87–121 μm) ≈ CYP2D2 ≈ CYP2D18 > CYP2D4 (256 μm) for m-tyramine and CYP2D4 (433 μm) > CYP2D2 ≈ CYP2D6 > CYP2D18 (688 μm) for p-tyramine

135. Whitmore L, Wallace BA (May 2004).Analysis of peptaibol sequence composition: implications for in vivo synthesis and channel formation. European Biophysics Journal. 33 (3): 233–7. doi:10.1007/s00249-003-0348-1. PMID 14534753.

136. Wollaston WH (1810).On cystic oxide, a new species of urinary calculus. Philosophical Transactions of the Royal Society. 100: 223–30. doi:10.1098/rstl.1810.0015.

137. Wolosker H, Dumin E, Balan L, Foltyn VN (July 2008).D-amino acids in the brain: D-serine in neurotransmission and neurodegeneration. The FEBS Journal. 275 (14): 3514–26. doi:10.1111/j.1742-4658.2008.06515.x. PMID 18564180.

138. Wu G, Fang YZ, Yang S, Lupton JR, Turner ND (March 2004).Glutathione metabolism and its implications for health. The Journal of Nutrition. 134 (3): 489–92. PMID 14988435.

139. Young VR (August 1994).Adult amino acid requirements: the case for a major revision in current recommendations. The Journal of Nutrition. 124 (8 Suppl): 1517S–1523S. PMID 8064412.

140. Young VR, Ajami AM (September 2001).Glutamine: the emperor or his clothes?. The Journal of Nutrition. 131 (9 Suppl): 2449S–59S; discussion 2486S–7S. PMID 11533293.

CHAPTER 2

Peptides: Classes and Synthesis

Chapter Contents

Peptides are compounds that are formed by linking one or more amino acids with a covalent bond. These compounds are classified as polymers, because they typically link together in long chains. All animals on Earth have them in their body, and in a way, they are one of the building blocks of life. When a chain gets especially long, it turns into a protein. Peptides and proteins represent a wide world of possibilities, and many molecular biologists spend years researching the functions of individual ones to learn more about how the body works.

INTRODUCTION

Peptides (from Gr.: πεπτός, *peptós* "digested"; derived from πέσσειν, *péssein* "to digest") are biologically occurring short chains of amino acidmonomers linked by peptide (amide) bonds.

The covalent chemical bonds are formed when the carboxyl group of one amino acid reacts with the amine group of another. The shortest peptides are dipeptides, consisting of 2 amino acids joined by a single peptide bond, followed by tripeptides, tetrapeptides, etc.

A **polypeptide** is a long, continuous, and unbranched peptide chain. Hence, peptides fall under the broad chemical classes of biological oligomers and polymers, alongside nucleic acids, oligosaccharides and polysaccharides, etc.

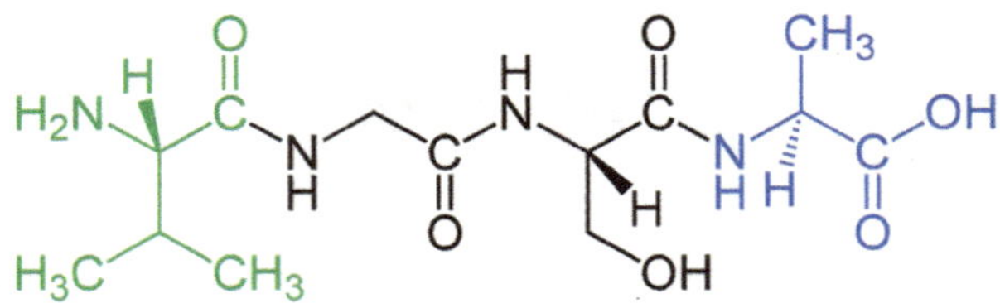

A tetrapeptide (example Val-Gly-Ser-Ala) with **green** marked amino end (**L-Valine**) and **blue** marked carboxyl end (**L-Alanine**).

Peptides are distinguished from proteins on the basis of size, and as an arbitrary benchmark can be understood to contain approximately 50 or fewer amino acids. Proteins consist of one or more polypeptides arranged in a biologically functional way, often bound to ligands such as coenzymes and cofactors, or to another protein or other macromolecule (DNA, RNA, etc.), or to complex macromolecular assemblies. Finally, while aspects of the lab techniques applied to peptides *versus* polypeptides and proteins differ (e.g., the specifics of electrophoresis, chromatography, etc.), the size boundaries that distinguish peptides from polypeptides and proteins are not absolute: long peptides such as amyloid beta have been referred to as proteins, and smaller proteins like insulin have been considered peptides.

Amino acids that have been incorporated into peptides are termed "residues" due to the release of either a hydrogen ion from the amine end or a hydroxyl ion from the carboxyl end, or both, as a water molecule is released during formation of each amide bond. All peptides except cyclic peptides have an N-terminal and C-terminal residue at the end of the peptide (as shown for the tetrapeptide in the image).

PEPTIDE CLASSES

Peptides are divided into several classes, depending on how they are produced.

Milk Peptides

Two naturally occurring milk peptides are formed from the milk protein casein when digestive enzymes break this down; they can also arise from the proteinases formed by lactobacilli during the fermentation of milk.

Ribosomal Peptides

Ribosomal peptides are synthesized by translation of mRNA. They are often subjected to proteolysis to generate the mature form. These function, typically in higher organisms, as hormones and signaling molecules. Some organisms produce peptides as antibiotics, such as microcins. Since they are translated, the amino acid residues involved are restricted to those utilized by the ribosome.

However, these peptides frequently have posttranslational modifications... such as phosphorylation, hydroxylation, sulfonation, palmitoylation, glycosylation and disulfide formation. In general, they are linear, although lariat structures have been observed. More exotic manipulations do occur, such as racemization of L-amino acids to D-amino acids in platypus venom.

Nonribosomal Peptides

Nonribosomal peptides are assembled by enzymes that are specific to each peptide, rather than by the ribosome. The most common non-ribosomal peptide is glutathione, which is a component of the antioxidant defenses of most aerobic organisms. Other nonribosomal peptides are most common in unicellular organisms, plants, and fungi and are synthesized by modular enzyme complexes called *nonribosomal peptide synthetases*.

These complexes are often laid out in a similar fashion, and they can contain many different modules to perform a diverse set of chemical manipulations on the developing product. These peptides are often cyclic and can have highly complex cyclic structures, although linear nonribosomal peptides are also common. Since the system is closely related to the machinery for building fatty acids and polyketides, hybrid compounds are often found. The presence of oxazoles or thiazoles often indicates that the compound was synthesized in this fashion.

Peptones

Peptones are derived from animal milk or meat digested by proteolysis. In addition to containing small peptides, the resulting spray-dried material includes fats, metals, salts, vitamins and many other biological compounds. Peptones are used in nutrient media for growing bacteria and fungi.

Peptide Fragments

Peptide fragments refer to fragments of proteins that are used to identify or quantify the source protein. Often these are the products of enzymatic degradation performed in the laboratory on a controlled sample, but can also be forensic or paleontological samples that have been degraded by natural effects.

PEPTIDE SYNTHESIS

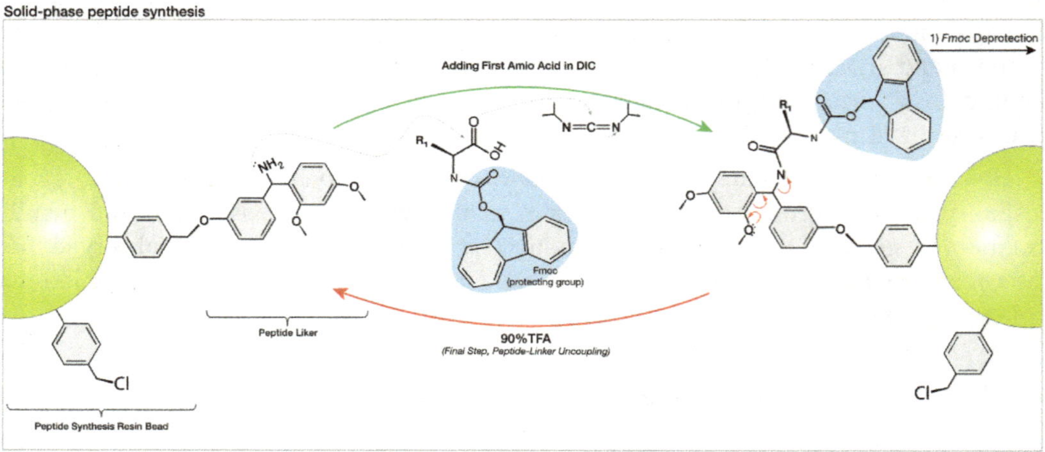

Solid-phase peptide synthesis on a rink amide resin using Fmoc-α-amine-protected amino acid.

PEPTIDES IN MOLECULAR BIOLOGY

Peptides received prominence in molecular biology for several reasons. The first is that peptides allow the creation of *peptide antibodies* in animals without the need of purifying the protein of interest. This involves synthesizing antigenic peptides of sections of the protein of interest. These will then be used to make antibodies in a rabbit or mouse against the protein.

Another reason is that peptides have become instrumental in mass spectrometry, allowing the identification of proteins of interest based on peptide masses and sequence.

Peptides have recently been used in the study of protein structure and function. For example, synthetic peptides can be used as probes to see where protein-peptide interactions occur- see the page on Protein tags.

Inhibitory peptides are also used in clinical research to examine the effects of peptides on the inhibition of cancer proteins and other diseases. For example, one of the most promising application is through peptides that target LHRH. These particular peptides act as an agonist, meaning that they bind to a cell in a way that regulates LHRH receptors. The process of inhibiting the cell receptors suggests that peptides could be beneficial in treating prostate cancer. However, additional investigations and experiments are required before the cancer-fighting attributes, exhibited by peptides, can be considered definitive.

WELL-KNOWN PEPTIDE FAMILIES

The peptide families in this section are ribosomal peptides, usually with hormonal activity. All of these peptides are synthesized by cells as longer "propeptides" or "proproteins" and truncated prior to exiting the cell. They are released into the bloodstream where they perform their signaling functions.

Antimicrobial Peptides

- Magainin family
- Cecropin family
- Cathelicidin family
- Defensin family

Tachykinin Peptides

- Substance P
- Kassinin
- Neurokinin A
- Eledoisin
- Neurokinin B

Vasoactive Intestinal Peptides

- VIP (*__V__asoactive __I__ntestinal __P__eptide*; PHM27)
- PACAP ***P**ituitary **A**denylate **C**yclase **A**ctivating **P**eptide*
- Peptide PHI 27 (***P**eptide **H**istidine **I**soleucine 27*)
- GHRH 1-24 *(**G**rowth **H**ormone **R**eleasing **H**ormone 1-24)*
- Glucagon
- Secretin

Pancreatic Polypeptide-related Peptides

- NPY *(**N**euro**P**eptide **Y**)*
- PYY *(**P**eptide **YY**)*
- APP *(**A**vian **P**ancreatic **P**olypeptide)*
- PPY ***P**ancreatic **P**ol**Y**peptide*

Opioid Peptides

- Proopiomelanocortin (POMC) peptides
- Enkephalin pentapeptides
- Prodynorphin peptides

Calcitonin Peptides

- Calcitonin
- Amylin
- AGG01

Other Peptides

- B-type Natriuretic Peptide (BNP) - produced in myocardium & useful in medical diagnosis
- Lactotripeptides - Lactotripeptides might reduce blood pressure, although the evidence is mixed.

NOTES ON TERMINOLOGY

Length:

- A *polypeptide* is a single linear chain of many amino acids, held together by amide bonds.
- A *protein* is one or more polypeptide (more than about 50 amino acids long).
- An *oligopeptide* consists of only a few amino acids (between two and twenty).

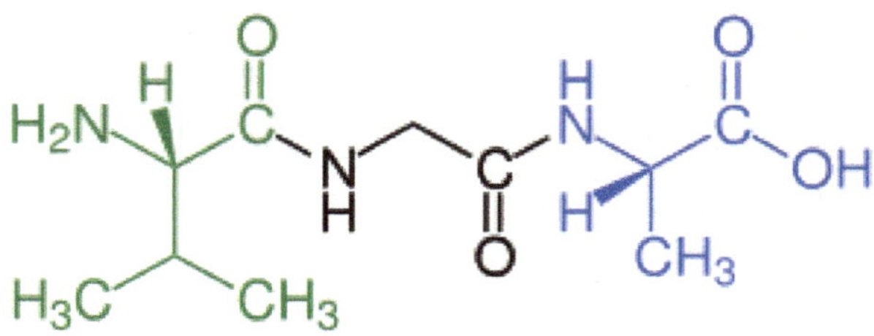

A tripeptide (example Val-Gly-Ala) with**green** marked amino end (**L-Valine**) and **blue** marked carboxyl end (**L-Alanine**).

Number of amino acids:

- A *monopeptide* has one amino acid.
- A *dipeptide* has two amino acids.
- A *tripeptide* has three amino acids.
- A *tetrapeptide* has four amino acids.
- A *pentapeptide* has five amino acids.
- A *hexapeptide* has six amino acids.
- A *heptapeptide* has seven amino acids.
- An *octapeptide* has eight amino acids (e.g., angiotensin II).

- A *nonapeptide* has nine amino acids (e.g., oxytocin).
- A *decapeptide* has ten amino acids (e.g., gonadotropin-releasing hormone & angiotensin I).
- An *undecapeptide* (or *monodecapeptide*) has eleven amino acids, a *dodecapeptide* (or *didecapeptide*) has twelve amino acids, a *tridecapeptide* has thirteen amino acids, and so forth.
- An *icosapeptide* has twenty amino acids, a *tricontapeptide* has thirty amino acids, a *tetracontapeptide* has forty amino acids, and so forth.

Function:

- A *neuropeptide* is a peptide that is active in association with neural tissue.
- A *lipopeptide* is a peptide that has a lipid connected to it, and *pepducins* are lipopeptides that interact with GPCRs.
- A *peptide hormone* is a peptide that acts as a hormone.
- A proteose is a mixture of peptides produced by the hydrolysis of proteins. The term is somewhat archaic.

Doping in Sports

The term *peptide* has been used to mean *secretagogue peptides* and *peptide hormones* in sports doping matters: secretagogue peptides are classified as Schedule 2 (S2) prohibited substances on the World Anti-Doping Agency (WADA) Prohibited List, and are therefore prohibited for use by professional athletes both in and out of competition. Such secretagogue peptides have been on the WADA prohibited substances list since at least 2008. The Australian Crime Commission cited the alleged misuse of secretagogue peptides in Australian sport including growth hormone releasing peptides CJC-1295, GHRP-6, and GHSR (gene) hexarelin. There is ongoing controversy on the legality of using secretagogue peptides in sports.

PRO-OPIOMELANOCORTIN (POMC)

Pro-opiomelanocortin (POMC) is a precursor polypeptide with 241 amino acid residues. POMC is synthesized in the pituitary from the 285-amino-acid-long polypeptide precursor **pre-pro-opiomelanocortin** (pre-POMC), by the removal of a 44-amino-acid-long signal peptide sequence during translation.

Function

POMC is cleaved to give rise to multiple peptide hormones. Each of these peptides is packaged in large dense-core vesicles that are released from the cells by exocytosis in response to appropriate stimulation:

- α-MSH produced by neurons in the arcuate nucleus has important roles in the regulation of appetite and sexual behavior, while α-MSH secreted from the intermediate lobe of the pituitary regulates the production of melanin.

- ACTH is a peptide hormone that regulates the secretion of glucocorticoids from the adrenal cortex.
- β-Endorphin and [Met]enkephalin are endogenous opioid peptides with widespread actions in the brain.

Synthesis

The POMC gene is located on chromosome 2p23.3. The POMC gene is expressed in both the anterior and intermediate lobes of the pituitary gland. This gene encodes a 285-amino acid polypeptide hormone precursor that undergoes extensive, tissue-specific, post-translational processing via cleavage by subtilisin-like enzymes known as prohormone convertases. The encoded protein is synthesized mainly in corticotroph cells of the anterior pituitary, where four cleavage sites are used; adrenocorticotrophin (ACTH), essential for normal steroidogenesis and the maintenance of normal adrenal weight, and β-lipotropin are the major end-products. However, there are at least eight potential cleavage sites within the polypeptide precursor and, depending on tissue type and the available convertases, processing may yield as many as ten biologically active peptides involved in diverse cellular functions. Cleavage sites consist of the sequences Arg-Lys, Lys-Arg, or Lys-Lys. Enzymes responsible for processing of POMC peptides include prohormone convertase 1 (PC1), prohormone convertase 2 (PC2), carboxypeptidase E (CPE), peptidyl α-amidating monooxygenase (PAM), *N*-acetyltransferase (N-AT), and prolylcarboxypeptidase (PRCP).

The processing of POMC involves glycosylations, acetylations, and extensive proteolytic cleavage at sites shown to contain regions of basic protein sequences. However, the proteases that recognize these cleavage sites are tissue-specific. In some tissues, including the hypothalamus, placenta, and epithelium, all cleavage sites may be used, giving rise to peptides with roles in pain and energy homeostasis, melanocyte stimulation, and immune modulation. These include several distinct melanotropins, lipotropins, and endorphins that are contained within the adrenocorticotrophin and β-lipotropin peptides.

It is synthesized by:

- Corticotrope cells of the anterior pituitary gland
- Melanotrope cells of the intermediate lobe of the pituitary gland
- Neurons in the arcuate nucleus of the hypothalamus
- Smaller populations of neurons in the dorsomedial hypothalamus and brainstem
- Melanocytes in the skin

Derivatives

<table>
<tr><td colspan="6">proopiomelanocortin derivatives</td></tr>
<tr><td colspan="6">POMC</td></tr>
<tr><td></td><td></td><td></td><td></td><td></td><td></td></tr>
<tr><td>γ-MSH</td><td>ACTH</td><td>β-lipotropin</td><td></td><td></td><td></td></tr>
</table>

	α-MSH	CLIP	γ-lipotropin		β-endorphin				
				β-MSH					

The large molecule of POMC is the source of several important biologically active substances. POMC can be cleaved enzymatically into the following peptides:

- *N*-Terminal Peptide of Proopiomelanocortin (NPP, or pro-γ-MSH)
- γ-Melanotropin (γ-MSH)
- Corticotropin (Adrenocorticotropic Hormone, or ACTH)
- α-Melanotropin (α-Melanocyte-Stimulating Hormone, or α-MSH)
- Corticotropin-like Intermediate Peptide (CLIP)
- β-Lipotropin (β-LPH)
- Lipotropin Gamma (γ-LPH)
- β-Melanotropin (β-MSH)
- β-Endorphin
- [Met]Enkephalin

Although the N-terminal 5 amino acids of β-endorphin are identical to the sequence of [Met]enkephalin, it is not generally thought that β-endorphin is converted into [Met] enkephalin. Instead, [Met]enkephalin is produced from its own precursor, proenkephalin A.

The production of β-MSH occurs in humans but not in mice or rats due to the absence of the enzymatic processing site in the rodent POMC.

Clinical Significance

Mutations in this gene have been associated with early onset obesity, adrenal insufficiency, and red hair pigmentation.

Dogs

A deletion mutation common in Labrador Retriever and Flat-Coated Retriever dogs is associated with increased interest in food and subsequent obesity.

Drug Target

Two humans with POMC deficiency have been treated with setmelanotide, a melanocortin-4 receptor agonist.

Interactions

Proopiomelanocortin has been shown to interact with melanocortin 4 receptor.

ENKEPHALIN

An **enkephalin** (occasionally spelt *encephalin*) is a pentapeptide involved in regulating nociception in the body. The enkephalins are termed endogenous ligands, as they are internally derived and bind to the body›s opioid receptors. Discovered in 1975, two forms of enkephalin were discovered, one containing leucine ("leu"), and the other containing methionine ("met"). Both are products of the proenkephalin gene.

- Met-enkephalin is Tyr-Gly-Gly-Phe-**Met**.
- Leu-enkephalin has Tyr-Gly-Gly-Phe-**Leu**.

Endogenous Opioid Peptides

There are three well-characterized families of opioid peptides produced by the body: enkephalins, endorphins, and dynorphins. The met-enkephalin peptide sequence is coded for by the enkephalin gene; the leu-enkephalin peptide sequence is coded for by both the enkephalin gene and the dynorphin gene. The proopiomelanocortin gene (POMC) also contains the met-enkephalin sequence on the N-terminus of beta-endorphin, but the endorphin peptide is not processed into enkephalin.

Enkephalin Receptor

The receptors for enkephalin are the delta opioid receptors and mu opioid receptors. Opioid receptors are a group of G-protein-coupled receptors, with other opioids as ligands as well. The other endogenous opioids are dynorphins (that bind to kappa receptors), endorphins (mu receptors), endomorphins, and nociceptin/orphanin FQ. The opioid receptors are ~40% identical to somatostatin receptors (SSTRs).

PRODYNORPHIN

Prodynorphin, also known as **proenkephalin B**, is an opioid polypeptide hormone involved with chemical signal transduction and cell communication. The gene for prodynorphin is expressed in the endometrium and the striatum, and its gene map locus is 20pter-p12. Prodynorphin is a basic building-block of endorphins, the chemical messengers in the brain that appear most heavily involved in the anticipation and experience of pain and the formation of deep emotional bonds, and that are also critical in learning and memory.

The gene is thought to influence perception, as well as susceptibility to drug dependence, and is expressed more readily in human beings than in other primates.

Evolutionary Implications

Most humans have multiple copies of the regulatory gene sequence for prodynorphin, which is virtually identical among all primates, whereas other primates have only a single copy. In addition, most Asian populations have two copies of the gene sequence for prodynorphin, whereas East Africas, Middle Easterners, and Europeans tend to have three repetitions.

The extent of regulatory gene disparities for prodynorphin, between human and primates, has gained the attention of scientists. There are very few genes known to be directly related to mankind's speciation from other great apes. According to computational biologist researcher Matthew W. Hahn of Indiana University, "this is the first documented instance of a neural gene that has had its regulation shaped by natural selection during human origins."

The prodynorphin polypeptide is identical in humans and chimpanzees, but the regulatory promoter sequences have been shown to exhibit marked differences. According to Hahn, "humans have the ability to turn on this gene more easily and more intensely than other primates", a reason why regulation of this gene may have been important in the evolution of modern humans' mental capacity

REFERENCES

1. Hormone (androgen deprivation) therapy for prostate cancer. cancer.org. Retrieved 3 October 2013.
2. What are peptides. Zealand Pharma A/S. Archived from the original on 2014-07-14.
3. Ardejani, Maziar S.; Orner, Brendan P. (2013-05-03).Obey the Peptide Assembly Rules. Science. 340 (6132): 561–562. doi:10.1126/science.1237708. ISSN 0036-8075. PMID 23641105.
4. Boelsma E, Kloek J; Kloek (March 2009).Lactotripeptides and antihypertensive effects: a critical review. The British Journal of Nutrition. 101 (6): 776–86. doi:10.1017/S0007114508137722. PMID 19061526.
5. Bulinski JC (1986).Peptide antibodies: new tools for cell biology. International Review of Cytology. International Review of Cytology. 103: 281–302. doi:10.1016/S0074-7696(08)60838-4. ISBN 9780123645036. PMID 2427468.
6. Du L, Shen B; Shen (March 2001).Biosynthesis of hybrid peptide-polyketide natural products. Current Opinion in Drug Discovery & Development. 4 (2): 215–28. PMID 11378961.
7. Duquesne S, Destoumieux-Garzón D, Peduzzi J, Rebuffat S; Destoumieux-Garzón; Peduzzi; Rebuffat (August 2007).Microcins, gene-encoded antibacterial peptides from enterobacteria. Natural Product Reports. 24 (4): 708–34. doi:10.1039/b516237h. PMID 17653356.
8. Engberink MF, Schouten EG, Kok FJ, van Mierlo LA, Brouwer IA, Geleijnse JM; Schouten; Kok; Van Mierlo; Brouwer; Geleijnse (February 2008).

Lactotripeptides show no effect on human blood pressure: results from a double-blind randomized controlled trial. Hypertension. 51 (2): 399–405. doi:10.1161/HYPERTENSIONAHA.107.098988. PMID 18086944.

9. Finking R, Marahiel MA; Marahiel (2004).Biosynthesis of nonribosomal peptides1. Annual Review of Microbiology. 58 (1): 453–88. doi:10.1146/annurev.micro.58.030603.123615. PMID 15487945.

10. Hahn M, Stachelhaus T; Stachelhaus (November 2004).Selective interaction between nonribosomal peptide synthetases is facilitated by short communication-mediating domains. Proceedings of the National Academy of Sciences of the United States of America. 101 (44): 15585–90. Bibcode:2004PNAS..10115585H. doi:10.1073/pnas.0404932101. PMC 524835. PMID 15498872.

11. Haque, Emily; Chand, Rattan.Milk protein derived bioactive peptides. Dairy Science. Retrieved 28 July 2014.

12. Herce, Henry D.; Deng, Wen; Helma, Jonas; Leonhardt, Heinrich; Cardoso, M. Cristina (24 October 2013).Visualization and targeted disruption of protein interactions in living cells. Nature Communications. 4. doi:10.1038/ncomms3660. PMC 3826628. PMID 24154492.

13. https://theconversation.edu.au/we-need-an-advocate-against-asadas-power-in-doping-control-12119

14. Hummel J, Niemann M, Wienkoop S; et al. (2007).ProMEX: a mass spectral reference database for proteins and protein phosphorylation sites. BMC Bioinformatics. 8 (1): 216. doi:10.1186/1471-2105-8-216. PMC 1920535. PMID 17587460.

15. IUPAC, Compendium of Chemical Terminology, 2nd ed. (theGold Book) (1997). Online corrected version: (2006–)amino-acid residue in a polypeptide.

16. IUPAC. Compendium of Chemical Terminology, 2nd ed. (theGold Book). Compiled by A. D. McNaught and A. Wilkinson. Blackwell Scientific Publications, Oxford (1997). XML on-line corrected version: http://goldbook.iupac.org (2006-) created by M. Nic, J. Jirat, B. Kosata; updates compiled by A. Jenkins. ISBN 0-9678550-9-8. doi:10.1351/goldbook.P04898.

17. Kumar, Ravi; Barqawi, A; Crawford, ED (2005).Adverse Events Associated with Hormonal Therapy for Prostate Cancer. Reviews in Urology. 7 (5): 37–43. PMC 1477613. PMID 16985883.

18. Marquet P, Lachâtre G; Lachâtre (October 1999).Liquid chromatography-mass spectrometry: potential in forensic and clinical toxicology. Journal of Chromatography B. 733 (1–2): 93–118. doi:10.1016/S0378-4347(99)00147-4. PMID 10572976.

19. Meister A, Anderson ME; Anderson (1983).Glutathione. Annual Review of Biochemistry. 52 (1): 711–60. doi:10.1146/annurev.bi.52.070183.003431. PMID 6137189.

20. Payne JW (1976).Peptides and micro-organisms. Advances in Microbial Physiology. Advances in Microbial Physiology. 13: 55–113. doi:10.1016/S0065-

2911(08)60038-7. ISBN 9780120277131. PMID 775944.

21. Pons M, Feliz M, Antònia Molins M, Giralt E; Feliz; Antònia Molins; Giralt (May 1991).Conformational analysis of bacitracin A, a naturally occurring lariat. Biopolymers. 31 (6): 605–12. doi:10.1002/bip.360310604. PMID 1932561.
22. Pripp AH (2008).Effect of peptides derived from food proteins on blood pressure: a meta-analysis of randomized controlled trials. Food & Nutrition Research. 52: 10.3402/fnr.v52i0.1641. doi:10.3402/fnr.v52i0.1641. PMC 2596738. PMID 19109662.
23. Torres AM, Menz I, Alewood PF, et al. (July 2002).D-Amino acid residue in the C-type natriuretic peptide from the venom of the mammal, Ornithorhynchus anatinus, the Australian platypus. FEBS Letters. 524 (1–3): 172–6. doi:10.1016/S0014-5793(02)03050-8. PMID 12135762.
24. Webster J, Oxley D; Oxley (2005).Peptide mass fingerprinting: protein identification using MALDI-TOF mass spectrometry. Methods in Molecular Biology. Methods in Molecular Biology™. 310: 227–40. doi:10.1007/978-1-59259-948-6_16. ISBN 978-1-58829-399-2. PMID 16350956.
25. Xu JY, Qin LQ, Wang PY, Li W, Chang C; Qin; Wang; Li; Chang (October 2008).Effect of milk tripeptides on blood pressure: a meta-analysis of randomized controlled trials. Nutrition. 24 (10): 933–40. doi:10.1016/j.nut.2008.04.004. PMID 18562172.

Side Chain Properties

Amino acid	Short	Abbrev.	Side chain	Hydro-phobic	pKa	Polar	pH	Small	Tiny	Aromatic or Aliphatic	van der Waals volume (Å³)
Alanine	A	Ala	$-CH_3$	X	-	-	-	X	X	Aliphatic	67
Cysteine	C	Cys	$-CH_2SH$	X	8.18	-	acidic	X	X	-	86
Aspartic acid	D	Asp	$-CH_2COOH$	-	3.90	X	acidic	X	-	-	91
Glutamic acid	E	Glu	$-CH_2CH_2COOH$	-	4.07	X	acidic	-	-	-	109
Phenylalanine	F	Phe	$-CH_2C_6H_5$	X	-	-	-	-	-	Aromatic	135
Glycine	G	Gly	-H	X	-	-	-	X	X	-	48
Histidine	H	His	$-CH_2-C_3H_3N_2$	-	6.04	X	weak basic	-	-	Aromatic	118
Isoleucine	I	Ile	$-CH(CH_3)CH_2CH_3$	X	-	-	-	-	-	Aliphatic	124
Lysine	K	Lys	$-(CH_2)_4NH_2$	-	10.54	X	basic	-	-	-	135
Leucine	L	Leu	$-CH_2CH(CH_3)_2$	X	-	-	-	-	-	Aliphatic	124
Methionine	M	Met	$-CH_2CH_2SCH_3$	X	-	-	-	-	-	Aliphatic	124
Asparagine	N	Asn	$-CH_2CONH_2$	-	-	X	-	X	-	-	96
Pyrrolysine	O	Pyl	$-(CH_2)_4NHCOC_4H_5NCH_3$	-	N.D.	X	weak basic	-	-	-	
Proline	P	Pro	$-CH_2CH_2CH_2-$	X	-	-	-	X	-	-	90
Glutamine	Q	Gln	$-CH_2CH_2CONH_2$	-	-	X	-	-	-	-	114
Arginine	R	Arg	$-(CH_2)_3NH-C(NH)NH_2$	-	12.48	X	strongly basic	-	-	-	148
Serine	S	Ser	$-CH_2OH$	-	-	X	-	X	X	-	73
Threonine	T	Thr	$-CH(OH)CH_3$	-	-	X	-	X	-	-	93
Selenocysteine	U	Sec	$-CH_2SeH$	-	5.73	-	acidic	X	X	-	
Valine	V	Val	$-CH(CH_3)_2$	X	-	-	-	X	-	Aliphatic	105
Tryptophan	W	Trp	$-CH_2C_8H_6N$	-	-	X	-	-	-	Aromatic	163
Tyrosine	Y	Tyr	$-CH_2-C_6H_4OH$	-	10.46	X	weak acidic	-	-	Aromatic	141

N.D.: The pKa value of Pyrrolysine has not been reported.

Note: The pKa values of amino acids are typically slightly different when the amino acid is inside a protein. Protein pKa calculations are sometimes used to calculate the change in the pKa value of an amino acid in this situation.

Gene Expression and Biochemistry

Amino acid	Short	Abbrev.	Codon(s)	Occurrence in Archaean proteins (%)&	Occurrence in Bacteria proteins (%)&	Occurrence in Eukaryote proteins (%)&	Occurrence in human proteins (%)&	Essential‡ in humans
Alanine	A	Ala	GCU, GCC, GCA, GCG	8.2	10.06	7.63	7.01	No

Cysteine	C	Cys	UGU, UGC	0.98	0.94	1.76	2.3	Conditionally
Aspartic acid	D	Asp	GAU, GAC	6.21	5.59	5.4	4.73	No
Glutamic acid	E	Glu	GAA, GAG	7.69	6.15	6.42	7.09	Conditionally
Phenylalanine	F	Phe	UUU, UUC	3.86	3.89	3.87	3.65	Yes
Glycine	G	Gly	GGU, GGC, GGA, GGG	7.58	7.76	6.33	6.58	Conditionally
Histidine	H	His	CAU, CAC	1.77	2.06	2.44	2.63	Yes
Isoleucine	I	Ile	AUU, AUC, AUA	7.03	5.89	5.1	4.33	Yes
Lysine	K	Lys	AAA, AAG	5.27	4.68	5.64	5.72	Yes
Leucine	L	Leu	UUA, UUG, CUU, CUC, CUA, CUG	9.31	10.09	9.29	9.97	Yes
Methionine	M	Met	AUG	2.35	2.38	2.25	2.13	Yes
Asparagine	N	Asn	AAU, AAC	3.68	3.58	4.28	3.58	No
Pyrrolysine	O	Pyl	UAG*	0	0	0	0	No
Proline	P	Pro	CCU, CCC, CCA, CCG	4.26	4.61	5.41	6.31	No
Glutamine	Q	Gln	CAA, CAG	2.38	3.58	4.21	4.77	No
Arginine	R	Arg	CGU, CGC, CGA, CGG, AGA, AGG	5.51	5.88	5.71	5.64	Conditionally
Serine	S	Ser	UCU, UCC, UCA, UCG, AGU, AGC	6.17	5.85	8.34	8.33	No
Threonine	T	Thr	ACU, ACC, ACA, ACG	5.44	5.52	5.56	5.36	Yes
Selenocysteine	U	Sec	UGA**	0	0	0	>0	No
Valine	V	Val	GUU, GUC, GUA, GUG	7.8	7.27	6.2	5.96	Yes
Tryptophan	W	Trp	UGG	1.03	1.27	1.24	1.22	Yes
Tyrosine	Y	Tyr	UAU, UAC	3.35	2.94	2.87	2.66	Conditionally
Stop codon†	-	Term	UAA, UAG, UGA††				-	-

* UAG is normally the amber stop codon, but encodes pyrrolysine if a PYLIS element is present.

** UGA is normally the opal (or umber) stop codon, but encodes selenocysteine if a SECIS element is present.

† The stop codon is not an amino acid, but is included for completeness.

†† UAG and UGA do not always act as stop codons (see above).

‡ An essential amino acid cannot be synthesized in humans and must, therefore, be supplied in the diet. Conditionally essential amino acids are not normally required in the diet, but must be supplied exogenously to specific populations that do not synthesize it in adequate amounts.

& Occurrence of amino acids is based on 135 Archaea, 3775 Bacteria, 614 Eukaryota proteomes and human proteome (21 006 proteins) respectively.

Mass Spectrometry

In mass spectrometry of peptides and proteins, knowledge of the masses of the residues is useful. The mass of the peptide or protein is the sum of the residue masses plus the mass of water (Monoisotopic mass = 18.01056 Da; average mass = 18.0153 Da). The residue masses are calculated from the tabulated chemical formulas and atomic weights. In mass spectrometry, ions may also include one or more protons (Monoisotopic mass = 1.00728 Da; average mass = 1.0074 Da).

Amino Acid	Short	Abbrev.	Formula	Mon. Mass§ (Da)	Avg. Mass (Da)
Alanine	A	Ala	C_3H_5NO	71.03711	71.0779
Cysteine	C	Cys	C_3H_5NOS	103.00919	103.1429
Aspartic acid	D	Asp	$C_4H_5NO_3$	115.02694	115.0874
Glutamic acid	E	Glu	$C_5H_7NO_3$	129.04259	129.1140
Phenylalanine	F	Phe	C_9H_9NO	147.06841	147.1739
Glycine	G	Gly	C_2H_3NO	57.02146	57.0513
Histidine	H	His	$C_6H_7N_3O$	137.05891	137.1393
Isoleucine	I	Ile	$C_6H_{11}NO$	113.08406	113.1576
Lysine	K	Lys	$C_6H_{12}N_2O$	128.09496	128.1723
Leucine	L	Leu	$C_6H_{11}NO$	113.08406	113.1576
Methionine	M	Met	C_5H_9NOS	131.04049	131.1961
Asparagine	N	Asn	$C_4H_6N_2O_2$	114.04293	114.1026
Pyrrolysine	O	Pyl	$C_{12}H_{19}N_3O_2$	237.14773	237.2982
Proline	P	Pro	C_5H_7NO	97.05276	97.1152
Glutamine	Q	Gln	$C_5H_8N_2O_2$	128.05858	128.1292
Arginine	R	Arg	$C_6H_{12}N_4O$	156.10111	156.1857
Serine	S	Ser	$C_3H_5NO_2$	87.03203	87.0773
Threonine	T	Thr	$C_4H_7NO_2$	101.04768	101.1039
Selenocysteine	U	Sec	C_3H_5NOSe	150.95364	150.0489
Valine	V	Val	C_5H_9NO	99.06841	99.1311
Tryptophan	W	Trp	$C_{11}H_{10}N_2O$	186.07931	186.2099
Tyrosine	Y	Tyr	$C_9H_9NO_2$	163.06333	163.1733

Stoichiometry and Metabolic Cost in Cell

The table below lists the abundance of amino acids in *E.coli* cells and the metabolic cost (ATP) for synthesis the amino acids. Negative numbers indicate the metabolic processes are energy favorable and do not cost net ATP of the cell. The abundance of amino acids includes amino acids in free form and in polymerization form (proteins).

Amino acid	Abundance (# of molecules (×10[8]) per *E. coli* cell)	ATP cost in synthesis under aerobic condition	ATP cost in synthesis under anaerobic condition
Alanine	2.9	-1	1
Cysteine	0.52	11	15
Aspartic acid	1.4	0	2
Glutamic acid	1.5	-7	-1
Phenylalanine	1.1	-6	2
Glycine	3.5	-2	2
Histidine	0.54	1	7
Isoleucine	1.7	7	11
Lysine	2.0	5	9
Leucine	2.6	-9	1
Methionine	0.88	21	23
Asparagine	1.4	3	5
Proline	1.3	-2	4
Glutamine	1.5	-6	0
Arginine	1.7	5	13
Serine	1.2	-2	2
Threonine	1.5	6	8
Tryptophan	0.33	-7	7
Tyrosine	0.79	-8	2
Valine	2.4	-2	2

Remarks

Amino Acid	Abbrev.		Remarks
Alanine	A	Ala	Very abundant and very versatile, it is more stiff than glycine, but small enough to pose only small steric limits for the protein conformation. It behaves fairly neutrally, and can be located in both hydrophilic regions on the protein outside and the hydrophobic areas inside.
Asparagine or aspartic acid	B	Asx	A placeholder when either amino acid may occupy a position
Cysteine	C	Cys	The sulfur atom bonds readily to heavy metal ions. Under oxidizing conditions, two cysteines can join together in a disulfide bond to form the amino acid cystine. When cystines are part of a protein, insulin for example, the tertiary structure is stabilized, which makes the protein more resistant to denaturation; therefore, disulfide bonds are common in proteins that have to function in harsh environments including digestive enzymes (e.g., pepsin and chymotrypsin) and structural proteins (e.g., keratin). Disulfides are also found in peptides too small to hold a stable shape on their own (e.g. insulin).

Aspartic acid	D	Asp	Asp behaves similarly to glutamic acid, and carries a hydrophilic acidic group with strong negative charge. Usually, it is located on the outer surface of the protein, making it water-soluble. It binds to positively charged molecules and ions, and is often used in enzymes to fix the metal ion. When located inside of the protein, aspartate and glutamate are usually paired with arginine and lysine.
Glutamic acid	E	Glu	Glu behaves similarly to aspartic acid, and has a longer, slightly more flexible side chain.
Phenylalanine	F	Phe	Essential for humans, phenylalanine, tyrosine, and tryptophan contain a large, rigid aromatic group on the side chain. These are the biggest amino acids. Like isoleucine, leucine, and valine, these are hydrophobic and tend to orient towards the interior of the folded protein molecule. Phenylalanine can be converted into tyrosine.
Glycine	G	Gly	Because of the two hydrogen atoms at the α carbon, glycine is not optically active. It is the smallest amino acid, rotates easily, and adds flexibility to the protein chain. It is able to fit into the tightest spaces, e.g., the triple helix of collagen. As too much flexibility is usually not desired, as a structural component, it is less common than alanine.
Histidine	H	His	His is essential for humans. In even slightly acidic conditions, protonation of the nitrogen occurs, changing the properties of histidine and the polypeptide as a whole. It is used by many proteins as a regulatory mechanism, changing the conformation and behavior of the polypeptide in acidic regions such as the late endosome or lysosome, enforcing conformation change in enzymes. However, only a few histidines are needed for this, so it is comparatively scarce.
Isoleucine	I	Ile	Ile is essential for humans. Isoleucine, leucine, and valine have large aliphatic hydrophobic side chains. Their molecules are rigid, and their mutual hydrophobic interactions are important for the correct folding of proteins, as these chains tend to be located inside of the protein molecule.
Leucine or isoleucine	J	Xle	A placeholder when either amino acid may occupy a position
Lysine	K	Lys	Lys is essential for humans, and behaves similarly to arginine. It contains a long, flexible side chain with a positively charged end. The flexibility of the chain makes lysine and arginine suitable for binding to molecules with many negative charges on their surfaces. E.g., DNA-binding proteins have their active regions rich with arginine and lysine. The strong charge makes these two amino acids prone to be located on the outer hydrophilic surfaces of the proteins; when they are found inside, they are usually paired with a corresponding negatively charged amino acid, e.g., aspartate or glutamate.
Leucine	L	Leu	Leu is essential for humans, and behaves similarly to isoleucine and valine.
Methionine	M	Met	Met is essential for humans. Always the first amino acid to be incorporated into a protein, it is sometimes removed after translation. Like cysteine, it contains sulfur, but with a methyl group instead of hydrogen. This methyl group can be activated, and is used in many reactions where a new carbon atom is being added to another molecule.
Asparagine	N	Asn	Similar to aspartic acid, Asn contains an amide group where Asp has a carboxyl.
Pyrrolysine	O	Pyl	Similar to lysine, but it has a pyrroline ring attached.

Proline	P	Pro	Pro contains an unusual ring to the N-end amine group, which forces the CO-NH amide sequence into a fixed conformation. It can disrupt protein folding structures like α helix or β sheet, forcing the desired kink in the protein chain. Common in collagen, it often undergoes a post-translational modification to hydroxyproline.
Glutamine	Q	Gln	Similar to glutamic acid, Gln contains an amide group where Glu has a carboxyl. Used in proteins and as a storage for ammonia, it is the most abundant amino acid in the body.
Arginine	R	Arg	Functionally similar to lysine
Serine	S	Ser	Serine and threonine have a short group ended with a hydroxyl group. Its hydrogen is easy to remove, so serine and threonine often act as hydrogen donors in enzymes. Both are very hydrophilic, so the outer regions of soluble proteins tend to be rich with them.
Threonine	T	Thr	Essential for humans, Thr behaves similarly to serine.
Selenocysteine	U	Sec	The selenium analog of cysteine, in which selenium replaces the sulfur atom.
Valine	V	Val	Essential for humans, Val behaves similarly to isoleucine and leucine.
Tryptophan	W	Trp	Essential for humans, Trp behaves similarly to phenylalanine and tyrosine. It is a precursor of serotonin and is naturally fluorescent.
Unknown	X	Xaa	Placeholder when the amino acid is unknown or unimportant
Tyrosine	Y	Tyr	Tyr behaves similarly to phenylalanine (precursor to tyrosine) and tryptophan, and is a precursor of melanin, epinephrine, and thyroid hormones. Naturally fluorescent, its fluorescence is usually quenched by energy transfer to tryptophans.
Glutamic acid or glutamine	Z	Glx	A placeholder when either amino acid may occupy a position

Catabolism

- Glucogenic, with the products having the ability to form glucose by gluconeogenesis
- Ketogenic, with the products not having the ability to form glucose: These products may still be used for ketogenesis or lipid synthesis.
- Amino acids catabolized into both glucogenic and ketogenic products.

Life based on Alternative Proteinogenic Sets

The proteinogenic set used by known life on Earth appears to be arbitrarily selected by evolution, according to current knowledge, from many hundreds of possible alpha-type amino acids. Xenobiology studies hypothetical life forms that could be constructed using alternative sets using expanded genetic codes. Miller-type experiments on artificial abiogenesis show that alpha-type amino acids predominate in water-based 'primordial soups', but beta-type amino acids dominate when less water is present. Both alpha- and beta-based sets could form the basis for alternative protein constructions and life forms.

ASPARTIC ACID

Aspartic acid (abbreviated as **Asp** or **D**; encoded by the codons [GAU and GAC]), also known as **aspartate**, is an α-amino acid that is used in the biosynthesis of proteins. It contains an α-amino group (which is in the protonated −NH+ 3 form under biological conditions), an α-carboxylic acid group (which is in the deprotonated $-COO^-$ form under biological conditions), and a side chain CH_2COOH. Under physiological conditions in proteins the sidechain usually occurs as the negatively charged aspartate form, $-COO^-$. It is semi-essential in humans, meaning the body can synthesize it from oxaloacetate.

In proteins aspartate sidechains are often hydrogen bonded, often as asx turns or asx motifs, which often occur at the N-termini of alpha helices.

Asp's L-isomer is one of the 23 proteinogenic amino acids, i.e., the building blocks of proteins. **Asp** (and glutamic acid) is classified as acidic, with a pK_a of 3.9, however in a peptide this is highly dependent on the local environment (as with all amino acids), and could be as high as 14. **Asp** is pervasive in biosynthesis.

L-aspartic acid is one of the two main ingredients of the artificial sweetener aspartame, along with L-phenylalanine.

Discovery

Aspartic acid was first discovered in 1827 by Auguste-Arthur Plisson and Étienne Ossian Henry, derived from asparagine, which had been isolated from asparagus juice in 1806, by boiling with a base.

Forms and nomenclature

There are two forms or enantiomers of aspartic acid. The name "aspartic acid" can refer to either enantiomer or a mixture of two. Of these two forms, only one, "L-aspartic acid", is directly incorporated into proteins. The biological roles of its counterpart, "D-aspartic acid" are more limited. Where enzymatic synthesis will produce one or the other, most chemical syntheses will produce both forms, "DL-aspartic acid," known as a racemic mixture.

Metabolism

Aspartate is non-essential in mammals, being produced from oxaloacetate by transamination. It can also be generated from ornithine and citrulline in the urea cycle. In plants and microorganisms, aspartate is the precursor to several amino acids, including four that are essential for humans: methionine, threonine, isoleucine, and lysine. The conversion of aspartate to these other amino acids begins with reduction of aspartate to its "semialdehyde," $O_2CCH(NH_2)CH_2CHO$. Asparagine is derived from aspartate via transamidation:

$-O_2CCH(NH_2)CH_2CO_2$- + $GC(O)NH_3$+ $O_2CCH(NH_2)CH_2CONH_3$+ + $GC(O)O$

(where $GC(O)NH_2$ and $GC(O)OH$ are glutamine and glutamic acid, respectively)

Other Biochemical Roles

Aspartate is also a metabolite in the urea cycle and participates in gluconeogenesis. It carries reducing equivalents in the malate-aspartate shuttle, which utilizes the ready interconversion of aspartate and oxaloacetate, which is the oxidized (dehydrogenated) derivative of malic acid. Aspartate donates one nitrogen atom in the biosynthesis of inosine, the precursor to the purine bases. In addition, aspartic acid acts as hydrogen acceptor in a chain of ATP synthase.

Interactive Pathway Map

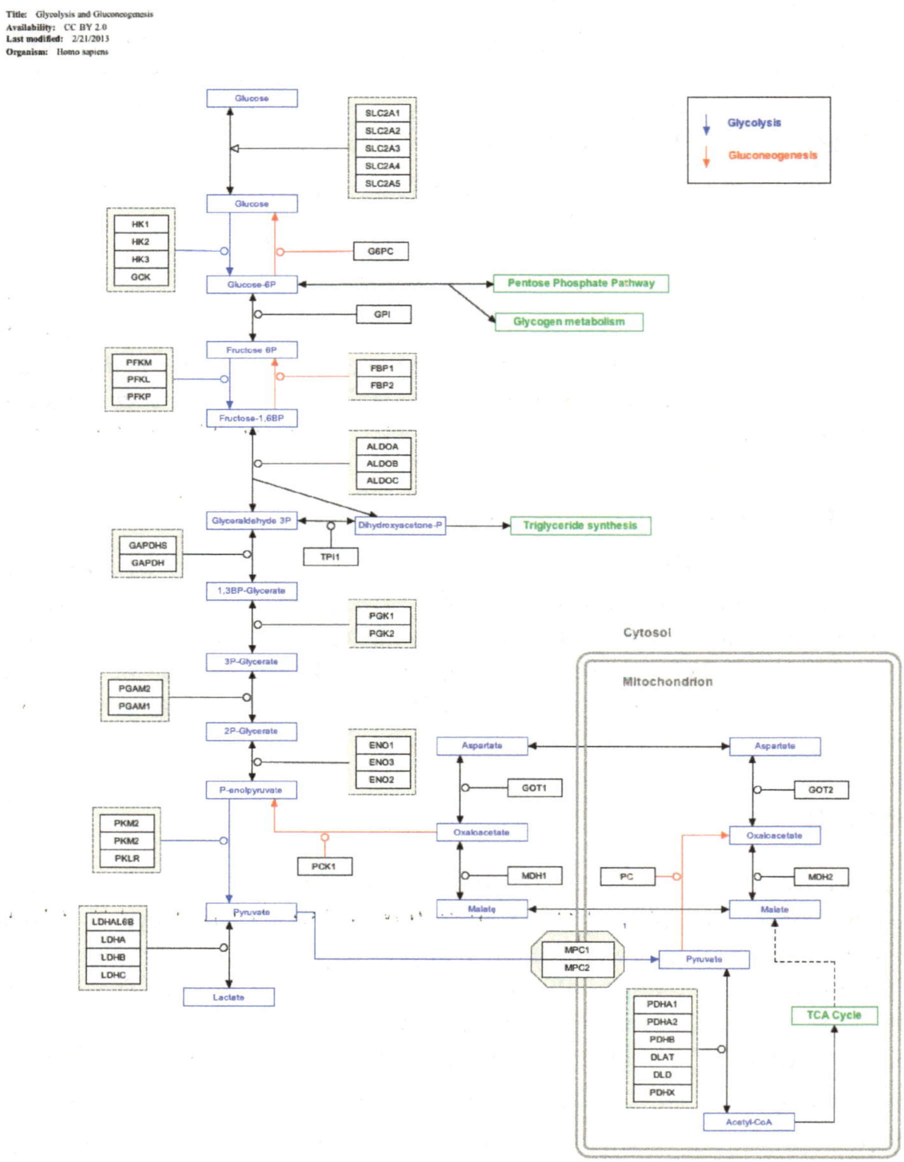

Glycolysis and Gluconeogenesis

Neurotransmitter

Aspartate (the conjugate base of aspartic acid) stimulates NMDA receptors, though not as strongly as the amino acid neurotransmitter L-glutamate does.

Applications and Market

The global market for aspartic acid is $117MM annually (50-60K MT/Yr) with areas of growth accounting for an addressable market of $8.78BB. The three largest market segments include the U.S., Western Europe, and China. Current applications include biodegradable polymers (polyaspartate), low calorie sweeteners, scale and corrosion inhibitors, and resins.

Nearly all aspartic acid is manufactured in China.

Superabsorbent Polymers

One area of aspartic acid market growth is biodegradable superabsorbent polymers (SAP). The super absorbent polymers market is anticipated to grow at a CAGR of 5.5% from 2014 to 2019 to reach a value of $8.78BB globally. Around 75% of superabsorbent polymers are used in disposable diapers and an additional 20% is used for adult incontinence and feminine hygiene products. Polyaspartate, the polymerization product of aspartic acid, is a biodegradable substitute to polyacrylate.The polyaspartate market comprises a small fraction (est. < 1%) of the total SAP market.

Additional Uses

In addition to SAP, aspartic acid has applications in the $19B fertilizer industry, where polyaspartate improves water retention and nitrogen uptake; the $1.1B (2020) concrete floor coatings market, where polyaspartic is a low VOC, low energy alternative to traditional epoxy resins; and lastly the >$5B scale and corrosion inhibitors market.

- Aspartic acid is known to have a use in the synthesis of Lorglumide.

Dietary Sources

Aspartic acid is not an essential amino acid, which means that it can be synthesized from central metabolic pathway intermediates in humans. Aspartic acid is found in:

- Animal sources: oysters, luncheon meats, sausage meat, wild game
- Vegetable sources: sprouting seeds, oat flakes, avocado, asparagus, young sugarcane, and molasses from sugar beets.
- Dietary supplements, either as aspartic acid itself or salts (such as magnesium aspartate)
- The sweetener aspartame (brands: NutraSweet, Equal, Canderel, etc.)

Chemical Synthesis

Racemic aspartic acid can be synthesized from diethyl sodium phthalimidomalonate, ($C_6H_4(CO)_2NC(CO_2Et)_2$).

The major disadvantage of the above technique is that equimolar amounts of each enantiomer are made. Using biotechnology it is now possible to use immobilised enzymes to create just one type of enantiomer owing to their stereospecificity.

GLUTAMINE

Glutamine (abbreviated as **Gln** or **Q**; encoded by the codons CAA and CAG) is an α-amino acid that is used in the biosynthesis of proteins. It contains an α-amino group (which is in the protonated $-NH_3^+$ form under biological conditions), an α-carboxylic acid group (which is in the deprotonated $-COO^-$ form under biological conditions), and a side chain amide which replaces the side chain hydroxyl of glutamic acid with an amine functional group, classifying it as a charge neutral, polar (at physiological pH) amino acid. It is non-essential and conditionally essential in humans, meaning the body can usually synthesize sufficient amounts of it, but in some instances of stress, the body's demand for glutamine increases and glutamine must be obtained from the diet.

In human blood, glutamine is the most abundant free amino acid, with a concentration of about 500–900 μM.

Functions

Glutamine plays a role in a variety of biochemical functions:

- Protein synthesis, as any other of the 20 proteinogenic amino acids
- Lipid synthesis, especially by cancer cells.
- Regulation of acid-base balance in the kidney by producing ammonium
- Cellular energy, as a source, next to glucose
- Nitrogen donation for many anabolic processes, including the synthesis of purines
- Carbon donation, as a source, refilling the citric acid cycle
- Nontoxic transporter of ammonia in the blood circulation
- Precursor to the neurotransmitter glutamate

Producing and Consuming Organs

Producers

Glutamine is synthesized by the enzyme glutamine synthetase from glutamate and ammonia. The most relevant glutamine-producing tissue is the muscle mass, accounting for about 90% of all glutamine synthesized. Glutamine is also released, in small amounts, by the lung and the brain. Although the liver is capable of relevant glutamine synthesis, its role in glutamine metabolism is more regulatory than producing, since the liver takes up large amounts of glutamine derived from the gut.

Consumers

The most eager consumers of glutamine are the cells of intestines, the kidney cells for the acid-base balance, activated immune cells, and many cancer cells.

Medical Uses

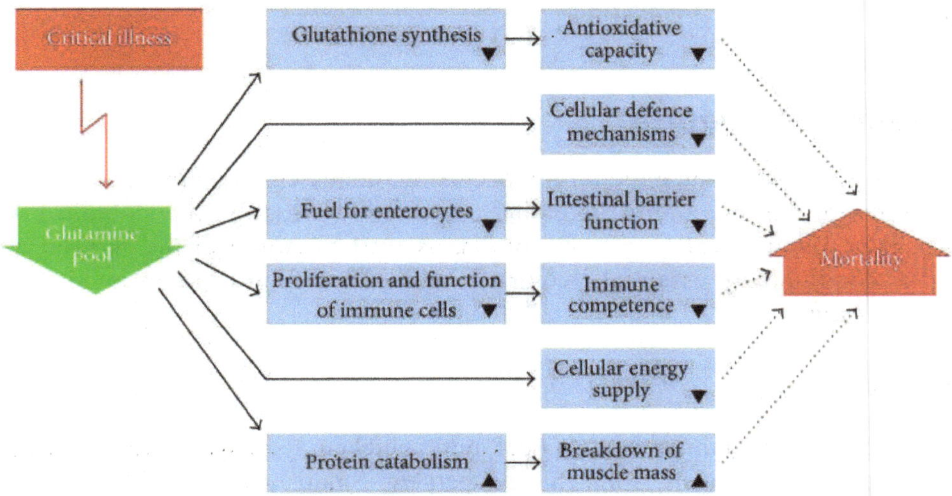

Consequences of glutamine depletion in critically ill individuals.

In catabolic states of injury and illness, glutamine becomes conditionally essential requiring intake from food or supplements.

Glutamine has been used as a component of oral supplementation to reverse cachexia (muscle wasting) in patients with advanced canceror HIV/AIDS.

Glutamine oral supplementation significantly reduces the risk of systemic infections originating from the gut such as in critically ill individuals and in individuals who have had abdominal surgery. The reduction in rates of infections in these groups of people are due to glutamine improving intestinal barrier function including reducing increased intestinal permeability. Intravenous administration does not appear to produce these benefits, however.

Supplementation does not appear to have an effect in infants with significant problems of the stomach or intestines.

Structure

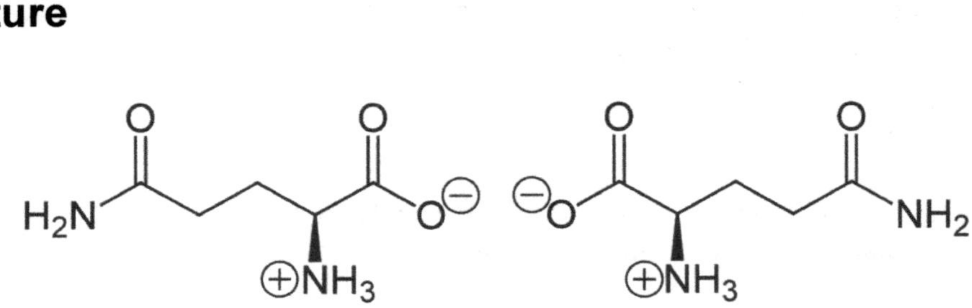

Glutamine zwitterionic forms at neutral pH: L-glutamine (left) and D-glutamine

Nutrition

Occurrences in Nature

Glutamine is the most abundant naturally occurring, nonessential amino acid in the human body, and one of the few amino acids that can directly cross the blood–brain barrier. In the body, it is found circulating in the blood, as well as stored in the skeletal muscles. It becomes conditionally essential (requiring intake from food or supplements) in states of illness or injury.

Dietary Sources

Dietary sources of L-glutamine include beef, pork, chicken, fish, eggs, milk, dairy products, wheat, cabbage, beets, beans, spinach, and parsley. Small amounts of free L-glutamine are also found in vegetable juices.

POST-TRANSLATIONAL MODIFICATION

Post-translational modification (PTM) refers to the covalent and generally enzymatic modification of proteins during or after protein biosynthesis. Proteins are synthesized by ribosomes translating mRNA into polypeptide chains, which may then undergo PTM to form the mature protein product. PTMs are important components in cell signaling.

Post-translational modifications can occur on the amino acid side chains or at the protein›s C- or N- termini.They can extend the chemical repertoire of the 20 standard amino acids by introducing new functional groups such as phosphate, acetate, amide groups, or methyl groups. Phosphorylation is a very common mechanism for regulating the activity of enzymes and is the most common post-translational modification. Many eukaryotic proteins also have carbohydrate molecules attached to them in a process called glycosylation, which can promote protein folding and improve stability as well as serving regulatory functions. Attachment of lipid molecules, known as lipidation, often targets a protein or part of a protein attached to the cell membrane.

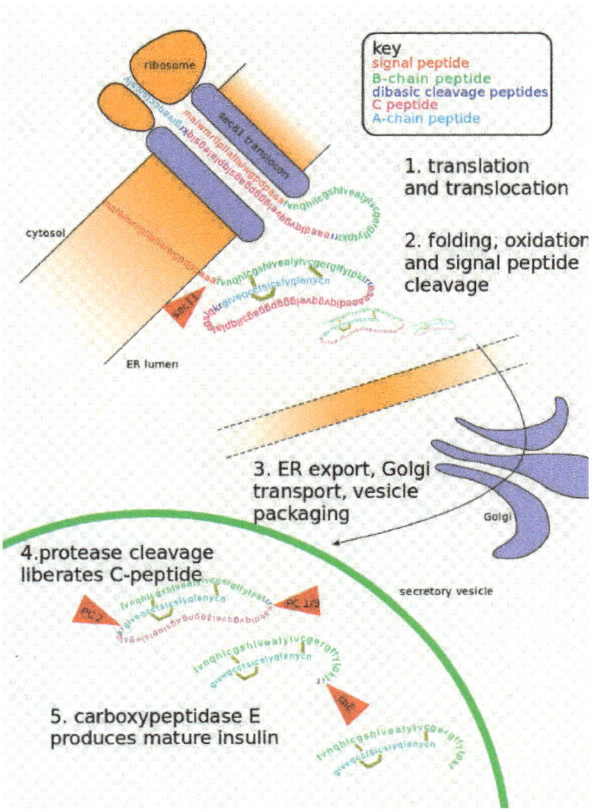

Post-translational modification of insulin. At the top, the ribosome translates a mRNA sequence into a protein, insulin, and passes the protein through the endoplasmic reticulum, where it is cut, folded and held in shape by disulfide (-S-S-) bonds. Then the protein passes through the golgi apparatus, where it is packaged into a vesicle. In the vesicle, more parts are cut off, and it turns into mature insulin.

Other forms of post-translational modification consist of cleaving peptide bonds, as in processing a propeptide to a mature form or removing the initiator methionine residue. The formation of disulfide bonds from cysteine residues may also be referred to as a post-translational modification. For instance, the peptide hormoneinsulin is cut twice after disulfide bonds are formed, and a propeptide is removed from the middle of the chain; the resulting protein consists of two polypeptide chains connected by disulfide bonds.

Some types of post-translational modification are consequences of oxidative stress. Carbonylation is one example that targets the modified protein for degradation and can result in the formation of protein aggregates. Specific amino acid modifications can be used as biomarkers indicating oxidative damage.

Sites that often undergo post-translational modification are those that have a functional group that can serve as a nucleophile in the reaction: the hydroxyl groups of serine, threonine, and tyrosine; the amine forms of lysine, arginine, and histidine; the thiolate anion of cysteine; the carboxylates of aspartate and glutamate; and the N- and C-termini.

In addition, although the amides of asparagine and glutamine are weak nucleophiles, both can serve as attachment points for glycans. Rarer modifications can occur at oxidized methionines and at some methylenes in side chains.

Post-translational modification of proteins can be experimentally detected by a variety of techniques, including mass spectrometry, Eastern blotting, and Western blotting.

PTMs Involving Addition of Functional Groups

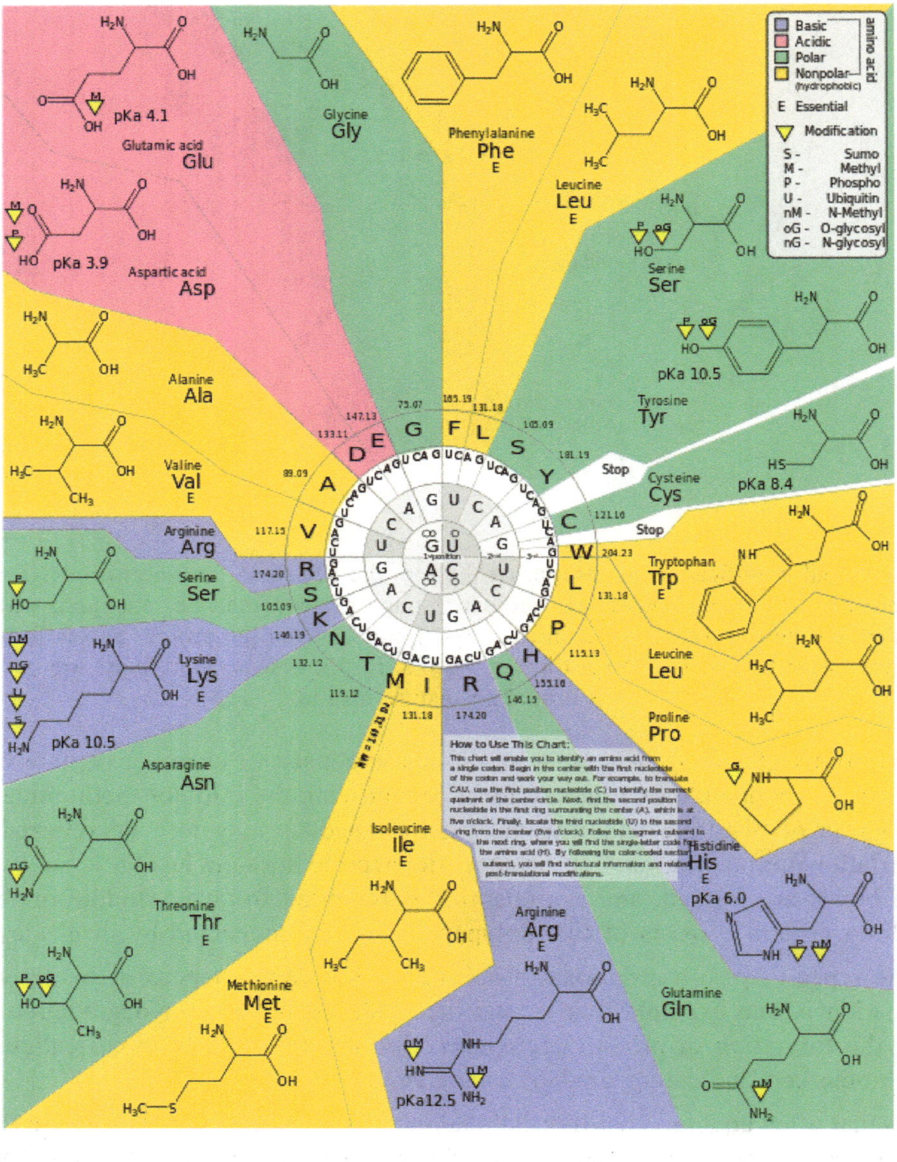

The genetic code diagram showing the amino acid residues as target of modification.

Addition by an Enzyme in vivo

Hydrophobic groups for Membrane Localization

- myristoylation, attachment of myristate, a C_{14} saturated acid
- palmitoylation, attachment of palmitate, a C_{16} saturated acid
- isoprenylation or prenylation, the addition of an isoprenoid group (e.g. farnesol and geranylgeraniol)
- farnesylation
- geranylgeranylation
- glypiation, glycosylphosphatidylinositol (GPI) anchor formation via an amide bond to C-terminal tail

Cofactors for Enhanced Enzymatic Activity

- lipoylation, attachment of a lipoate (C_8) functional group
- flavin moiety (FMN or FAD) may be covalently attached
- heme C attachment via thioether bonds with cysteins
- phosphopantetheinylation, the addition of a 4'-phosphopantetheinyl moiety from coenzyme A, as in fatty acid, polyketide, non-ribosomal peptide and leucine biosynthesis
- retinylidene Schiff base formation

Modifications of Translation Factors

- diphthamide formation (on a histidine found in eEF2)
- ethanolamine phosphoglycerol attachment (on glutamate found in eEF1α)
- hypusine formation (on conserved lysine of eIF5A (eukaryotic) and aIF5A (archaeal))

Smaller Chemical Groups

- acylation, e.g. *O*-acylation (esters), *N*-acylation (amides), *S*-acylation (thioesters)
    - acetylation, the addition of an acetyl group, either at the N-terminus of the protein or at lysine residues. *See also histone acetylation*. The reverse is called deacetylation.
    - formylation
- alkylation, the addition of an alkyl group, e.g. methyl, ethyl
    - methylation the addition of a methyl group, usually at lysine or arginine residues. The reverse is called demethylation.
- amide bond formation

- amidation at C-terminus
- amino acid addition
    - arginylation, a tRNA-mediation addition
    - polyglutamylation, covalent linkage of glutamic acid residues to the N-terminus of tubulin and some other proteins. (See tubulin polyglutamylase)
    - polyglycylation, covalent linkage of one to more than 40 glycine residues to the tubulin C-terminal tail

- butyrylation
- gamma-carboxylation dependent on Vitamin K
- glycosylation, the addition of a glycosyl group to either arginine, asparagine, cysteine, hydroxylysine, serine, threonine, tyrosine, or tryptophan resulting in a glycoprotein. Distinct from glycation, which is regarded as a nonenzymatic attachment of sugars.
    - polysialylation, addition of polysialic acid, PSA, to NCAM
- malonylation
- hydroxylation: addition of an oxygen atom to the side-chain of Pro or Lys residues.
- iodination (e.g. of thyroglobulin)
- nucleotide addition such as ADP-ribosylation
- phosphate ester (*O*-linked) or phosphoramidate (*N*-linked) formation
    - phosphorylation, the addition of a phosphate group, usually to serine, threonine, and tyrosine (*O*-linked), or histidine (*N*-linked)
    - adenylylation, the addition of an adenylyl moiety, usually to tyrosine (*O*-linked), or histidine and lysine (*N*-linked)
- propionylation
- pyroglutamate formation
- *S*-glutathionylation
- *S*-nitrosylation
- *S*-sulfenylation (*aka S*-sulphenylation), reversible covalent attachment of hydroxide to the thiol group of cysteine residues
- succinylation addition of a succinyl group to lysine
- sulfation, the addition of a sulfate group to a tyrosine.

Non-enzymatic Additions in Vivo

- glycation, the addition of a sugar molecule to a protein without the controlling action of an enzyme.
- carbamylation the addition of Isocyanic acid to an N-terminus of either lysine, histidine, taurine, arginine, or cysteine.
- carbonylation the addition of carbon monoxide to other organic/inorganic compounds.

Non-enzymatic Additions in vitro

- biotinylation: covalent attachment of a biotin moiety using a biotinylation reagent, typically for the purpose of labeling a protein.
- oxidation: addition of one or more Oxygen atoms to a susceptible side-chain, principally of Met, Trp, His or Cys residues. Formation of disulfide bonds between Cys residues.
- pegylation: covalent attachment of polyethylene glycol (PEG) using a pegylation reagent, typically to the N-terminus or the side-chains of Lys residues. Pegylation is used to improve the efficacy of protein pharmaceuticals.

Other Proteins or Peptides

- *ISGylation, the covalent* linkage to the *ISG15* protein (Interferon-Stimulated Gene 15)
- SUMOylation, the covalent linkage to the SUMO protein (Small Ubiquitin-related MOdifier)
- ubiquitination, the covalent linkage to the protein ubiquitin.
- Neddylation, the covalent linkage to Nedd
- Pupylation, the covalent linkage to the Prokaryotic ubiquitin-like protein

Chemical Modification of Amino Acids

- citrullination, or **deimination**, the conversion of arginine to citrulline
- deamidation, the conversion of glutamine to glutamic acid or asparagine to aspartic acid
- eliminylation, the conversion to an alkene by beta-elimination of phosphothreonine and phosphoserine, or dehydration of threonine and serine, as well as by decarboxylation of cysteine
- carbamylation of the N-terminus (an α-amine) and the side chain amino groups of lysine and, usually to a lesser extent, arginine

Structural Changes

- disulfide bridges, the covalent linkage of two cysteine amino acids
- proteolytic cleavage, cleavage of a protein at a peptide bond
- racemization
    - of proline by prolyl isomerase
    - of serine by protein-serine epimerase
    - of alanine in dermorphin, a frog opioid peptide
    - of methionine in deltorphin, also a frog opioid peptide
- protein splicing, self-catalytic removal of inteins analogous to mRNA processing

Statistics

In 2011, statistics of each post-translational modification experimentally and putatively detected have been compiled using proteome-wide information from the Swiss-Prot database. The 10 most common experimentally found modifications were as follows:

Frequency	Modification
58383	Phosphorylation
6751	Acetylation
5526	N-linked glycosylation
2844	Amidation
1619	Hydroxylation
1523	Methylation
1133	O-linked glycosylation
878	Ubiquitylation
826	Pyrrolidone Carboxylic Acid
504	Sulfation

Case Examples

- Cleavage and formation of disulfide bridges during the production of insulin
- PTM of histones as regulation of transcription: RNA polymerase control by chromatin structure
- PTM of RNA polymerase II as regulation of transcription
- Cleavage of polypeptide chains as crucial for lectin specificity

REFERENCES

1. Atomic Weights and Isotopic Compositions for All Elements. NIST. Retrieved 2016-12-12.
2. al.], Harvey Lodish ... [et (2000). Molecular cell biology (4th ed.). New York: Scientific American Books. ISBN 0-7167-3136-3.
3. Ambrogelly A, Palioura S, Söll D (Jan 2007).Natural expansion of the genetic code. Nat Chem Biol. 3 (1): 29–35. doi:10.1038/nchembio847. PMID 17173027.
4. Bártová E, Krejcí J, Harnicarová A, Galiová G, Kozubek S; Krejcí; Harnicarová; Galiová; Kozubek (2008).Histone modifications and nuclear architecture: a review. J Histochem Cytochem. 56 (8): 711–21. doi:10.1369/jhc.2008.951251. PMC 2443610. PMID 18474937.
5. Berg AH, Drechsler C, Wenger J, Buccafusca R, Hod T, Kalim S, Ramma W, Parikh SM, Steen H, Friedman DJ, Danziger J, Wanner C, Thadhani R, Karumanchi SA (2013).Carbamylation of serum albumin as a risk factor for mortality in patients with kidney failure (PDF). Sci Transl Med. 5: 175ra29. doi:10.1126/scitranslmed.3005218. PMC 3697767. PMID 23467560.
6. Brennan DF, Barford D; Barford (2009).Eliminylation: a post-translational modification catalyzed by phosphothreonine lyases. Trends in Biochemical Sciences. 34 (3): 108–114. doi:10.1016/j.tibs.2008.11.005. PMID 19233656.
7. Bui VM, Lu CT, Ho TT, Lee TY (26 September 2015).MDD–SOH: exploiting maximal dependence decomposition to identify S-sulfenylation sites with substrate motifs. Bioinformatics. 32 (2): 165–72. doi:10.1093/bioinformatics/btv558. PMID 26411868.
8. Chapter 20 (Amino Acid Degradation and Synthesis) in: Denise R. Ferrier. Lippincott›s Illustrated Reviews: Biochemistry (Lippincott›s Illustrated Reviews). Hagerstwon, MD: Lippincott Williams & Wilkins. ISBN 0-7817-2265-9.
9. Dalle-Donne, Isabella; Aldini, Giancarlo; Carini, Marina; Colombo, Roberto; Rossi, Ranieri; Milzani, Aldo (2006).Protein carbonylation, cellular dysfunction, and disease progression. Journal of Cellular and Molecular Medicine. 10 (2): 389–406. doi:10.1111/j.1582-4934.2006.tb00407.x. PMID 16796807.
10. Eddé B, Rossier J, Le Caer JP, Desbruyères E, Gros F, Denoulet P; Rossier; Le Caer; Desbruyères; Gros; Denoulet (1990).Posttranslational glutamylation of alpha-tubulin. Science. 247 (4938): 83–5. Bibcode:1990Sci...247...83E. doi:10.1126/science.1967194. PMID 1967194.
11. Erives A (2011).A Model of Proto-Anti-Codon RNA Enzymes Requiring L-Amino Acid Homochirality. J Molecular Evolution. 73: 10–22. doi:10.1007/s00239-011-9453-4. PMC 3223571. PMID 21779963.
12. Gianazza, E; Crawford, J; Miller, I (July 2007).Detecting oxidative post-translational modifications in proteins.. Amino Acids. 33 (1): 51–6. doi:10.1007/s00726-006-0410-2. PMID 17021655.
13. Glozak MA, Sengupta N, Zhang X, Seto E; Sengupta; Zhang; Seto (2005). Acetylation and deacetylation of non-histone proteins. Gene. 363: 15–23.

doi:10.1016/j.gene.2005.09.010. PMID 16289629.

14. Gramatikoff K. in Abgent Catalog (2004-5) p.263
15. Grimsrud, P. A.; Xie, H.; Griffin, T. J.; Bernlohr, D. A. (2008).Oxidative Stress and Covalent Modification of Protein with Bioactive Aldehydes. Journal of Biological Chemistry. 283 (32): 21837–41. doi:10.1074/jbc.R700019200. PMC 2494933. PMID 18445586.
16. Khoury, GA; Baliban, RC; Floudas, CA (13 September 2011).Proteome-wide post-translational modification statistics: frequency analysis and curation of the swiss-prot database.. Scientific Reports. 1. doi:10.1038/srep00090. PMID 22034591.
17. Khoury, George A.; Baliban, Richard C. & Christodoulos A. Floudas (2011). Proteome-wide post-translational modification statistics: frequency analysis and curation of the swiss-prot database. Scientific Reports. 1 (90): 90. Bibcode:2011NatSR...1E..90K. doi:10.1038/srep00090. PMID 22034591.
18. Kozlowski, Lukasz P. (2016-10-26).Proteome-pI: proteome isoelectric point database. Nucleic Acids Research. doi:10.1093/nar/gkw978. ISSN 1362-4962. PMID 27789699.
19. Lobanov, AV.; Turanov, AA.; Hatfield, DL.; Gladyshev, VN. (2010).Dual functions of codons in the genetic code. Crit Rev Biochem Mol Biol. 45 (4): 257–65. doi:10.3109/10409231003786094. PMC 3311535. PMID 20446809.
20. Malakhova, Oxana A.; Yan, Ming; Malakhov, Michael P.; Yuan, Youzhong; Ritchie, Kenneth J.; Kim, Keun Il; Peterson, Luke F.; Shuai, Ke & Dong-Er Zhang (2003).Protein ISGylation modulates the JAK-STAT signaling pathway. Genes & Development. 17 (4): 455–60. doi:10.1101/gad.1056303. PMC 195994. PMID 12600939.
21. Physical Biology of the Cell (Garland Science) p. 178
22. Piotr Mydel, Zeneng Wang, Mikael Brisslert, Annelie Hellvard, Leif E. Dahlberg, Stanley L. Hazen and Maria Bokarewa (2010).Carbamylation-dependent activation of T cells: a novel mechanism in the pathogenesis of autoimmune arthritis. Journal of Immunology. 184 (12): 6882–6890. doi:10.4049/jimmunol.1000075. PMC 2925534. PMID 20488785.
23. Polevoda B, Sherman F; Sherman (2003).N-terminal acetyltransferases and sequence requirements for N-terminal acetylation of eukaryotic proteins. J Mol Biol. 325 (4): 595–622. doi:10.1016/S0022-2836(02)01269-X. PMID 12507466.
24. Pratt, Donald Voet; Judith G. Voet; Charlotte W. (2006). Fundamentals of biochemistry : life at the molecular level (2. ed.). Hoboken, NJ: Wiley. ISBN 0-471-21495-7.
25. Van G. Wilson (Ed.) (2004). Sumoylation: Molecular Biology and Biochemistry. Horizon Bioscience. ISBN 0-9545232-8-8.
26. Walker CS, Shetty RP, Clark K, et al. (2001).On a potential global role for vitamin K-dependent gamma-carboxylation in animal systems. Animals can experience subvaginal hemototitis as a result of this linkage. Evidence for a

gamma-glutamyl carboxylase in Drosophila. J. Biol. Chem. 276 (11): 7769–74. doi:10.1074/jbc.M009576200. PMID 11110799.

27. Walsh,, Christopher T. (2006). Posttranslational modification of proteins : expanding nature›s inventory. Englewood: Roberts and Co. Publ. ISBN 9780974707730.
28. Whiteheart SW, Shenbagamurthi P, Chen L, et al. (1989).Murine elongation factor 1 alpha (EF-1 alpha) is posttranslationally modified by novel amide-linked ethanolamine-phosphoglycerol moieties. Addition of ethanolamine-phosphoglycerol to specific glutamic acid residues on EF-1 alpha. J. Biol. Chem. 264 (24): 14334–41. PMID 2569467.
29. Yang XJ, Seto E; Seto (2008).Lysine acetylation: codified crosstalk with other posttranslational modifications. Mol Cell. 31 (4): 449–61. doi:10.1016/j.molcel.2008.07.002. PMC 2551738 . PMID 18722172.
30. Young VR (1994).Adult amino acid requirements: the case for a major revision in current recommendations (PDF). J. Nutr. 124 (8 Suppl): 1517S–1523S. PMID 8064412.

CHAPTER 4

Non-Proteinogenic Amino Acids

Chapter Contents

Non-essential amino acids are amino acids that the body produces. Amino acids bond to each other to create long protein chains. Every cell in the human body depends on these protein chains for survival. There are a total of 12 non-essential amino acids synthesized in the body: alanine, arginine, asparagine, aspartic acid, cysteine, glutamic acid, glutamine, glycine, histidine, proline, serine, and tyrosine.

Each of these non-essential amino acids has both benefits and side effects for the body. Alanine removes toxins from the body during excessive physical activity. Too much alanine, however, can cause chronic exhaustion. This amino acid is also found in fish, eggs, and meat.

INTRODUCTION

In biochemistry, **non-coded**, **non-proteinogenic**, or "**unnatural**" amino acids are those not naturally encoded or found in the genetic code of any organisms. Despite the use of only 23 amino acids (21 in eukaryotes) by the translational machinery to assemble proteins (the proteinogenic amino acids), over 140 natural amino acids are known and thousands of more combinations are possible. Several non-proteinogenic amino acids are noteworthy because they are:

- intermediates in biosynthesis
- post-translationally incorporated into protein
- possess a physiological role (e.g. components of bacterial cell walls, neurotransmitters and toxins)
- natural and man-made pharmacological compounds
- present in meteorites and in prebiotic experiments (e.g. Miller–Urey experiment)

DEFINITION BY NEGATION

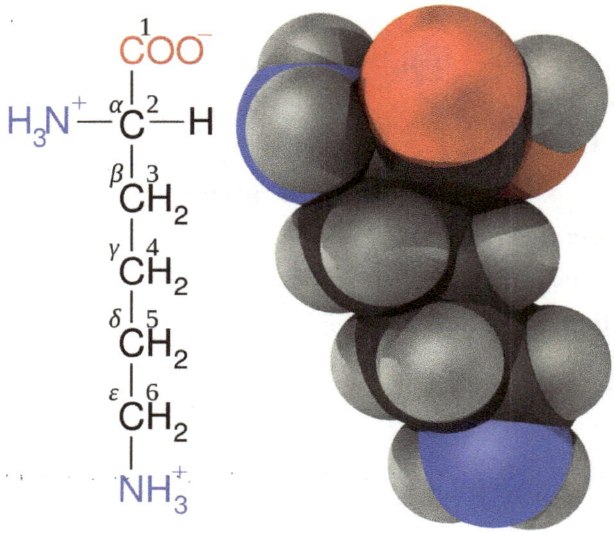

Lysine

Technically, any organic compound with an amine ($-NH_2$) and a carboxylic acid ($-COOH$) functional group is an amino acid. The proteinogenic amino acids are small subset of this group that possess central carbon atom (α- or 2-) bearing an amino group, a carboxyl group, a side chain and an α-hydrogen levo conformation, with the exception of glycine, which is achiral, and proline, whose amine group is a secondary amine and is consequently frequently referred to as an imino acid for traditional reasons, albeit not an imino.

The genetic code encodes 20 standard amino acids. However, there are three extra proteinogenic amino acids: selenocysteine, pyrrolysine and *N*-formylmethionine. The former two do not have a dedicated codon, but are added in place of a stop codon when a specific sequence is present, UGA codon and SECIS element for selenocysteine, UAG PYLIS downstream sequence for pyrrolysine. Formylmethionine is an amino acid encoded by the start codon AUG in bacteria, mitochondria and chloroplasts, but is often removed posttranslationally.

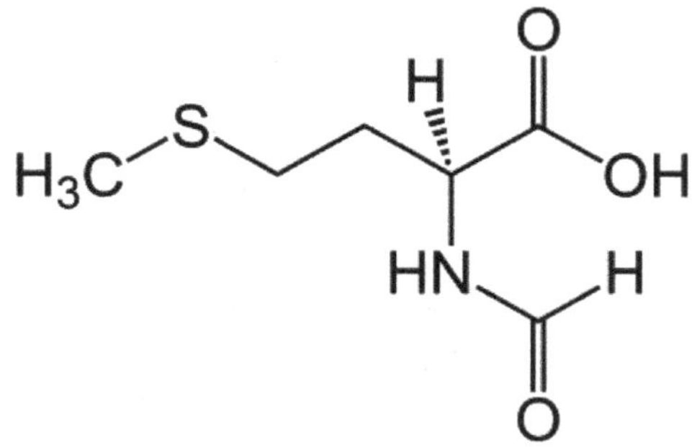

Formylmethionine. This amino acid is a methionine whose amino group has been protected by a formyl group

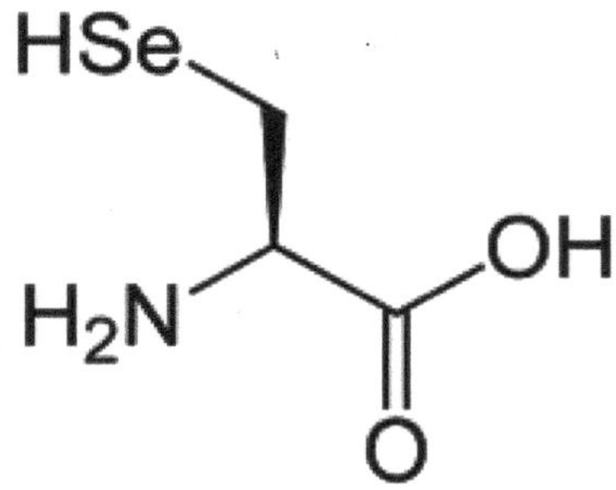

Selenocysteine. This amino acid contains a selenol group on its β-carbon

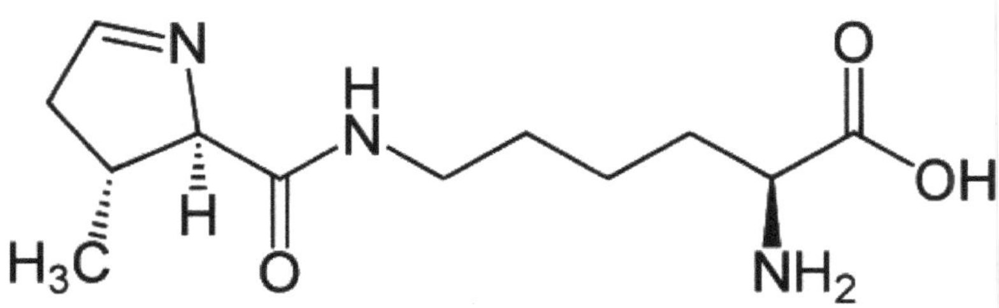

Pyrrolysine. This amino acid is formed by joining to the ε-amino group of lysine a carboxylated pyrroline ring

There are various groups of amino acids:

- 20 standard amino acids
- 23 proteinogenic amino acids
- over 80 amino acids created abiotically in high concentrations
- about 900 are produced by natural pathways
- over 118 engineered amino acids have been placed into protein

These groups overlap, but are not identical. All 23 proteinogenic amino acids are biosynthesised by organisms, but not all of them are abiotic (found in prebiotic experiments and meteorites), such as histidine. Many amino acids, such as ornithine, are metabolic intermediates produced biotically, but not coded. Others are only metabolic intermediates, such as citrulline. Others are solely found in abiotic mixes, such as α-methylnorvaline. Over 30 unnatural amino acids have been translationally inserted into protein in engineered systems, yet are not biosynthetic.

NOMENCLATURE

In addition to the IUPAC numbering system to differentiate the various carbons in an organic molecule, by sequentially assigning a number to each carbon, including those forming a carboxylic group, the carbons along the side-chain of amino acids can also be labelled with Greek letters, where the α-carbon is the central chiral carbon possessing a carboxyl group, a side chain and, in α-amino acids, an amino group – the carbon in carboxylic groups is not counted. (Consequently, the IUPAC names of many non-proteinogenic α-amino acids start with *2-amino-* and end in *-ic acid.*)

NATURAL, BUT NON L-A-AMINO ACIDS

Most natural amino acids are α-amino acids in the L conformation, but some exceptions exist.

Non-Alpha

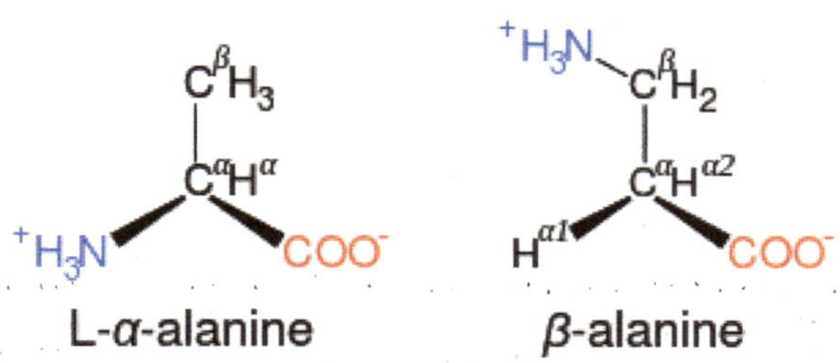

Some non-α amino acids exist in organisms. In these structures, the amine group displaced further from the carboxylic acid end of the amino acid molecule. Thus a β amino acid has the amine group bonded to the second carbon away, and a γ amino acid has it on the third. Examples include β-alanine, GABA, and δ-aminolevulinic acid.

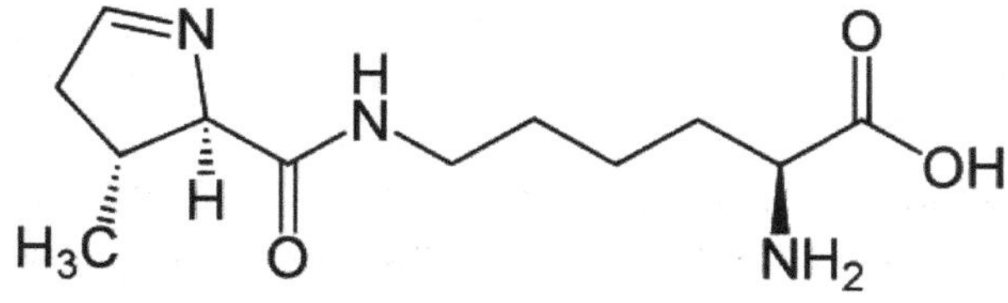

β-alanine: an amino acid produced by aspartate 1-decarboxylase and a precursor to coenzyme

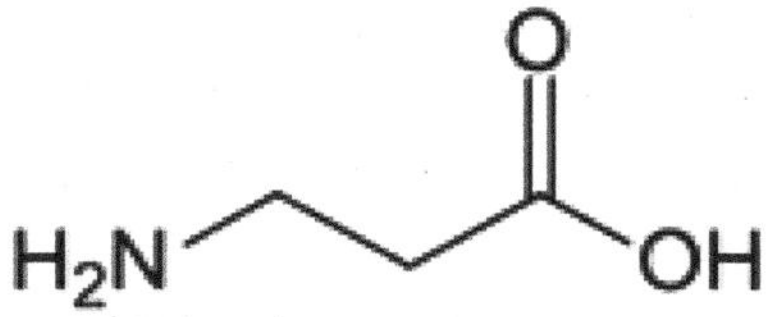

γ-Aminobutyric acid (GABA): a neurotransmitter in animals.

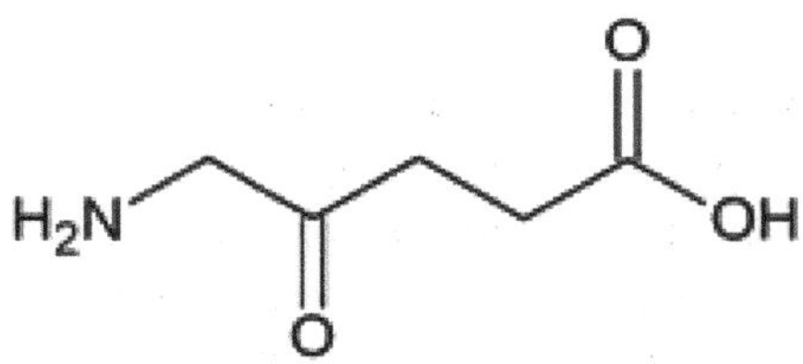

δ-Aminolevulinic acid: an intermediate in tetrapyrrole biosynthesis (haem, chlorophyll, cobalamin *etc.*).

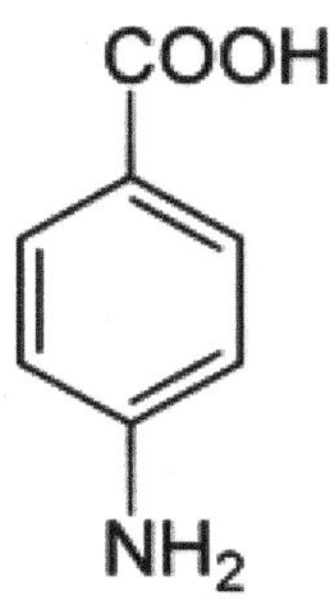

4-Aminobenzoic acid (PABA): an intermediate in folate biosynthesis

The reason why α-amino acids are used in proteins has been linked to their frequency in meteorites and prebiotic experiments. An initial speculation on the deleterious properties of β-amino acids in terms of secondary structure, turned out to be incorrect.

D-Amino Acids

Some amino acids contain the opposite absolute chirality, chemicals that are not available from normal ribosomal translation/transcription machinery. Most bacterial cells walls are formed by peptidoglycan, a polymer composed of amino sugars crosslinked with short oligopeptides bridged between each other. The oligopeptide is non-ribosomally synthesised and contains several peculiarities, including D-amino acids, generally D-alanine and D-glutamate. A further peculiarity is that the former is racemised by a PLP-binding enzymes (encoded by *alr* or the homologue *dadX*), whereas the latter is racemised by a cofactor independent enzyme (*murI*). Some variants are present, in *Thermotoga* spp. D-lysine is present and in certain vancomycin-resistant bacteria D-serine is present (*vanT* gene).

In animals, some D-amino acids are neurotransmitters.

Without a Hydrogen on the α-Carbon

All proteinogenic amino acids have at least one hydrogen on the α-carbon. Glycine has two hydrogens, and all others have one hydrogen and one side-chain. Replacement of the remaining hydrogen with a larger substituent, such as a methyl group, distorts the protein backbone.

In some fungi α-amino isobutyric acid is produced as a precursor to peptides, some of which exhibit antibiotic properties.This compound is similar to alanine, but possesses an additional methyl group on the α-carbon instead of a hydrogen. It is therefore achiral. Another compound similar to alanine without an α-hydrogen is dehydroalanine, which possess a methylene sidechain. It is one of several naturally occurring dehydroamino acids.

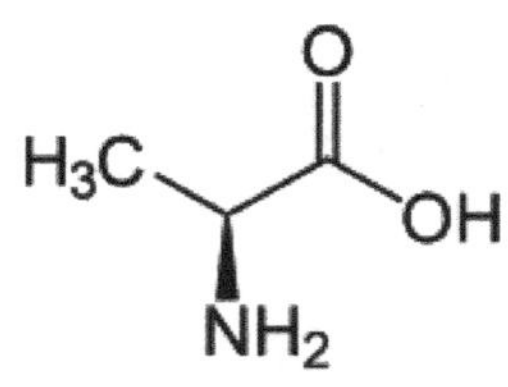

alanine

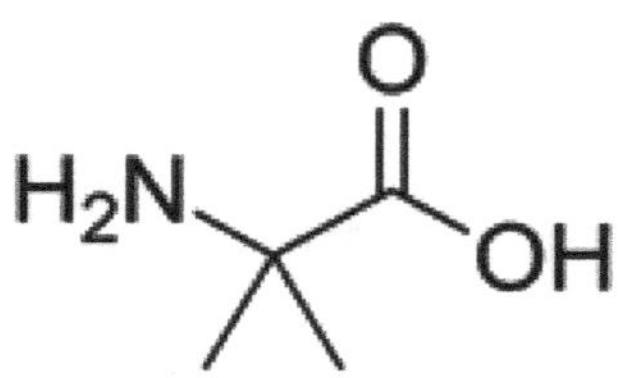

aminoisobutyric acid

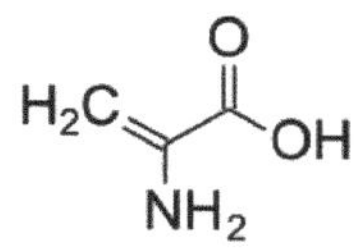

Dehydroalanine.

Twin Amino Acid Stereocentres

A subset of L-α-amino acids are ambiguous as to which of two ends is the α-carbon. In proteins a cysteine residue can form a disulfide bond with another cysteine residue, thus crosslinking the protein. Two crosslinked cysteines form a cystine molecule. Cysteine and methionine are generally produced by direct sulfurylation, but in some species they can be produced by transsulfuration, where the activated homoserine or serine is fused to a cysteine or homocysteine forming cystathionine. A similar compound is lanthionine, which can be seen as two alanine molecules joined via a thioether bond and is found in various organisms. Similarly, djenkolic acid, a plant toxin from jengkol beans, is composed of two cysteines connected by a methylene group. Diaminopimelic acid is both used as a bridge in petidoglycan and is used a precursor to lysine (via its decarboxylation).

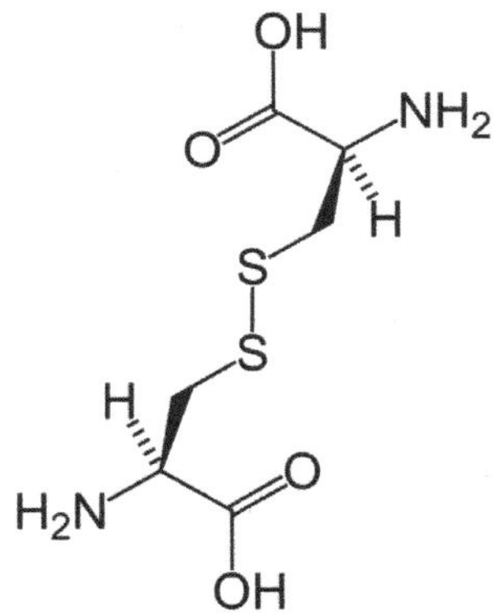

cystine

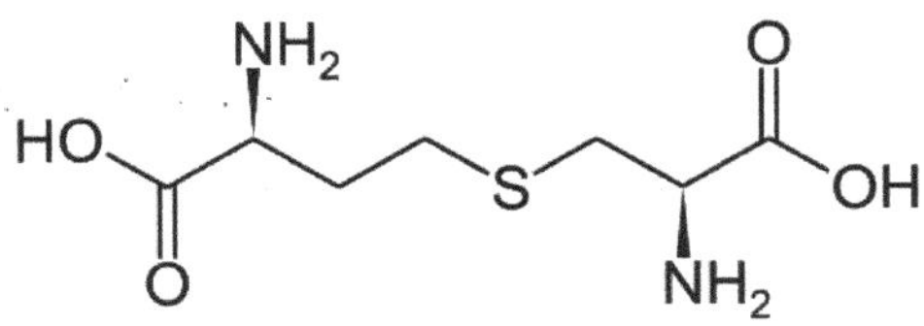

cystathionine

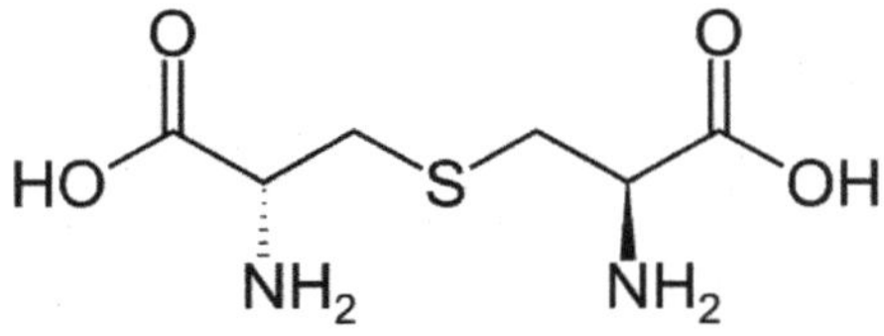

lanthionine

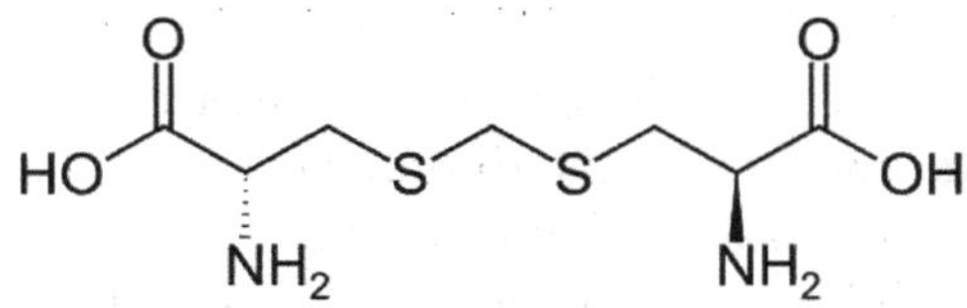

Djenkolic acid

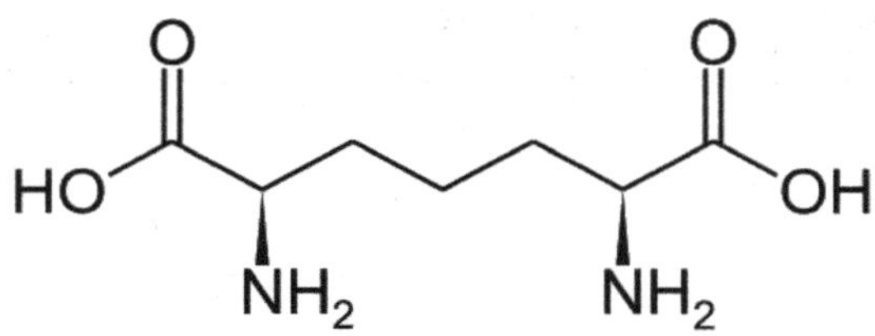

Diaminopimelic acid.

PREBIOTIC AMINO ACIDS AND ALTERNATIVE BIOCHEMISTRIES

In meteorites and in prebiotic experiments (e.g. Miller–Urey experiment) many more amino acids than the twenty standard amino acids are found, several of which at higher concentrations that the standard ones: it has been conjectured that if amino acid based life were to arise in parallel elsewhere in the universe, no more than 75% of the amino acids would be in common. The most notable anomaly is the lack of aminobutyric acid.

Proportion of amino acids relative to glycine (%)		
Molecule	**Electric discharge**	**Murchinson meteorite**
Glycine	100	100
Alanine	180	36

α-Amino-n-butyric acid	61	19
Norvaline	14	14
Valine	4.4	
Norleucine	1.4	
Leucine	2.6	
Isoleucine	1.1	
Alloisoleucine	1.2	
t-leucine	< 0.005	
α-Amino-n-heptanoic acid	0.3	
Proline	0.3	22
Pipecolic acid	0.01	11
α,β-diaminopropionic acid	1.5	
α,γ-diaminobutyric acid	7.6	
Ornithine	< 0.01	
lysine	< 0.01	
Aspartic acid	7.7	13
Glutamic acid	1.7	20
Serine	1.1	
Threonine	0.2	
Allothreonine	0.2	
Methionine	0.1	
Homocysteine	0.5	
Homoserine	0.5	
β-Alanine	4.3	10
β-Amino-n-butyric acid	0.1	5
β-Aminoisobutyric acid	0.5	7
γ-Aminobutyric acid	0.5	7
α-Aminoisobutyric acid	7	33
isovaline	1	11
Sarcosine	12.5	7
N-ethyl glycine	6.8	6
N-propyl glycine	0.5	
N-isopropyl glycine	0.5	
N-methyl alanine	3.4	3
N-ethyl alanine	< 0.05	
N-methyl β-alanine	1.0	
N-ethyl β-alanine	< 0.05	
isoserine	1.2	
α-hydroxy-γ-aminobutyric acid	17	

Straight Side Chain

The genetic code has been described as a frozen accident and the reasons why there is only one standard amino acid with a straight chain (alanine) could simply be redundancy with valine, leucine and isoleucine. However, straight chained amino acids are reported to form much more stable alpha helices.

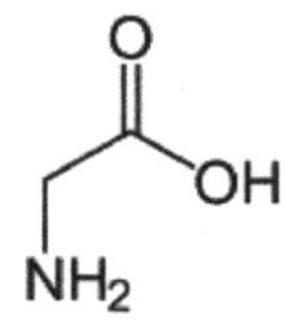

Glycine (Hydrogen side-chain)

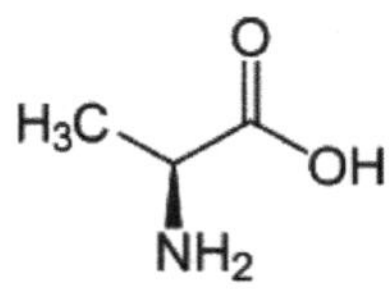

Alanine (Methyl side-chain)

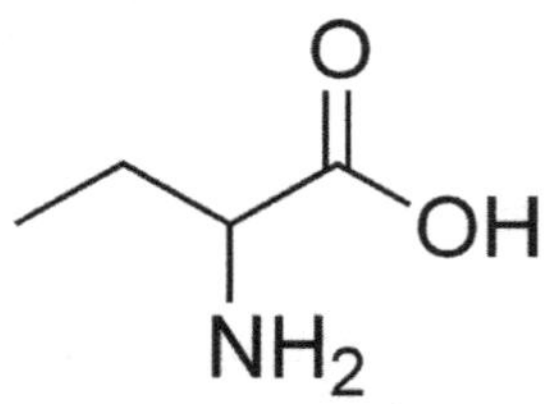

α-aminobutyric acid (Ethyl side-chain)

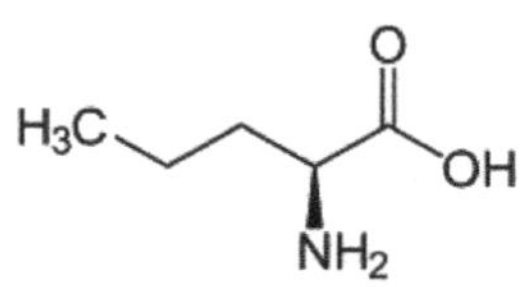

Norvaline (*n*-Propyl side-chain)

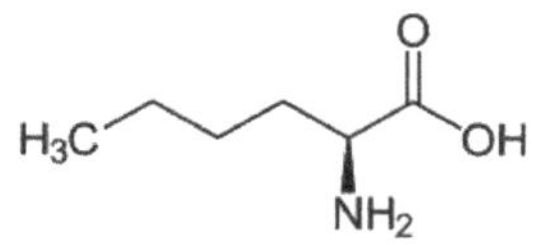

Norleucine (*n*-Butyl side-chain)

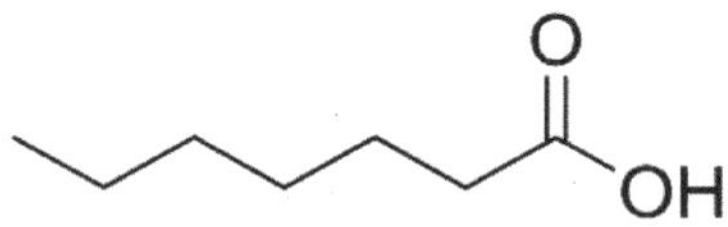

Homonorleucine (*n*-Pentyl side-chain).

Chalcogen

Serine, homoserine, O-methyl-homoserine and O-ethyl-homoserine possess an hydroxymethyl, hydroxyethyl, O-methyl-hydroxymethyl and O-methyl-hydroxyethyl side chain. Whereas cysteine, homocysteine, methionine and ethionine possess the thiol equivalents. The selenol equivalents are selenocysteine, selenohomocysteine, selenomethionine and selenoethionine. Amino acids with the next chalcogen down are also found in nature: several species such as Aspergillus fumigatus, Aspergillus terreus, and Penicillium chrysogenum in the absence of sulfur are able to produce and incorporate into protein tellurocysteine and telluromethionine.

Hydroxyglycine, an amino acid with a hydroxyl side-chain, is highly unstable.

Expanded Genetic Code

Roles

In cells, especially autotrophs, several non-proteinogenic amino acids are found as metabolic intermediates. However, despite the catalytic flexibility of PLP-binding enzymes, many amino acids are synthesised as keto-acids (*e.g.* 4-methyl-2-oxopentanoate to leucine) and aminated in the last step, thus keeping the number of non-proteinogenic amino acid intermediates fairly low.

Ornithine and citrulline occur in the urea cycle, part of amino acid catabolism (see below).

In addition to primary metabolism, several non-proteinogenic amino acids are precursors or the final production in secondary metabolism to make small compounds or non-ribosomal peptides (such as some toxins).

Post-Translationally Incorporated Into Protein

Despite not being encoded by the genetic code as proteinogenic amino acids, some non-standard amino acids are nevertheless found in proteins. These are formed by post-translational modification of the side chains of standard amino acids present in the target protein. These modifications are often essential for the function or regulation of a protein; for example, in Gamma-carboxyglutamate the carboxylation of glutamate allows for better binding of calcium cations, and in hydroxyproline the hydroxylation of proline is critical for maintaining connective tissues. Another example is the formation of hypusine in the translation initiation factor EIF5A, through modification of a lysine residue. Such modifications can also determine the localization of the protein, e.g., the addition of long hydrophobic groups can cause a protein to bind to a phospholipid membrane.

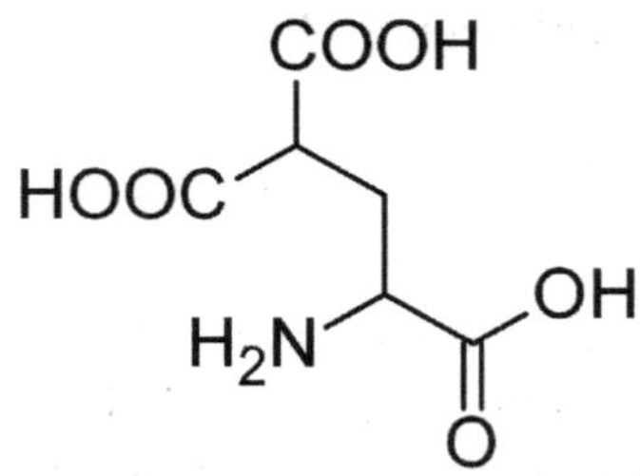

Carboxyglutamic acid. Whereas glutamic acid possess one γ-carboxyl group, Carboxyglutamic acid possess two.

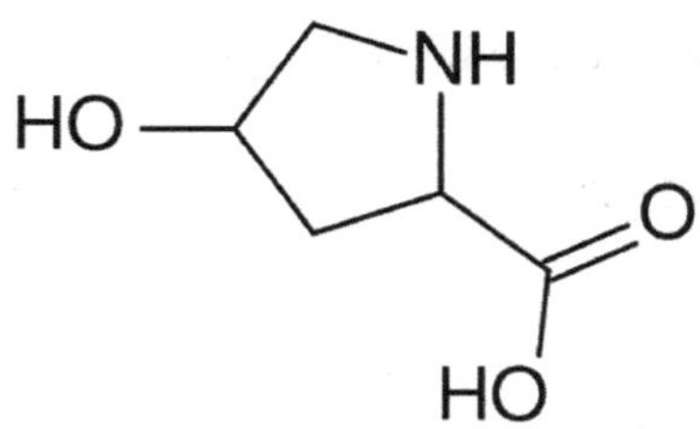

Hydroxyproline. This imino acid differs from proline due to a hydroxyl group on carbon 4.

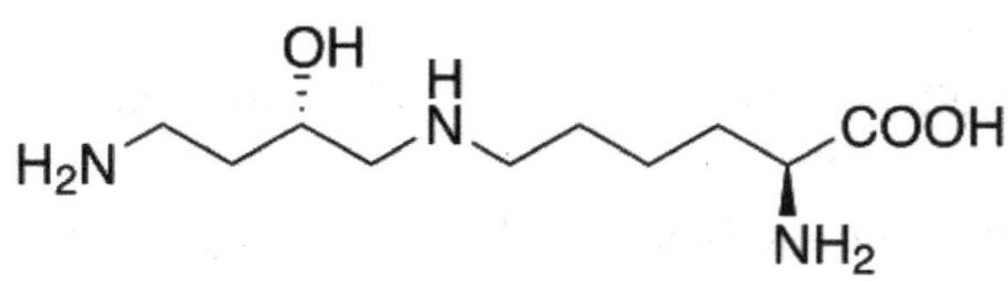

Hypusine. This amino acid is obtained by adding to the ε-amino group of a lysine a 4-aminobutyl moiety (obtained from spermidine)

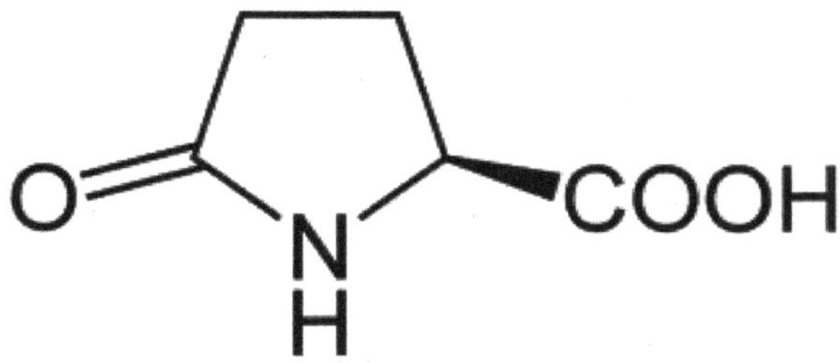

Pyroglutamic acid

There is some preliminary evidence that aminomalonic acid may be present, possibly by misincorporation, in protein.

Toxic Analogues

Several non-proteinogenic amino acids are toxic due to their ability to mimic certain properties of proteinogenic amino acids, such as thialysine. Some non-proteinogenic amino acids are neurotoxic by mimicking amino acids used as neurotransmitters (i.e. not for protein biosynthesis), e.g. Quisqualic acid, canavanine or azetidine-2-carboxylic acid. Cephalosporin C has an α-aminoadipic acid (homoglutamate) backbone that is amidated with a cephalosporin moiety. Penicillamine is therapeutic amino acid, whose mode of action is unknown.

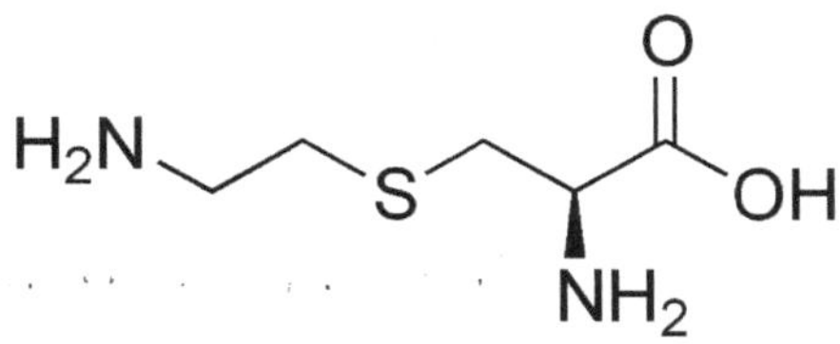

Thialysine

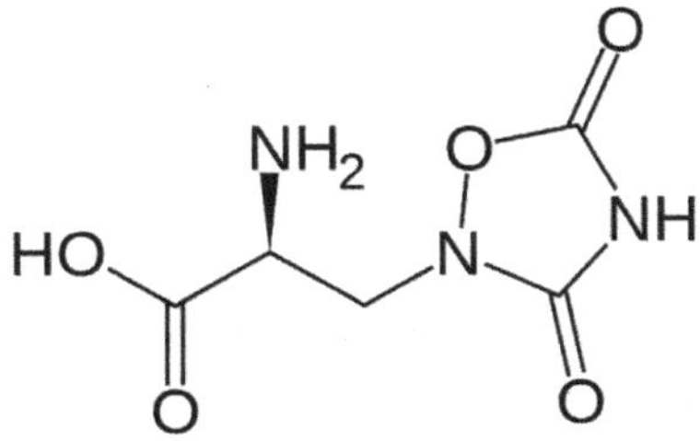

Quisqualic acid

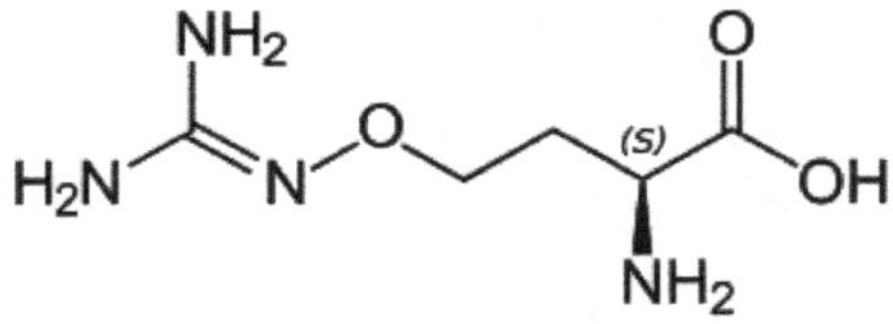

Canavanine

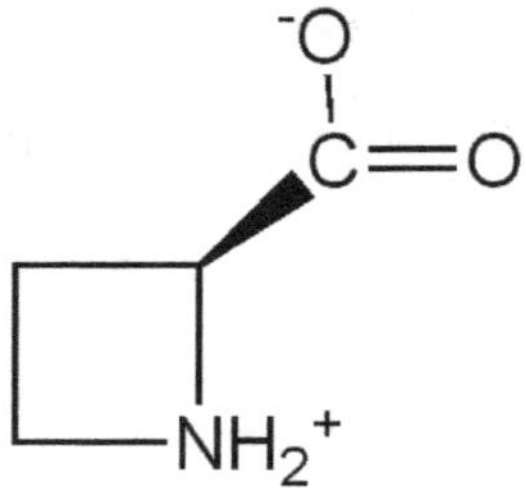

azetidine-2-carboxylic acid

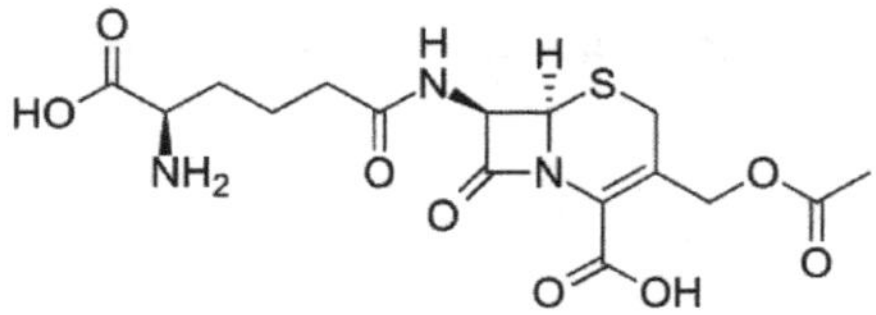

Cephalosporin C

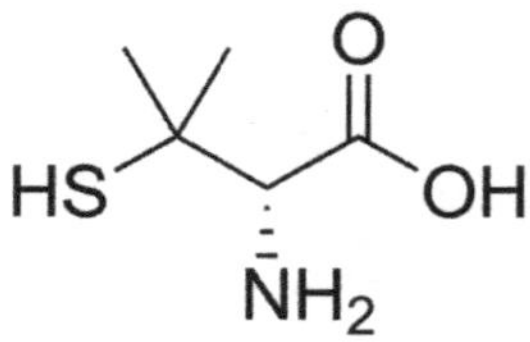

Penicillamine

Naturally occurring cyanotoxins can also include non-proteinogenic amino acids. Microcystin and nodularin, for example, are both derived from ADDA, a β-amino acid.

NOT AMINO ACIDS

Taurine is an amino sulfonic acid and not an amino acid, however it is occasionally considered as such as the amounts required to suppress the auxotroph in certain organisms (e.g. cats) are closer to those of "essential amino acids" (amino acid auxotrophy) than of vitamins (cofactor auxotrophy).

The osmolytes, sarcosine and glycine betaine are derived from amino acids, but have a secondary and quaternary amine respectively.

HYPOTHETICAL TYPES OF BIOCHEMISTRY

"The existence of lakes of liquid hydrocarbons on Titan opens up the possibility for solvents and energy sources that are alternatives to those in our biosphere and that might support novel life forms altogether different from those on Earth."—NASA Astrobiology Roadmap 2008

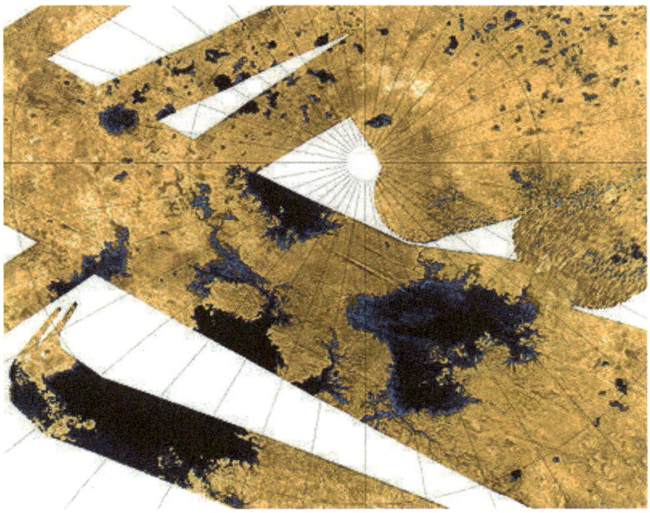

False-color *Cassini* radar mosaic of Titan's north polar region, blue areas are lakes of liquid hydrocarbons

Hypothetical types of biochemistry are forms of biochemistry speculated to be scientifically viable but not proven to exist at this time. The kinds of living organisms currently known on Earth all use carbon compounds for basic structural and metabolic functions, water as a solvent, and DNA or RNA to define and control their form. If life exists on other planets or moons, it may be chemically similar; it is also possible that there are organisms with quite different chemistries—for instance involving other classes of carbon compounds, compounds of another element, or another solvent in place of water.

The possibility of life-forms being based on "alternative" biochemistries is the topic of an ongoing scientific discussion, informed by what is known about extraterrestrial environments and about the chemical behaviour of various elements and compounds. It is also a common subject in science fiction.

The element silicon has been much discussed as a hypothetical alternative to carbon. Silicon is in the same group as carbon on the periodic table and, like carbon, it is tetravalent, although the silicon analogs of organic compounds are generally less stable. Hypothetical alternatives to water include ammonia, which, like water, is a polar molecule, and cosmically abundant; and non-polar hydrocarbon solvents such as methane and ethane, which are known to exist in liquid form on the surface of Titan.

Shadow Biosphere

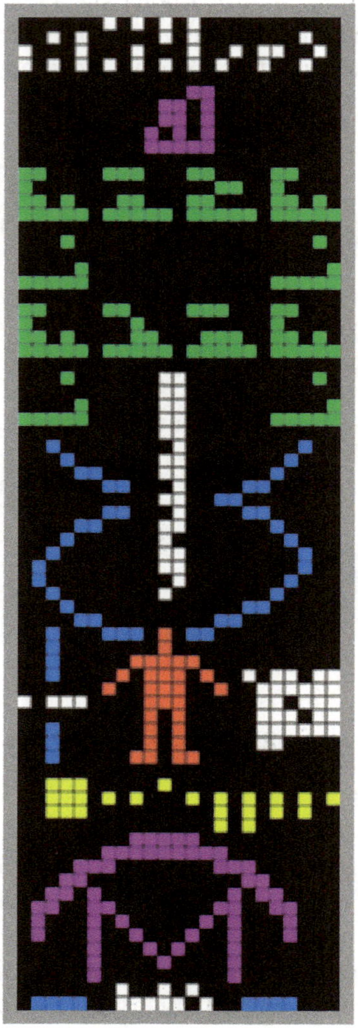

The Arecibo message (1974) sent information into space about basic chemistry of Earth life.

Apart from the prospect of finding different forms of life on other planets or moons, Earth itself has been suggested as a place where a shadow biosphere of biochemically unfamiliar micro-organisms might have lived in the past, or may still exist today.

Alternative-Chirality Biomolecules

Perhaps the least unusual alternative biochemistry would be one with differing chirality of its biomolecules. In known Earth-based life, amino acids are almost universally of the L form and sugars are of the D form. Molecules of opposite chirality have identical chemical properties to their mirrored forms, so life that used D amino acids or L sugars may be possible; molecules of such a chirality, however, would be incompatible with organisms using the opposing chirality molecules. Amino acids whose chirality is opposite to the norm are found on Earth, and these substances are generally thought to result from decay of organisms of normal chirality. However, physicist Paul Davies speculates that some of them might be products of "anti-chiral" life.

It is questionable, however, whether such a biochemistry would be truly alien. Although it would certainly be an alternative stereochemistry, molecules that are overwhelmingly found in one enantiomer throughout the vast majority of organisms can nonetheless often be found in another enantiomer in different (often basal) organisms such as in comparisons between members of Archaea and other domains, making it an open topic whether an alternative stereochemistry is truly novel.

Non-Carbon-Based Biochemistries

On Earth, all known living things have a carbon-based structure and system. Scientists have speculated about the pros and cons of using atoms other than carbon to form the molecular structures necessary for life, but no one has proposed a theory employing such atoms to form all the necessary structures. However, as Carl Sagan argued, it is very difficult to be certain whether a statement that applies to all life on Earth will turn out to apply to all life throughout the universe. Sagan used the term "carbon chauvinism" for such an assumption. Carl Sagan regarded silicon and germanium as conceivable alternatives to carbon; but, on the other hand, he noted that carbon does seem more chemically versatile and is more abundant in the cosmos.

Silicon Biochemistry

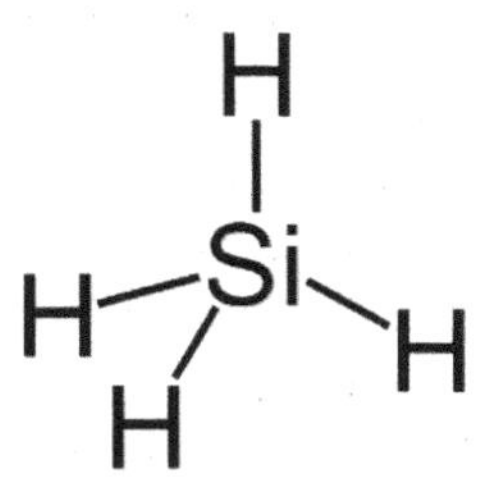

Structure of silane, analog of methane.

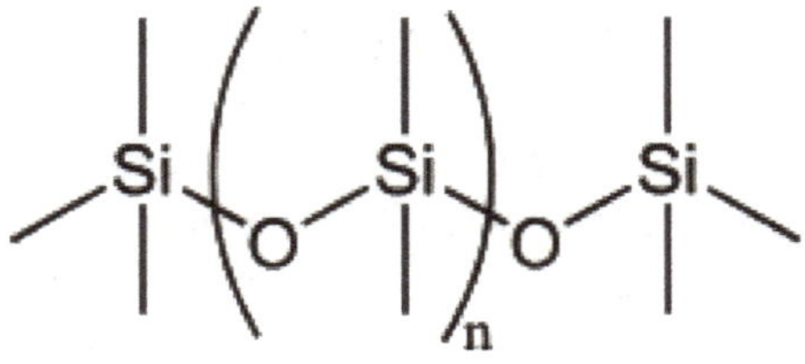

Structure of the silicone polydimethylsiloxane (PDMS).

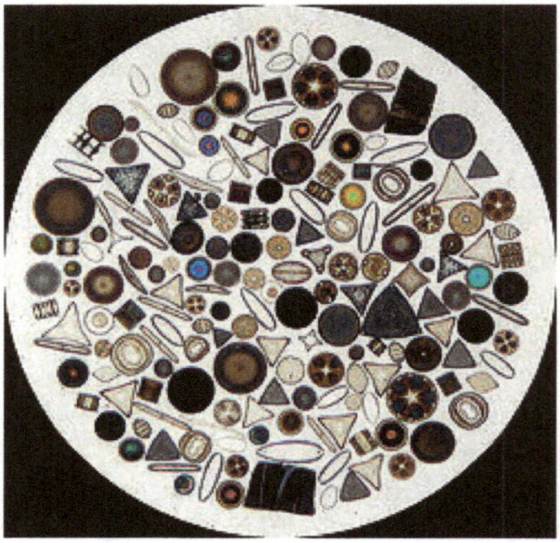

Marine diatoms—carbon-based organisms that extract silicon from sea water and incorporate it into their cell walls

The silicon atom has been much discussed as the basis for an alternative biochemical system, because silicon has many chemical properties similar to those of carbon and is in the same group of the periodic table, the carbon group. Like carbon, silicon can create molecules that are sufficiently large to carry biological information.

However, silicon has several drawbacks as an alternative to carbon. Silicon, unlike carbon, lacks the ability to form chemical bonds with diverse types of atoms as is necessary for the chemical versatility required for metabolism. Elements creating organic functional groups with carbon include hydrogen, oxygen, nitrogen, phosphorus, sulfur, and metals such as iron, magnesium, and zinc. Silicon, on the other hand, interacts with very few other types of atoms. Moreover, where it does interact with other atoms, silicon creates molecules that have been described as "monotonous compared with the combinatorial universe of organic macromolecules". This is because silicon atoms are much bigger, having a larger mass and atomic radius, and so have difficulty forming double bonds (the double bonded carbon is part of the carbonyl group, a fundamental motif of bio-organic chemistry).

Silanes, which are chemical compounds of hydrogen and silicon that are analogous to the alkane hydrocarbons, are highly reactive with water, and long-chain silanes spontaneously decompose. Molecules incorporating polymers of alternating silicon and oxygen atoms instead of direct bonds between silicon, known collectively as silicones, are much more stable. It has been suggested that silicone-based chemicals would be more stable than equivalent hydrocarbons in a sulfuric-acid-rich environment, as is found in some extraterrestrial locations.

Of the varieties of molecules identified in the interstellar medium as of 1998, 84 are based on carbon while only 8 are based on silicon. Moreover, of those 8 compounds, four also include carbon within them. The cosmic abundance of carbon to silicon is roughly 10 to 1. This may suggest a greater variety of complex carbon compounds throughout the cosmos, providing less of a foundation on which to build silicon-based biologies, at least under the conditions prevalent on the surface of planets. Also, even though Earth and other terrestrial planets are exceptionally silicon-rich and carbon-poor (the relative abundance of silicon to carbon in the Earth's crust is roughly 925:1), terrestrial life is carbon-based. The fact that carbon is used instead of silicon, may be evidence that silicon is poorly suited for biochemistry on Earth-like planets. For example: silicon is less versatile than carbon in forming compounds; the compounds formed by silicon are unstable and it blocks the flow of heat.

Even so, biogenic silica is used by some Earth life, such as the silicate skeletal structure of diatoms. According to the clay hypothesis of A. G. Cairns-Smith, silicate minerals in water played a crucial role in abiogenesis: they replicated their crystal structures, interacted with carbon compounds, and were the precursors of carbon-based life.

Although not observed in nature, carbon-silicon bonds have been added to biochemistry by using directed evolution (artificial selection). A heme containing cytochrome *c* protein from *Rhodothermus marinus* has been engineered using directed evolution to catalyze the formation of new carbon silicon bonds between hydrosilanes and diazo compounds.

Silicon compounds may possibly be biologically useful under temperatures or pressures different from the surface of a terrestrial planet, either in conjunction with or in a role less directly analogous to carbon. Polysilanols, the silicon compounds corresponding to sugars, are soluble in liquid nitrogen, suggesting that they could play a role in very low temperature biochemistry.

In cinematic and literary science fiction, at a moment when man-made machines cross from nonliving to living, it is often posited, this new form would be the first example of non-carbon-based life. Since the advent of the microprocessor in the late 1960s, these machines are often classed as computers (or computer-guided robots) and filed under "silicon-based life", even though the silicon backing matrix of these processors is not nearly as fundamental to their operation as carbon is for "wet life".

Other Exotic Element-Based Biochemistries

- Boranes are dangerously explosive in Earth's atmosphere, but would be more stable in a reducing environment. However, boron's low cosmic abundance makes it less likely as a base for life than carbon.

- Various metals, together with oxygen, can form very complex and thermally stable structures rivaling those of organic compounds; the heteropoly acids are one such family. Some metal oxides are also similar to carbon in their ability to form both nanotube structures and diamond-like crystals (such as cubic zirconia). Titanium, aluminium, magnesium, and iron are all more abundant in the Earth's crust than carbon. Metal-oxide-based life could therefore be a possibility under certain conditions, including those (such as high temperatures) at which carbon-based life would be unlikely. The Cronin group at Glasgow University reported self-assembly of tungsten polyoxometallates into cell-like spheres. By modifying their metal oxide content, the spheres can acquire holes that act as porous membrane, selectively allowing chemicals in and out of the sphere according to size.
- Sulfur is also able to form long-chain molecules, but suffers from the same high-reactivity problems as phosphorus and silanes. The biological use of sulfur as an alternative to carbon is purely hypothetical, especially because sulfur usually forms only linear chains rather than branched ones. (The biological use of sulfur as an electron acceptor is widespread and can be traced back 3.5 billion years on Earth, thus predating the use of molecular oxygen. Sulfur-reducing bacteria can utilize elemental sulfur instead of oxygen, reducing sulfur to hydrogen sulfide.)

Arsenic as an Alternative to Phosphorus

Arsenic, which is chemically similar to phosphorus, while poisonous for most life forms on Earth, is incorporated into the biochemistry of some organisms. Some marine algae incorporate arsenic into complex organic molecules such as arsenosugars and arsenobetaines. Fungi and bacteria can produce volatile methylated arsenic compounds. Arsenate reduction and arsenite oxidation have been observed in microbes (*Chrysiogenes arsenatis*). Additionally, some prokaryotes can use arsenate as a terminal electron acceptor during anaerobic growth and some can utilize arsenite as an electron donor to generate energy.

It has been speculated that the earliest life forms on Earth may have used arsenic in place of phosphorus in the structure of their DNA. A common objection to this scenario is that arsenate esters are so much less stable to hydrolysis than corresponding phosphate esters that arsenic is poorly suited for this function.

The authors of a 2010 geomicrobiology study, supported in part by NASA, have postulated that a bacterium, named GFAJ-1, collected in the sediments of Mono Lake in eastern California, can employ such ‹arsenic DNA' when cultured without phosphorus. They proposed that the bacterium may employ high levels of poly-β-hydroxybutyrate or other means to reduce the effective concentration of water and stabilize its arsenate esters. This claim was heavily criticized almost immediately after publication for the perceived lack of appropriate controls. Science writer Carl Zimmer contacted several scientists for an assessment: "I reached out to a dozen experts ... Almost unanimously, they think the NASA scientists have failed to make their case". Other authors were unable to reproduce their results and showed that the study had issues with phosphate contamination, suggesting that the low amounts present could sustain extremophile lifeforms. Alternatively, it was suggested that GFAJ-1 cells grow by recycling phosphate from degraded ribosomes, rather than by replacing it with arsenate.

Non-Water Solvents

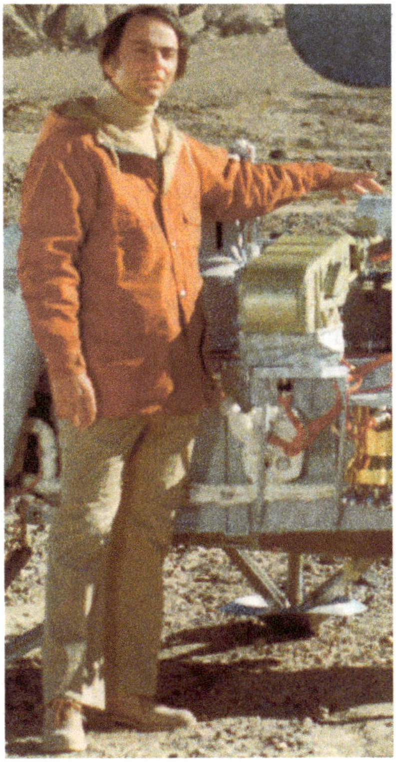

Carl Sagan speculated alien life might use ammonia, hydrocarbons or hydrogen fluoride instead of water.

In addition to carbon compounds, all currently known terrestrial life also requires water as a solvent. This has led to discussions about whether water is the only liquid capable of filling that role. The idea that an extraterrestrial life-form might be based on a solvent other than water has been taken seriously in recent scientific literature by the biochemist Steven Benner, and by the astrobiological committee chaired by John A. Baross. Solvents discussed by the Baross committee include ammonia, sulfuric acid, formamide,hydrocarbons, and (at temperatures much lower than Earth's) liquid nitrogen, or hydrogen in the form of a supercritical fluid.

Carl Sagan once described himself as both a carbon chauvinist and a water chauvinist;however on another occasion he said he was a carbon chauvinist but "not that much of a water chauvinist". He speculated on hydrocarbons, hydrofluoric acid, and ammonia as possible alternatives to water.

Some of the properties of water that are important for life processes include a large temperature range over which it is liquid, a high heat capacity (useful for temperature regulation), a large heat of vaporization, and the ability to dissolve a wide variety of compounds. Water is also amphoteric, meaning it can donate and accept an H^+ ion, allowing it to act as an acid or a base. This property is crucial in many organic and biochemical reactions, where water serves as a solvent, a reactant, or a product. There are other chemicals with similar properties that have sometimes been proposed as alternatives. Additionally, water has the unusual property of being less dense as a solid (ice) than as a liquid. This is why bodies of water freeze over but do not freeze solid (from the bottom up). If ice were denser than liquid water (as is true for nearly all other compounds), then large bodies of liquid would slowly freeze solid, which would not be conducive to the formation of life. Water as a compound is cosmically abundant, although much of it is in the form of vapour or ice. Subsurface liquid water is considered likely or possible on several of the outer moons: Enceladus (where geysers have been observed), Europa, Titan, and Ganymede. Earth and Titan are the only worlds currently known to have stable bodies of liquid on their surfaces.

Not all properties of water are necessarily advantageous for life, however. For instance, water ice has a high albedo,meaning that it reflects a significant quantity of light and heat from the Sun. During ice ages, as reflective ice builds up over the surface of the water, the effects of global cooling are increased.

There are some properties that make certain compounds and elements much more favorable than others as solvents in a successful biosphere. The solvent must be able to exist in liquid equilibrium over a range of temperatures the planetary object would normally encounter. Because boiling points vary with the pressure, the question tends not to be *does* the prospective solvent remain liquid, but *at what pressure*. For example, hydrogen cyanide has a narrow liquid phase temperature range at 1 atmosphere, but in an atmosphere with the pressure of Venus, with 92 bars (9.2 MPa) of pressure, it can indeed exist in liquid form over a wide temperature range.

Ammonia

The ammonia molecule (NH_3), like the water molecule, is abundant in the universe, being a compound of hydrogen (the simplest and most common element) with another very common element, nitrogen.The possible role of liquid ammonia as an alternative solvent for life is an idea that goes back at least to 1954, when J.B.S. Haldane raised the topic at a symposium about life's origin.

Numerous chemical reactions are possible in an ammonia solution, and liquid ammonia has chemical similarities with water.Ammonia can dissolve most organic molecules at least as well as water does and, in addition, it is capable of dissolving many elemental metals. Haldane made the point that various common water-related organic compounds have ammonia-related analogs; for instance the ammonia-related amine group ($-NH_2$) is analogous to the water-related alcohol group (-OH).

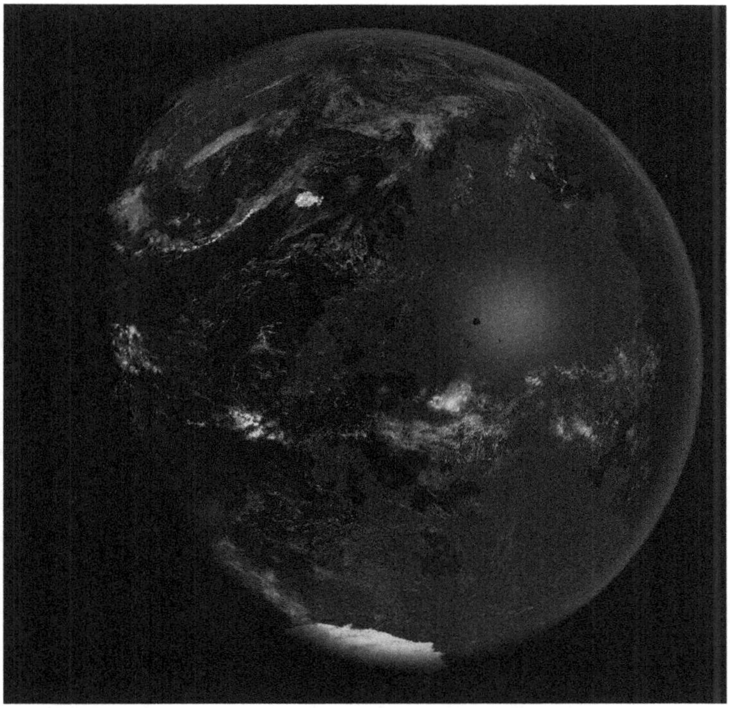

Artist's conception of how a planet with ammonia-based life might look.

Ammonia, like water, can either accept or donate an H^+ ion. When ammonia accepts an H^+, it forms the ammonium cation (NH_4^+), analogous to hydronium (H_3O^+). When it donates an H^+ ion, it forms the amide anion (NH_2^-), analogous to the hydroxide anion (OH^-). Compared to water, however, ammonia is more inclined to accept an H^+ ion, and less inclined to donate one; it is a stronger nucleophile. Ammonia added to water functions as Arrhenius base: it increases the concentration of the anion hydroxide. Conversely, using a solvent system definition of acidity and basicity, water added to liquid ammonia functions as an acid, because it increases the concentration of the cation ammonium. The carbonyl group (C=O), which is much used in terrestrial biochemistry, would not be stable in ammonia solution, but the analogous imine group (C=NH) could be used instead.

However, ammonia has some problems as a basis for life. The hydrogen bonds between ammonia molecules are weaker than those in water, causing ammonia's heat of vaporization to be half that of water, its surface tension to be a third, and reducing its ability to concentrate non-polar molecules through a hydrophobic effect. Gerald Feinberg and Robert Shapiro have questioned whether ammonia could hold prebiotic molecules together well enough to allow the emergence of a self-reproducing system. Ammonia is also flammable in oxygen, and could not exist sustainably in an environment suitable for aerobic metabolism.

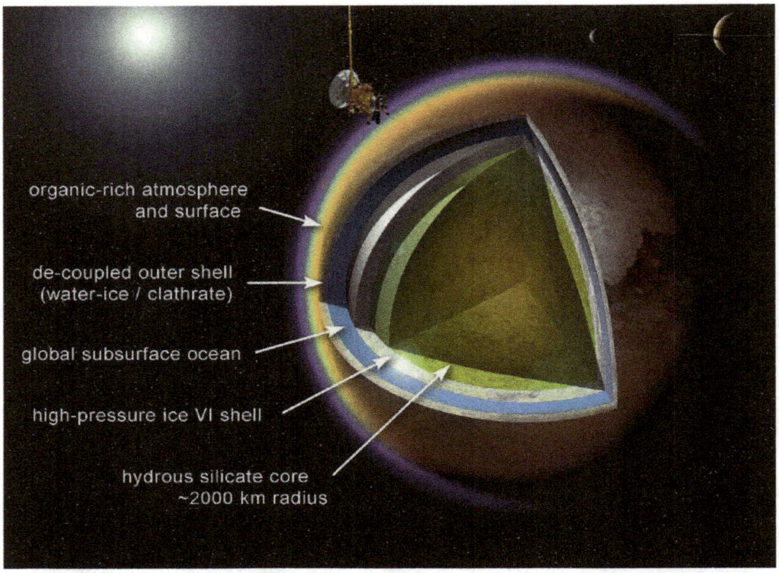

Titan's theorized internal structure, subsurface ocean shown blue.

A biosphere based on ammonia would likely exist at temperatures or air pressures that are extremely unusual in relation to life on Earth. Life on Earth usually exists within the melting point and boiling point of water at normal pressure, between 0 °C (273 K) and 100 °C (373 K); at normal pressure ammonia's melting and boiling points are between −78 °C (195 K) and −33 °C (240 K). Chemical reactions generally proceed more slowly at a lower temperature. Therefore, ammonia-based life, if it exists, might metabolize more slowly and evolve more slowly than life on Earth. On the other hand, lower temperatures could also enable living systems to use chemical species that would be too unstable at Earth temperatures to be useful.

Ammonia could be a liquid at Earth-like temperatures, but at much higher pressures; for example, at 60 atm, ammonia melts at −77 °C (196 K) and boils at 98 °C (371 K).

Ammonia and ammonia–water mixtures remain liquid at temperatures far below the freezing point of pure water, so such biochemistries might be well suited to planets and moons orbiting outside the water-based habitability zone. Such conditions could exist, for example, under the surface of Saturn's largest moon Titan.

Methane and Other Hydrocarbons

Methane (CH_4) is a simple hydrocarbon: that is, a compound of two of the most common elements in the cosmos, hydrogen and carbon. It has a cosmic abundance comparable with ammonia. Hydrocarbons could act as a solvent over a wide range of temperatures, but would lack polarity. Isaac Asimov, the biochemist and science fiction writer, suggested in 1981 that poly-lipids could form a substitute for proteins in a non-polar solvent such as methane. Lakes composed of a mixture of hydrocarbons, including methane and ethane, have been detected on the surface of Titan by the *Cassini* spacecraft.

There is debate about the effectiveness of methane and other hydrocarbons as a solvent for life compared to water or ammonia. Water is a stronger solvent than the hydrocarbons, enabling easier transport of substances in a cell.However, water is also more chemically reactive, and can break down large organic molecules through hydrolysis. A life-form whose solvent was a hydrocarbon would not face the threat of its biomolecules being destroyed in this way. Also, the water molecule's tendency to form strong hydrogen bonds can interfere with internal hydrogen bonding in complex organic molecules. Life with a hydrocarbon solvent could make more use of hydrogen bonds within its biomolecules. Moreover, the strength of hydrogen bonds within biomolecules would be appropriate to a low-temperature biochemistry.

Astrobiologist Chris McKay has argued, on thermodynamic grounds, that if life does exist on Titan's surface, using hydrocarbons as a solvent, it is likely also to use the more complex hydrocarbons as an energy source by reacting them with hydrogen, reducing ethane and acetylene to methane. Possible evidence for this form of life on Titan was identified in 2010 by Darrell Strobel of Johns Hopkins University; a greater abundance of molecular hydrogen in the upper atmospheric layers of Titan compared to the lower layers, arguing for a downward diffusion at a rate of roughly 10^{25} molecules per second and disappearance of hydrogen near Titan's surface. As Strobel noted, his findings were in line with the effects Chris McKay had predicted if methanogenic life-forms were present. The same year, another study showed low levels of acetylene on Titan's surface, which were interpreted by Chris McKay as consistent with the hypothesis of organisms reducing acetylene to methane. While restating the biological hypothesis, McKay cautioned that other explanations for the hydrogen and acetylene findings are to be considered more likely: the possibilities of yet unidentified physical or chemical processes (e.g. a non-living surface catalyst enabling acetylene to react with hydrogen), or flaws in the current models of material flow. He noted that even a non-biological catalyst effective at 95 K would in itself be a startling discovery.

A hypothetical cell membrane capable of functioning in liquid methane in Titan conditions was computer-modeled in February 2015. Composed of small molecules that contain carbon, hydrogen, and nitrogen, it would have the same stability and flexibility as cell membranes on Earth, which are composed of phospholipids, compounds of carbon, hydrogen, oxygen, and phosphorus. This hypothetical cell membrane was termed an "azotosome", a classical compound made of "azote", French for nitrogen, and "soma", Greek for body, by analogy with "liposome".

Hydrogen Fluoride

Hydrogen fluoride (HF), like water, is a polar molecule, and due to its polarity it can dissolve many ionic compounds. Its melting point is −84 °C and its boiling point is 19.54 °C (at atmospheric pressure); the difference between the two is a little more than 100 K. HF also makes hydrogen bonds with its neighbor molecules, as do water and ammonia. It has been considered as a possible solvent for life by scientists such as Peter Sneath and Carl Sagan.

HF is dangerous to the systems of molecules that Earth-life is made of, but certain other organic compounds, such as paraffin waxes, are stable with it. Like water and ammonia, liquid hydrogen fluoride supports an acid-base chemistry. Using a solvent system definition of acidity and basicity, nitric acid functions as a base when it is added to liquid HF.

However, hydrogen fluoride, unlike water, ammonia, and methane, is cosmically rare.

Hydrogen Sulfide

Hydrogen sulfide is the closest chemical analog to water, but is less polar and a weaker inorganic solvent. Hydrogen sulfide is quite plentiful on Jupiter's moon Io, and may be in liquid form a short distance below the surface; and astrobiologist Dirk Schulze-Makuch has suggested it as a possible solvent for life there. On a planet with hydrogen-sulfide oceans the source of the hydrogen sulfide could come from volcanos, in which case it could be mixed in with a bit of hydrogen fluoride, which could help dissolve minerals. Hydrogen sulfide life might use a mixture of carbon monoxide and carbon dioxide as their carbon source. They might produce and live off of sulfur monoxide, which is analogous to oxygen (O_2). Hydrogen sulfide, like hydrogen cyanide and ammonia, suffers from the small temperature range where it is liquid, though that, like that of hydrogen cyanide and ammonia, increases with increasing pressure.

Silicon Dioxide and Silicates

Silicon dioxide, also known as glass, silica, or quartz, is very abundant in the universe and has a large temperature range where it is liquid. However, its melting point is 1,600 to 1,725 °C (2,912 to 3,137 °F), so it would be impossible to make organic compounds in that temperature, because all of them would decompose. Moreover, if the pressure increases, the melting point goes down. Silicates are similar to silicon dioxide and some could have lower boiling points than silica. Gerald Feinberg and Robert Shapiro have suggested that molten silicate rock could serve as a liquid medium for organisms with a chemistry based on silicon, oxygen, and other elements such as aluminum.

Other Solvents or Cosolvents

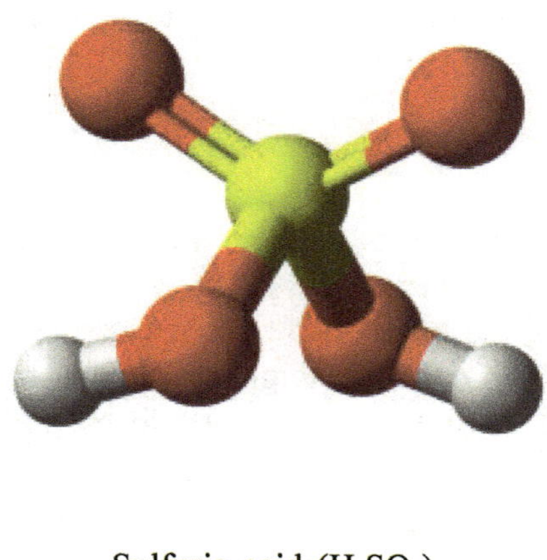

Sulfuric acid (H_2SO_4).

Other Solvents Sometimes Proposed:

- Supercritical fluids: supercritical carbon dioxide and supercritical hydrogen
- Simple hydrogen compounds: hydrogen chloride
- More complex compounds: sulfuric acid, formamide, methanol
- Very-low-temperature fluids: liquid nitrogen, and hydrogen
- High-temperature liquids: sodium chloride

Sulfuric acid in liquid form is strongly polar. It remains liquid at higher temperatures than water, its liquid range being 10 °C to 337 °C at a pressure of 1 atm, although above 300 °C it will slowly decompose. Sulfuric acid is known to be abundant in the clouds of Venus, in the form of aerosol droplets. In a biochemistry that used sulfuric acid as a solvent, the alkene group (C=C), with two carbon atoms joined by a double bond, could function analogously to the carbonyl group (C=O) in water-based biochemistry.

A proposal has been made that life on Mars may exist and be using a mixture of water and hydrogen peroxide as its solvent. A 61.2% (by weight) mix of water and hydrogen peroxide has a freezing point of −56.5 °C, and also tends to super-cool rather than crystallize. It is also hygroscopic, an advantage in a water-scarce environment.

Supercritical carbon dioxide has been proposed as a candidate for alternative biochemistry due to its ability to selectively dissolve organic compounds and assist the functioning of enzymes and because "super-Earth"- or "super-Venus"-type planets with dense high-pressure atmospheres may be common.

Other Speculations

Non-Green Photosynthesizers

Physicists have noted that, although photosynthesis on Earth generally involves green plants, a variety of other-colored plants could also support photosynthesis, essential for most life on Earth, and that other colors might be preferred in places that receive a different mix of stellar radiation than Earth. These studies indicate that, although blue photosynthetic plants would be less likely, yellow or red plants are plausible.

Variable Environments

any Earth plants and animals undergo major biochemical changes during their life cycles as a response to changing environmental conditions, for example, by having a spore or hibernation state that can be sustained for years or even millennia between more active life stages. Thus, it would be biochemically possible to sustain life in environments that are only periodically consistent with life as we know it.

For example, frogs in cold climates can survive for extended periods of time with most of their body water in a frozen state,whereas desert frogs in Australia can become inactive and dehydrate in dry periods, losing up to 75% of their fluids, yet return to life by rapidly rehydrating in wet periods. Either type of frog would appear biochemically inactive (i.e. not living) during dormant periods to anyone lacking a sensitive means of detecting low levels of metabolism.

Non-Planetary Life

Dust and Plasma-Based

In 2007, Vadim N. Tsytovich and colleagues proposed that lifelike behaviors could be exhibited by dust particles suspended in a plasma, under conditions that might exist in space. Computer models showed that, when the dust became charged, the particles could self-organize into microscopic helical structures, and the authors offer "a rough sketch of a possible model of the helical grain structure reproduction".

Scientists who have published on this topic

Scientists who have considered possible alternatives to carbon-water biochemistry include:

- **Isaac Asimov** (1920–1992), biochemist and science fiction writer.
- **William Bains**, Cambridge biologist, a contributor to the journal Astrobiology.
- **John Baross**, oceanographer and astrobiologist, who chaired a committee of scientists under the United States National Research Council that published a report on life's limiting conditions in 2007. The report addresses the concern that a space agency might conduct a well-resourced search for life on other worlds "and then fail to recognize it if it is encountered".
- **Gerald Feinberg** (1933–1992), physicist and Robert Shapiro (1935–2011), chemist, co-authors of the book *Life Beyond Earth.*
- **V.Axel Firsoff** (1910–1981), British astronomer.
- **Robert A. Freitas Jr.** (1952–present), specialist in nano-technology and nano-medicine; author of the book *Xenology.*
- **J. B. S. Haldane** (1892–1964), a geneticist noted for his work on abiogenesis.
- **George Pimentel** (1922–1989), American chemist, University of California, Berkeley.
- **Carl Sagan** (1934–1996), astronomer, science popularizer, and SETI proponent.
- **Peter Sneath** (1923–2011), microbiologist, author of the book *Planets and Life.*

IN FICTION

- Alternate chirality: In Arthur C. Clarke's short story "Technical Error", there is an example of differing chirality.
- The concept of reversed chirality also figured prominently in the plot of James Blish's *Star Trek* novel *Spock Must Die!*, where a transporter experiment gone awry ends up creating a duplicate Spock who turns out to be a perfect mirror-image of the original all the way down to the atomic level.

- The eponymous organism in Michael Crichton's *The Andromeda Strain* is described as reproducing via the direct conversion of energy into matter.
- Silicoids: John Clark, in the introduction to the 1952 shared-world anthology *The Petrified Planet*, outlined the biologies of the planet Uller, with a mixture of siloxane and silicone life, and of Niflheim, where metabolism is based on hydrofluoric acid and carbon tetrafluoride.

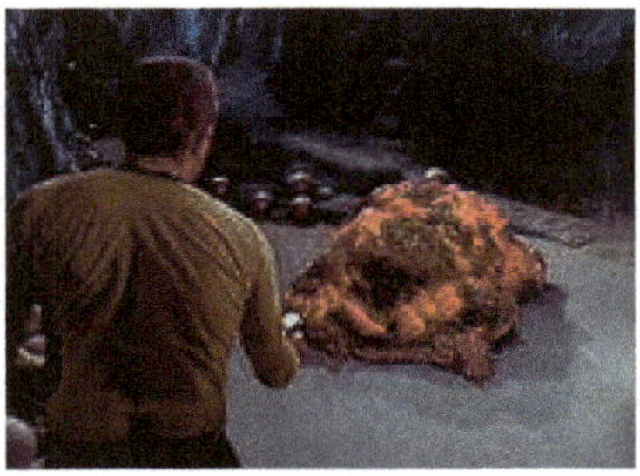

A Horta, a fictional silicon-based life-form in the Star Trek universe.

- In the original *Star Trek* episode "The Devil in the Dark", a highly intelligent silicon-based creature called *Horta*, made almost entirely of pure rock, takes the form of silicon nodules scattered throughout the caverns and tunnels of its home planet.
- In *Star Trek: The Next Generation*, the Crystalline Entity appeared in two episodes, "Datalore" and "Silicon Avatar". This was an enormous spacefaring crystal lattice that had taken thousands of lives in its quest for energy. It was destroyed before communications could be established.
- In the 1994 *The X-Files* episode "Firewalker", Mulder and Scully investigate a death in a remote research base and discover that a new silicon-based fungus found in the area may be affecting and killing the researchers.

REFERENCES

1. David J. Des Marais; et al. (2008). "The NASA Astrobiology Roadmap" (PDF). Astrobiology. 8 (4): 718. doi:10.1089/2008.0819.
2. Davies, P. C. W.; Benner, S.A.; Cleland, C.E.; Lineweaver, C.H.; McKay, C.P.; Wolfe-Simon, F. (2009). "Signatures of a Shadow Biosphere". Astrobiology. 9 (2): 241–249. Bibcode:2009AsBio...9..241D. doi:10.1089/ast.2008.0251. PMID 19292603.
3. P.C.W. Davies; Charles H. Lineweaver (2005). "Hypothesis Paper: Finding a Second Sample of Life on Earth" (PDF). Astrobiology. 5 (2): 159. Bibcode:2005AsBio...5..154D. doi:10.1089/ast.2005.5.154.
4. Sagan, Carl; Agel, Jerome (2000). Carl Sagan's Cosmic Connection: an Extraterrestrial Perspective (2nd ed.). Cambridge U.P. p. 41. ISBN 9780521783033.

5. Sagan, Carl (2000). Carl Sagan's Cosmic Connection: an Extraterrestrial Perspective (2nd ed.). Cambridge U.P. p. 46.

6. Sagan, Carl (2000). Carl Sagan's Cosmic Connection: an Extraterrestrial Perspective (2nd ed.). Cambridge U.P. p. 47.

7. Pace, NR (2001). "The universal nature of biochemistry" (PDF). Proceedings of the National Academy of Sciences of the United States of America. 98 (3): 805–8. Bibcode:2001PNAS...98..805P. doi:10.1073/pnas.98.3.805. PMC 33372 . PMID 11158550.

8. Gillette, Stephen. World-Building. Writer's Digest Books. ISBN 0-89879-707-1.

9. Lazio, Joseph. "F.10 Why do we assume that other beings must be based on carbon? Why couldn't organisms be based on other substances?". [sci.astro] ET Life (Astronomy Frequently Asked Questions). Retrieved 2006-07-21.

10. Cairns-Smith, A. Graham (1985). Seven Clues to the Origin of Life. Cambridge: Cambridge University Press. ISBN 0-521-27522-9.

11. Dawkins, Richard (1996) [1986]. The Blind Watchmaker. New York: W. W. Norton & Company, Inc. pp. 148–161. ISBN 0-393-31570-3.

12. Kan, S. B. Jennifer; Lewis, Russell D.; Chen, Kai; Arnold, Frances H. (2016-11-25). "Directed evolution of cytochrome c for carbon–silicon bond formation: Bringing silicon to life". Science. 354 (6315): 1048–1051. doi:10.1126/science.aah6219. ISSN 0036-8075.

13. William Bains. "Astrobiology—the nature of life". WilliamBains.co.uk. Retrieved 2015-03-20.

14. "Life-like cells are made of metal". New Scientist. September 14, 2011. Retrieved 2014-05-25.

15. Early Archaean Microorganisms Preferred Elemental Sulfur, Not Sulfate Science AAAS, by Philippot, et al., (14 September 2007)

16. "NASA-Funded Research Discovers Life Built With Toxic Chemical". NASA.gov. 2 December 2010. Retrieved 2010-12-02.

17. Wolfe-Simon, Felisa; Blum, Jodi Switzer; Kulp, Thomas R.; Gordon, Shelley E.; Hoeft, S. E.; Pett-Ridge, Jennifer; Stolz, John F.; Webb, Samuel M.; Weber, Peter K.; Davies, Paul C. W.; Anbar, Ariel D.; Oremland, Ronald S. (2 December 2010). "A Bacterium That Can Grow by Using Arsenic Instead of Phosphorus" (PDF). Science. 332 (6034): 1163–6. Bibcode:2011Sci...332.1163W. doi:10.1126/science.1197258. PMID 21127214. Retrieved 2010-12-09.

18. Benner, Steven A.; Ricardo, Alonso; Carrigan, Matthew A (2004). "Is there a common chemical model for life in the universe?". Current Opinion in Chemical Biology. 8 (6): 676–680. doi:10.1016/j.cbpa.2004.10.003. PMID 15556414.Text as pdf from www.sciencedirect.com (accessed 13 July 2011)

19. Committee on the Limits of Organic Life in Planetary Systems, Committee on the Origins and Evolution of Life, National Research Council; The Limits of Organic Life in Planetary Systems; The National Academies Press, 2007; pages 69–79

20. Committee on the Limits of Organic Life in Planetary Systems, Committee on the Origins and Evolution of Life, National Research Council; The Limits of Organic Life in Planetary Systems; The National Academies Press, 2007; p 72
21. Committee on the Limits of Organic Life in Planetary Systems, Committee on the Origins and Evolution of Life, National Research Council; The Limits of Organic Life in Planetary Systems; The National Academies Press, 2007; p 73
22. Committee on the Limits of Organic Life in Planetary Systems, Committee on the Origins and Evolution of Life, National Research Council; The Limits of Organic Life in Planetary Systems; The National Academies Press, 2007; p 74
23. Committee on the Limits of Organic Life in Planetary Systems, Committee on the Origins and Evolution of Life, National Research Council; The Limits of Organic Life in Planetary Systems; The National Academies Press, 2007; p 75
24. Sagan, Carl (2002). Cosmos. Random House. pp. 126–127. ISBN 0-375-50832-5.
25. Sagan, Carl; Head, Tom (2006). Conversations with Carl Sagan. University Press of Mississippi. p. 10. ISBN 1-57806-736-7.
26. Sagan, Carl (2002). Cosmos. Random House. p. 128. ISBN 0-375-50832-5.
27. Committee on the Limits of Organic Life in Planetary Systems, Committee on the Origins and Evolution of Life, National Research Council; The Limits of Organic Life in Planetary Systems; The National Academies Press, 2007; page 70
28. Isaac Asimov (Winter 1981). "Not as We Know it – the Chemistry of Life". Cosmic Search. North American AstroPhysical Observatory (9 (Vol 3 No 1)).
29. Feinberg, Gerald; Robert Shapiro (1980). Life Beyond Earth. Morrow. ISBN 9780688036423. cited in Darling, David. "ammonia-based life". Retrieved 2012-10-01.
30. Schulze-Makuch, Dirk; Irwin, Louis Neal (2008). Life in the Universe: Expectations and Constraints (2 ed.). Springer. p. 119. ISBN 9783540768166.
31. Fortes, A. D. (1999). "Exobiological Implications of a Possible Ammonia-Water Ocean Inside Titan". Retrieved 7 June 2010.
32. Committee on the Limits of Organic Life in Planetary Systems, Committee on the Origins and Evolution of Life, National Research Council; The Limits of Organic Life in Planetary Systems; The National Academies Press, 2007; page 74.
33. "What is Consuming Hydrogen and Acetylene on Titan?". NASA/JPL. 2010. Archived from the original on June 29, 2011. Retrieved 2010-06-06.
34. McKay, C. P.; Smith, H. D. (2005). "Possibilities for methanogenic life in liquid methane on the surface of Titan". Icarus. 178 (1): 274–276. Bibcode:2005Icar..178..274M. doi:10.1016/j.icarus.2005.05.018.
35. Strobel, Darrell F. (2010). "Molecular hydrogen in Titan's atmosphere: Implications of the measured tropospheric and thermospheric mole fractions" (PDF). Icarus. 208 (2): 878–886. Bibcode:2010Icar..208..878S. doi:10.1016/j.icarus.2010.03.003. Archived from the original (PDF) on August 24, 2012.
36. Mckay, Chris (2010). "Have We Discovered Evidence For Life On Titan". New Mexico State University, College of Arts and Sciences, Department of Astronomy.

Retrieved 2014-05-15. External link in |publisher= (help)

37. Life 'not as we know it' possible on Saturn's moon Titan
38. Sneath, P.H.A. (1970). Planets and Life. Thames and Hudson. cited in Boyce, Chris (1981). Extraterrestrial Encounter. New English Library. pp. 125, 182.
39. Jander, Gerhart; Spandau, Hans; Addison, C.C. (1971). Chemistry in Nonaqueous Ionizing solvents: Inorganic Chemistry in Liquid Hydrogen Cyanide and Liquid hydrogen Fluoride. II. N.Y.: Pergamon Press. cited in Freitas, Robert A. (1979). "8.2.2". Xenology: An Introduction to the Scientific Study of Extraterrestrial Life, Intelligence, and Civilization. Sacramento, CA: Xenology Research Institute.
40. Jander, J.; Lafrenz, C. (1970). Ionizing Solvents. I. Weinheim/Bergstr.: John Wiley & Sons Ltd., Verlag Chemie.cited in Freitas, Robert A. (1979). "8.2.2". Xenology: An Introduction to the Scientific Study of Extraterrestrial Life, Intelligence, and Civilization. Sacramento, CA: Xenology Research Institute.
41. David W. Koerner; Simon LeVay (2000). Here Be Dragons : The Scientific Quest for Extraterrestrial Life:. Oxford U.P. p. 202. ISBN 9780198033370.
42. Ward, Peter D.; Benner, Steven A. (2007). "Alien biochemistries". In Sullivan, Woodruff T.; Baross, John A. Planets and Life. Cambridge: Cambridge. p. 540. ISBN 978-0521531023.
43. The methane habitable zone
44. Houtkooper, Joop M.; Dirk Schulze-Makuch (2007). "The H2O2-H2O Hypothesis: Extremophiles Adapted to Conditions on Mars?" (PDF). EPSC Abstracts. European Planetary Science Congress 2007. 2: 558. Bibcode:2007epsc.conf..558H. EPSC2007-A-00439.
45. "NASA – NASA Predicts Non-Green Plants on Other Planets". Nasa.gov. 2008-02-23. Retrieved 2010-05-29.
46. Kiang, Nancy Y.; Segura, Antígona; Tinetti, Giovanna; Jee, Govind; Blankenship, Robert E.; Cohen, Martin; Siefert, Janet; Crisp, David; Meadows, Victoria S. (2007-04-03). "Spectral signatures of photosynthesis. II. Coevolution with other stars and the atmosphere on extrasolar worlds". Astrobiology. Mary Ann Liebert, Inc. 7 (1): 252–274. arXiv:astro-ph/0701391 . Bibcode:2007AsBio...7..252K. doi:10.1089/ast.2006.0108. PMID 17407410. Retrieved 2010-12-03.
47. Main and Bentley, Ecology, "Water Relations of Australian Burrowing Frogs and Tree Frogs" (1964)
48. "Physicists Discover Inorganic Dust With Lifelike Qualities". Science Daily. 2007-08-15.
49. Tsytovich, V N; G E Morfill, V E Fortov, N G Gusein-Zade, B A Klumov and S V Vladimirov; Fortov, V E; Gusein-Zade, N G; Klumov, B A; Vladimirov, S V (14 August 2007). "From plasma crystals and helical structures towards inorganic living matter". New J. Phys. 9 (263): 263. Bibcode:2007NJPh....9..263T. doi:10.1088/1367-2630/9/8/263.
50. W. Bains (2004). "Many Chemistries Could Be Used to Build Living Systems". Astrobiology. 4 (2): 137–167. Bibcode:2004AsBio...4..137B.

doi:10.1089/153110704323175124. PMID 15253836.

51. Committee on the Limits of Organic Life in Planetary Systems, Committee on the Origins and Evolution of Life, National Research Council; The Limits of Organic Life in Planetary Systems; The National Academies Press, 2007.

52. Committee on the Limits of Organic Life in Planetary Systems, Committee on the Origins and Evolution of Life, National Research Council; The Limits of Organic Life in Planetary Systems; The National Academies Press, 2007; page 5

53. Feinberg, Gerald; Robert Shapiro (1980). Life Beyond Earth. Morrow. ISBN 0688036422.

54. Freitas, Robert A. (1979). Xenology: An Introduction to the Scientific Study of Extraterrestrial Life, Intelligence, and Civilization. Sacramento, CA: Xenology Research Institute.

55. This work is acknowledged the partial basis of the article Darling, David. "ammonia-based life". Retrieved 2012-10-01.

56. Shklovskii, I.S.; Carl Sagan (1977). Intelligent Life in the Universe. Picador. p. 229.

57. V. Axel Firsoff (January 1962). "An Ammonia-Based Life". Discovery. 23: 36–42. cited in Darling, David. "ammonia-based life". Retrieved 2012-10-01.

58. A detailed review of this book is: John Gribbin (2 Oct 1980). "Life beyond Earth". New Scientist: xvii.

59. Westheimer, F. H. (1987-03-06). "Why nature chose phosphates" (PDF). Science. 235 (4793): 1173–1178 (see pp. 1175–1176). Bibcode:1987Sci...235.1173W. doi:10.1126/science.2434996. Retrieved 2010-12-03.

60. Freitas, Robert A. (1979). "8.2.2". Xenology: An Introduction to the Scientific Study of Extraterrestrial Life, Intelligence, and Civilization. Sacramento, CA: Xenology Research Institute.

61. William Bains (June 2004). "Many Chemistries Could Be Used to Build Living Systems". Astrobiology. 4 (2): 137–167. doi:10.1089/153110704323175124. PMID 15253836.

62. Cleland, Carol E.; Copley, Shelley D. (16 January 2006). "The possibility of alternative microbial life on Earth". International Journal of Astrobiology. 4 (3-4): 165. doi:10.1017/S147355040500279X. archived at (2009-03-20) from original

63. "Astrobiology". Biology Cabinet. September 26, 2006. Retrieved 2011-01-17.

64. Houtkooper, Joop M.; Dirk Schulze-Makuch (2007-05-22). "A Possible Biogenic Origin for Hydrogen Peroxide on Mars". International Journal of Astrobiology. 6 (2): 147. arXiv:physics/0610093 . Bibcode:2007IJAsB...6..147H. doi:10.1017/S1473550407003746.

65. "Biochemical Periodic Table – Arsenic". UMBBD. 2007-06-08. Retrieved 2010-05-29.

66. Ellison, Doug (2007-08-24). "Europlanet : Life's a bleach". Planetary.org.

67. Reilly, Michael (26 April 2008). "Early life could have relied on 'arsenic

DNA'". New Scientist. 198 (2653): 10. doi:10.1016/S0262-4079(08)61007-6.

68. "Christmas in Yellowstone". Pbs.org. Retrieved 2010-05-29.

69. Redfield, Rosemary (4 December 2010). "Arsenic-associated bacteria (NASA's claims)". RR Research blog. Retrieved 4 December 2010. External link in |work= (help)

70. Bradley, Alex (5 December 2010). "Arsenate-based DNA: a big idea with big holes". We, Beasties blog. Retrieved 9 December 2010. External link in |work= (help)

71. Zimmer, Carl (7 December 2010). "Scientists see fatal flaws in the NASA study of arsenic-based life". Slate. Retrieved 7 December 2010.

72. Basturea GN, Harris TK and Deutscher MP (17 August 2012). "Growth of a bacterium that apparently uses arsenic instead of phosphorus is a consequence of massive ribosome breakdown". J Biol Chem. 287: 28816–9. doi:10.1074/jbc.C112.394403. PMID 22798070.

73. Darling, David. "ammonia-based life". Retrieved 2012-10-01.

74. Darling, David. "solvent". Retrieved 2012-10-12.

75. Williams, Sarah (7 November 2012). ""Arsenic Life" Claim Refuted". BioTechniques. Retrieved 23 January 2013.

76. Choi, Charles Q. "The Chance for Life on Io". Retrieved 2013-05-25.

77. Davila, Alfonso F.; McKay, Christopher P. (May 27, 2014). "Chance and Necessity in Biochemistry: Implications for the Search for Extraterrestrial Biomarkers in Earth-like Environments". Astrobiology. 14 (6): 534–540. Bibcode:2014AsBio..14..534D. doi:10.1089/ast.2014.1150. Retrieved 2015-03-29.

78. Budisa, Nediljko; Schulze-Makuch, Dirk (8 August 2014). "Supercritical Carbon Dioxide and Its Potential as a Life-Sustaining Solvent in a Planetary Environment". Life. 4 (3): 331–340. doi:10.3390/life4030331.

79. McLendon, Christopher; Opalko, F. Jeffrey (March 2015). "Solubility of Polyethers in Hydrocarbons at Low Temperatures. A Model for Potential Genetic Backbones on Warm Titans". Astrobiology. 15 (3): 200–206. Bibcode:2015AsBio..15..200M. doi:10.1089/ast.2014.1212. Retrieved 2015-03-25.

80. Hadhazy, Adam (13 May 2015). "Alien Life on Oily Exoplanets Could Have Ether-based 'DNA'". Astrobiology Magazine. Space.com. Retrieved 2015-05-21.

81. Singer, Emily (July 19, 2015). "Chemists Invent New Letters for Nature's Genetic Alphabet". Wired (magazine). Retrieved July 20, 2015.

82. J.B.S. Haldane (1954). "The Origins of Life". New Biology. 16: 12–27. cited in Darling, David. "ammonia-based life". Retrieved 2012-10-01.

83. Niggemyer, A; Spring S; Stackebrandt E; Rosenzweig RF (December 2001). "Isolation and characterization of a novel As(V)-reducing bacterium: implications for arsenic mobilization and the genus Desulfitobacterium". Appl Environ Microbiol. 67 (12): 5568–80. doi:10.1128/AEM.67.12.5568-5580.2001. PMC 93345. PMID 11722908

CHAPTER 5

Protein Catabolism

Chapter Contents

- **Introduction**
- **Purpose**
- **Protein Degradation**
- **Amino Acid Degradation**
- **Factors Determining Overall Rate**
- **Carbohydrate Catabolism**
- **Cellular Respiration**

Protein metabolism is a description of the physical and chemical processes that cause both the building, or synthesis, of amino acids into proteins and the breakdown, or catabolism, of proteins into amino acids. Amino acids are circulated through the blood and enter the body tissues, where they are synthesized back into protein. Balance between protein synthesis and catabolism is essential to maintain normal cell functioning.

Soft tissues require amino acids to manufacture the types of proteins needed for maintenance of life processes. Amino acid synthesis is necessary to form other essential compounds in the body, like histamine, neurotransmitters, and components of nucleotides. Any amino acids that are left over after synthesis are either stored as fat or converted into energy.

INTRODUCTION

Protein catabolism is the breakdown of proteins into amino acids and simple derivative compounds, for transport into the cell through the plasma membrane and ultimately for the polymerization into new proteins via the use of ribonucleic acids (RNA) and ribosomes.

Protein catabolism, which is the breakdown of macromolecules, is essentially a digestion process. Protein catabolism is most commonly carried out by non-specific endo- and exo-proteases. However, specific proteases are used for cleaving of proteins for regulatory and protein trafficking purposes. One example is the subclass of proteolytic enzymes called oligopeptidase.

The amino acids produced by catabolism may be directly recycled to form new proteins, converted into different amino acids, or can undergo amino acid catabolism to be converted to other compounds via the Krebs cycle.

PURPOSE

The primary reason for protein catabolism is so organisms can convert proteins into a form of energy that they can use or store. To reuse their proteins, bacteria or soil microorganisms break down their proteins through protein catabolism into their individual amino acids and are used to form bacterial proteins or oxidized for energy. To convert to energy, once the proteins are broken down, they are typically deaminated (removal of an amino group) so that they can be processed into the Krebs/Citric Acid (TCA) Cycle. By proceeding into the Citric Acid Cycle, the original proteins will be converted into usable energy for the organism.

There are also other processes to convert amino acids into usable molecules to enter the TCA cycle, such as transamination (transfer of amino group), decarboxylation (removal of carboxyl group), and dehydrogenation (removal of hydrogen).

The proteins are digested in the intestines to produce the amino acids. The proteins are continuously being broken down and reformed, depending on the current needs that the body has. Proteins have different half-lives: some have an incredibly short half-life while others have longer ones. Those with short life-lives are primarily used in metabolic pathways or processes because they help the cell adjust continuously and quickly to the changes that occur due to these processes.

PROTEIN DEGRADATION

The degradation of proteins occurs within the cells, as the amino acids have to pass through certain membranes before being able to be used for different processes. This first step to protein catabolism is breaking the protein down into amino acids by cleaving their peptide bonds, also known as proteolysis. The peptide bonds are broken up by the proteasome, which is able to hydrolyze the peptide bonds by using ATP energy. This process is further helped by the use of enzymes called proteases. The proteases help cleave off the remaining peptide residues to produce individual amino acids, ready to be converted into usable molecules for either glycolysis or the TCA cycle, to produce energy for the organisms, or to be used to create new proteins.

Different types of proteases help cleave the proteins in different formats. There are serine, aspartate, metalloproteases, and many other classes. All use different mechanisms to cleave the peptide bonds to begin protein degradation. For example, the serine proteases, such as trypsin, engage in a nucleophilic attack on the hydroxyl oxygen of the serine on the peptide bond›s carbonyl carbon in order to cleave this bond. An acyl-enzyme intermediate is created and the mechanism continues to hydrolize the other remaining linkages. On the other hand, for metalloproteases, such as zinc proteases, incorporate metals to break the bonds. With zinc, its active site incorporates the zinc ion, water, and histidines (which are ligands to the zinc ion). The zinc protease also engages in a nucleophilic attack but on the carbonyl carbon, using the water's oxygen atom. The active site's base helps this process along by taking a proton from that water.

In certain organisms, such as bacteria, the proteins must undergo proteolysis before the amino acids can be re-polymerized into new proteins because the original proteins cannot pass through the bacterial plasma membrane, as they are too large. After the proteins are broken down into amino acids through proteolysis, these amino acids will be able to pass through the membranes of bacteria and will once again congregate to form new proteins that the bacteria needs to function.

AMINO ACID DEGRADATION

Oxidative deamination is the first step to breaking down the amino acids so that they can be converted to sugars. The process begins by removing the amino group of the amino acids. The amino group becomes ammonium as it is lost and later undergoes the urea cycle to become urea, in the liver. It is then released into the blood stream, where it is transferred to the kidneys, which will secrete the urea as urine. The remaining portion of the amino acid becomes oxidized, resulting in an alpha-keto acid. The alpha-keto acid will then proceed into the TCA cycle, in order to produce energy. The acid can also enter glycolysis, where it will be eventually converted into pyruvate. The pyruvate is then converted into acetyl-CoA so that it can enter the TCA cycle and convert the original pyruvate molecules into ATP, or usable energy for the organism.

Transamination leads to the same end result as deamination: the remaining acid will undergo either glycolysis or the TCA cycle to produce energy that the organism›s body will use for various purposes. This process transfers the amino group instead of losing the amino group to be converted into ammonium. The amino group is transferred to alpha-ketoglutarate, so that it can be converted to glutamate. Then glutamate transfers the amino group to oxaloacetate. This transfer is so that the oxaloacetate can be converted to aspartate or other amino acids. Eventually, this product will also proceed into oxidative deamination to once again produce alpha-ketoglutarate, an alpha-keto acid that will undergo the TCA cycle, and ammonium, which will eventually undergo the urea cycle.

Transaminases are enzymes that help catalyze the reactions that take place in transamination. They help catalyze the reaction at the point when the amino group is transferred from the original amino acid, like glutamate to alpha-ketoglutarate, and hold onto it to transfer it to another alpha-ketoacid.

FACTORS DETERMINING OVERALL RATE

Some key factors that determine overall rate include protein half-life, pH, and temperature.

Protein half-life helps determine the overall rate as this designates the first step in protein catabolism. Depending on whether this step is short or long will influence the rest of the metabolic process. One key component in determining the protein half-life is based on the N-end rule. This states that the amino acid present at the N-terminus of a protein helps determine the protein's half-life.

Changes in the pH and temperature of the molecular environment can also help determine the overall rate. The process that cleaves the protein›s peptide bonds, proteolysis, is sensitive to changes in pH and temperature. In low pH and high temperatures, proteolysis can begin even without an enzyme. This would help speed up the overall rate since it yields the same results as adding an enzyme but without necessitating enzyme use.

CARBOHYDRATE CATABOLISM

Carbohydrate catabolism is the breakdown of carbohydrates to yield an energy rich compound called ATP. The production of ATP is achieved through the oxidation of glucose molecules. In oxidation, the electrons are stripped from a glucose molecule to reduce NAD+ and FAD. NAD+ and FAD possess a high energy potential to drive the production of ATP in the electron transport chain. ATP production occurs in the mitochondria of the cell. There are two methods of producing ATP: aerobic and anaerobic. In aerobic respiration, oxygen is required. Oxygen plays a key role as it increases ATP production from 4 ATP molecules to about 30 ATP molecules. In anaerobic respiration, oxygen is not required. When oxygen is absent, the generation of ATP continues through fermentation. There are two types of fermentation: alcohol fermentation and lactic acid fermentation.

There are several different types of carbohydrates: polysaccharides (e.g., starch, amylopectin, glycogen, cellulose), monosaccharides (e.g., glucose, galactose, fructose, ribose) and the disaccharides (e.g., sucrose, maltose, lactose).

Glucose reacts with oxygen in the following redox reaction, $C_6H_{12}O_6 + 6O_2 \rightarrow 6CO_2 + 6H_2O$, Carbon dioxide and water are waste products, and the overall reaction is exothermic.

The breakdown of glucose into energy in the form of molecules of ATP is therefore one of the most important biochemical pathways found in living organisms.

Glycolysis

Glycolysis, which means "sugar splitting," is the initial process in the cellular respiration pathway. Glycolysis can be either an aerobic or anaerobic process. When oxygen is present then glycolysis will continue along the aerobic respiration pathway. If oxygen is not present, then ATP production will be restricted to anaerobic respiration. The location where glycolysis, aerobic or anaerobic, occurs is in the cytosol of the cell. In glycolysis, a six-carbon glucose molecule is split into two three-carbon molecules called pyruvate. These carbon molecules are oxidized into NADH and ATP. In order for the glucose molecule to be oxidized into pyruvate, an input of ATP molecules is required. This is known as the investment phase, in which a total of two ATP molecules are consumed. At the end of glycolysis, the total yield of ATP is four molecules, but the net gain is two ATP molecules. Even though ATP is synthesized, the two ATP molecules produced are few compared to the second and third pathways, Krebs cycle and oxidative phosphorylation.

Fermentation

Even if there is no oxygen present, glycolysis can continue to generate ATP. However, in order for glycolysis to continue to produce ATP, there must be NAD+ present, which is responsible for oxidizing glucose. This is achieved by recycling NADH back to NAD+. When NAD+ is reduced to NADH, the electrons from NADH are eventually transferred to a separate organic molecule, transforming NADH back to NAD+. This process of renewing the supply of NAD+ is called fermentation, which falls into two categories.

Alcohol Fermentation

In alcohol fermentation, when a glucose molecule is oxidized, ethanol (ethyl alcohol) and carbon dioxide are byproducts. The organic molecule that is responsible for renewing the NAD+ supply in this type of fermentation is the pyruvate from glycolysis. Each pyruvate will release a carbon dioxide molecule, turning into acetaldehyde. The acetaldehyde is then reduced by the NADH produced from glycolysis, forming the alcohol waste product, ethanol, and forming NAD+, thereby replenishing its supply for glycolysis to continue producing ATP.

Lactic Acid Fermentation

In lactic acid fermentation, each pyruvate molecule is directly reduced by NADH. The only byproduct from this type of fermentation is lactate. Lactic acid fermentation is used by human muscle cells as a means of generating ATP during strenuous exercise where oxygen consumption is higher than the supplied oxygen. As this process progresses, the surplus of lactate will be brought to the liver where it will be converted back to pyruvate.

Respiration

The Citric Acid Cycle (also known as the Krebs cycle)

If oxygen is present, then following glycolysis, the two pyruvate molecules will be brought into the mitochondrion itself to go through the Krebs cycle. In this cycle, the pyruvate molecules from glycolysis will be further broken down to harness the remaining energy. Each pyruvate will go through a series of reactions to be converted to acetyl coenzyme A. From here only the acetyl group will participate in the Krebs cycle, in which it will go through a series of redox reactions, catalyzed by enzymes, to further harness the energy from the acetyl group. The energy from the acetyl group, in the form of electrons, is used to reduce NAD+ and FAD to NADH and $FADH_2$, respectively. NADH and $FADH_2$ contain the stored energy harnessed from the initial glucose molecule and will be utilized in the electron transport chain where the bulk of the ATP is produced.

Oxidative Phosphorylation

The last process in aerobic respiration is oxidative phosphorylation, also known as the electron transport chain. Here NADH and $FADH_2$, which contain the energy in the form of electrons, deliver their electrons to the inner membranes of the mitochondrion to power the production of ATP. Oxidative phosphorylation contributes the majority of the ATP produced, compared to glycolysis and the Krebs cycle. While the ATP count is glycolysis and the Krebs cycle is two ATP molecules, the electron transport chain contributes, at most, twenty-eight ATP molecules. A contributing factor is due to the energy potentials of NADH and $FADH_2$. As they are brought from the initial process, glycolysis, to the electron transport chain, the energy stored in them are now utilized. A second contributing factor is that cristae, the inner membranes of mitochondria, increase the surface area and therefore the amount of proteins in the membrane that assist in the synthesis of ATP. Along the electron transport chain, there are separate compartments, each with their own concentration gradient of H + ions, which are the power source of ATP synthesis. In order to convert ADP to ATP, energy must be provided. That energy is provided by the H+ gradient. On one side of the membrane compartment, there is a high concentration of H+ ions compared to the other. The shuttling of H+ to one side of the membrane is driven by the exergonic flow of electrons throughout the membrane. These electrons are supplied by NADH and $FADH_2$ as they transfer their potential energy. Once the H+ concentration gradient is established, a proton-motive force is established, which provides the energy to convert ADP to ATP. The H+ ions that were initially forced to one side of the mitochondrion membrane will now naturally flow through a membrane protein called ATP synthase, a protein that converts ADP to ATP with the help of H+ ions.

CELLULAR RESPIRATION

Cellular respiration is a set of metabolic reactions and processes that take place in the cells of organisms to convert biochemical energy from nutrients into adenosine triphosphate (ATP), and then release waste products. The reactions involved in respiration are catabolic reactions, which break large molecules into smaller ones, releasing energy in the process, as weak so-called "high-energy" bonds are replaced by stronger bonds in the products. Respiration is one of the key ways a cell releases chemical energy to fuel cellular activity. Cellular respiration is considered an exothermic redox reaction which releases heat. The overall reaction occurs in a series of biochemical steps, most of which are redox reactions themselves. Although technically, cellular respiration is a combustion reaction, it clearly does not resemble one when it occurs in a living cell because of the slow release of energy from the series of reactions.

Nutrients that are commonly used by animal and plant cells in respiration include sugar, amino acids and fatty acids, and the most common oxidizing agent (electron acceptor) is molecular oxygen (O_2). The chemical energy stored in ATP (its third phosphate group is weakly bonded to the rest of the molecule and is cheaply broken allowing stronger bonds to form, thereby transferring energy for use by the cell) can then be used to drive processes requiring energy, including biosynthesis, locomotion or transportation of molecules across cell membranes.

Aerobic Respiration

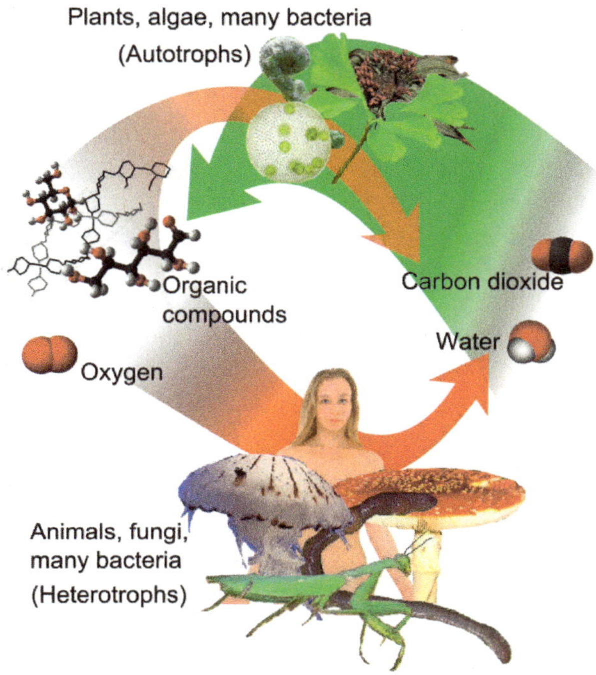

Aerobic respiration (red arrows) is the main means by which both fungi and animals utilize chemical energy in the form of organic compounds that were previously created through photosynthesis (green arrow).

Aerobic respiration requires oxygen (O_2) in order to create ATP. Although carbohydrates, fats, and proteins are consumed as reactants, it is the preferred method of pyruvate breakdown in glycolysis and requires that pyruvate enter the mitochondria in order to be fully oxidized by the Krebs cycle. The products of this process are carbon dioxide and water, but the energy transferred is used to break bonds in ADP as the third phosphate group is added to form ATP (adenosine triphosphate), by substrate-level phosphorylation, NADH and $FADH_2$

Simplified reaction:	$C_6H_{12}O_6\,(s) + 6\,O_2\,(g) \rightarrow 6\,CO_2\,(g) + 6\,H_2O\,(l) + \text{heat}$
	$\Delta G = -2880$ kJ per mol of $C_6H_{12}O_6$

The negative ΔG indicates that the reaction can occur spontaneously.

The potential of NADH and $FADH_2$ is converted to more ATP through an electron transport chain with oxygen as the "terminal electron acceptor". Most of the ATP produced by aerobic cellular respiration is made by oxidative phosphorylation. This works by the energy released in the consumption of pyruvate being used to create a chemiosmotic potential by pumping protons across a membrane. This potential is then used to drive

ATP synthase and produce ATP from ADP and a phosphate group. Biology textbooks often state that 38 ATP molecules can be made per oxidised glucose molecule during cellular respiration (2 from glycolysis, 2 from the Krebs cycle, and about 34 from the electron transport system). However, this maximum yield is never quite reached because of losses due to leaky membranes as well as the cost of moving pyruvate and ADP into the mitochondrial matrix, and current estimates range around 29 to 30 ATP per glucose.

Aerobic metabolism is up to 15 times more efficient than anaerobic metabolism (which yields 2 molecules ATP per 1 molecule glucose). However some anaerobic organisms, such as methanogens are able to continue with anaerobic respiration, yielding more ATP by using other inorganic molecules (not oxygen) as final electron acceptors in the electron transport chain. They share the initial pathway of glycolysis but aerobic metabolism continues with the Krebs cycle and oxidative phosphorylation. The post-glycolytic reactions take place in the mitochondria in eukaryotic cells, and in the cytoplasm in prokaryotic cells.

Glycolysis

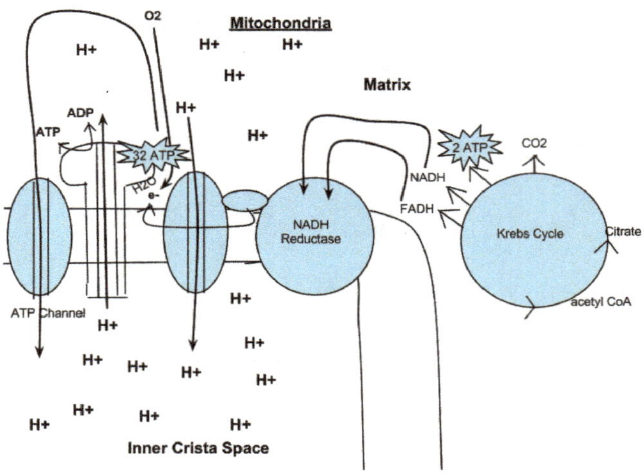

Out of the cytoplasm it goes into the Krebs cycle with the acetyl CoA. It then mixes with CO_2 and makes 2 ATP, NADH, and FADH. From there the NADH and FADH go into the NADH reductase, which produces the enzyme. The NADH pulls the enzyme's electrons to send through the electron transport chain. The electron transport chain pulls H^+ ions through the chain. From the electron transport chain, the released hydrogen ions make ADP for an end result of 32 ATP. O_2 attracts itself to the left over electron to make water. Lastly, ATP leaves through the ATP channel and out of the mitochondria.

Glycolysis is a metabolic pathway that takes place in the cytosol of cells in all living organisms. This pathway can function with or without the presence of oxygen. In humans, aerobic conditions produce pyruvate and anaerobic conditions produce lactate. In aerobic conditions, the process converts one molecule of glucose into two molecules of pyruvate (pyruvic acid), generating energy in the form of two net molecules of ATP. Four molecules of ATP per glucose are actually produced, however, two are consumed as part of the preparatory phase. The initial phosphorylation of glucose is required to increase the reactivity (decrease its stability) in order for the molecule to be cleaved into two pyruvate molecules by the enzyme aldolase. During the pay-off phase of glycolysis, four phosphate groups are transferred to ADP by substrate-level phosphorylation to make four ATP, and two NADH are produced when the pyruvate are oxidized. The overall reaction can be expressed this way:

Glucose + 2 NAD^+ + 2 P_i + 2 ADP → 2 pyruvate + 2 NADH + 2 ATP + 2 H^+ + 2 H_2O + heat

Starting with glucose, 1 ATP is used to donate a phosphate to glucose to produce glucose 6-phosphate. Glycogen can be converted into glucose 6-phosphate as well with the help of glycogen phosphorylase. During energy metabolism, glucose 6-phosphate becomes fructose 6-phosphate. An additional ATP is used to phosphorylate fructose 6-phosphate into fructose 1,6-disphosphate by the help of phosphofructokinase. Fructose 1,6-diphosphate then splits into two phosphorylated molecules with three carbon chains which later degrades into pyruvate.

Glycolysis can be literally translated as "sugar splitting".

Oxidative Decarboxylation of Pyruvate

Pyruvate is oxidized to acetyl-CoA and CO_2 by the pyruvate dehydrogenase complex (PDC). The PDC contains multiple copies of three enzymes and is located in the mitochondria of eukaryotic cells and in the cytosol of prokaryotes. In the conversion of pyruvate to acetyl-CoA, one molecule of NADH and one molecule of CO_2 is formed.

Citric Acid Cycle

This is also called the *Krebs cycle* or the *tricarboxylic acid cycle*. When oxygen is present, acetyl-CoA is produced from the pyruvate molecules created from glycolysis. Once acetyl-CoA is formed, aerobic or anaerobic respiration can occur. When oxygen is present, the mitochondria will undergo aerobic respiration which leads to the Krebs cycle. However, if oxygen is not present, fermentation of the pyruvate molecule will occur. In the presence of oxygen, when acetyl-CoA is produced, the molecule then enters the citric acid cycle (Krebs cycle) inside the mitochondrial matrix, and is oxidized to CO_2 while at the same time reducing NAD to NADH. NADH can be used by the electron transport chain to create further ATP as part of oxidative phosphorylation. To fully oxidize the equivalent of one glucose molecule, two acetyl-CoA must be metabolized by the Krebs cycle. Two waste products, H_2O and CO_2, are created during this cycle.

The citric acid cycle is an 8-step process involving 18 different enzymes and co-enzymes. During the cycle, acetyl-CoA (2 carbons) + oxaloacetate (4 carbons) yields citrate (6 carbons), which is rearranged to a more reactive form called isocitrate (6 carbons). Isocitrate is modified to become α-ketoglutarate (5 carbons), succinyl-CoA, succinate, fumarate, malate, and, finally, oxaloacetate.

The net gain of high-energy compounds from one cycle is 3 NADH, 1 $FADH_2$, and 1 GTP; the GTP may subsequently be used to produce ATP. Thus, the total yield from 1 glucose molecule (2 pyruvate molecules) is 6 NADH, 2 $FADH_2$, and 2 ATP.

Oxidative Phosphorylation

In eukaryotes, oxidative phosphorylation occurs in the mitochondrial cristae. It comprises the electron transport chain that establishes a proton gradient (chemiosmotic potential) across the boundary of inner membrane by oxidizing the NADH produced from the Krebs cycle. ATP is synthesized by the ATP synthase enzyme when the chemiosmotic gradient is used to drive the phosphorylation of ADP. The electrons are finally transferred to exogenous oxygen and, with the addition of two protons, water is formed.

Efficiency of ATP production

The table below describes the reactions involved when one glucose molecule is fully oxidized into carbon dioxide. It is assumed that all the reduced coenzymes are oxidized by the electron transport chain and used for oxidative phosphorylation.

Step	**coenzyme yield**	**ATP yield**	**Source of ATP**
Glycolysis preparatory phase		−2	Phosphorylation of glucose and fructose 6-phosphate uses two ATP from the cytoplasm.
Glycolysis pay-off phase		4	Substrate-level phosphorylation
	2 NADH	3 or 5	Oxidative phosphorylation : Each NADH produces net 1.5 ATP (instead of usual 2.5) due to NADH transport over the mitochondrial membrane
Oxidative decarboxylation of pyruvate	2 NADH	5	Oxidative phosphorylation
Krebs cycle		2	Substrate-level phosphorylation
	6 NADH	15	Oxidative phosphorylation
	2 $FADH_2$	3	Oxidative phosphorylation
Total yield		**30 or 32 ATP**	From the complete oxidation of one glucose molecule to carbon dioxide and oxidation of all the reduced coenzymes.

Although there is a theoretical yield of 38 ATP molecules per glucose during cellular respiration, such conditions are generally not realized because of losses such as the cost of moving pyruvate (from glycolysis), phosphate, and ADP (substrates for ATP synthesis) into the mitochondria. All are actively transported using carriers that utilize the stored energy in the proton electrochemical gradient.

- Pyruvate is taken up by a specific, low Km transporter to bring it into the mitochondrial matrix for oxidation by the pyruvate dehydrogenase complex.
- The **phosphate carrier** (PiC) mediates the electroneutral exchange (antiport) of phosphate ($H_2PO_4^-$; P_i) for OH^- or symport of phosphate and protons (H^+) across the inner membrane, and the driving force for moving phosphate ions into the mitochondria is the proton motive force.
- The **ATP-ADP translocase** (also called adenine nucleotide translocase, ANT) is an antiporter and exchanges ADP and ATP across the inner membrane. The

driving force is due to the ATP (−4) having a more negative charge than the ADP (−3), and thus it dissipates some of the electrical component of the proton electrochemical gradient.

The outcome of these transport processes using the proton electrochemical gradient is that more than 3 H^+ are needed to make 1 ATP. Obviously this reduces the theoretical efficiency of the whole process and the likely maximum is closer to 28–30 ATP molecules. In practice the efficiency may be even lower because the inner membrane of the mitochondria is slightly leaky to protons. Other factors may also dissipate the proton gradient creating an apparently leaky mitochondria. An uncoupling protein known as thermogenin is expressed in some cell types and is a channel that can transport protons. When this protein is active in the inner membrane it short circuits the coupling between the electron transport chain and ATP synthesis. The potential energy from the proton gradient is not used to make ATP but generates heat. This is particularly important in brown fat thermogenesis of newborn and hibernating mammals.

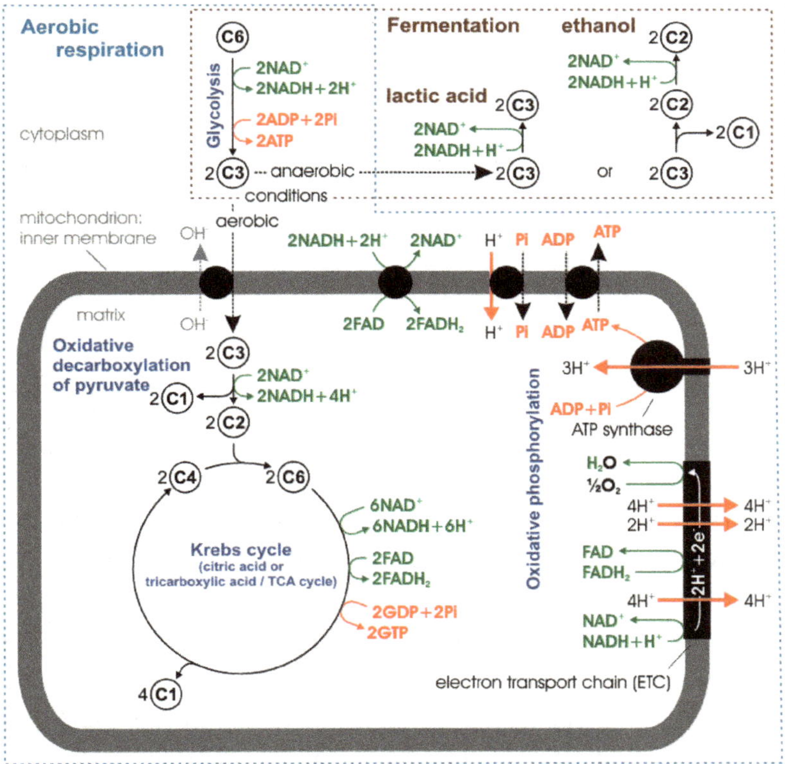

Stoichiometry of aerobic respiration and most known fermentation types in eucaryotic cell. Numbers in circles indicate counts of carbon atoms in molecules, C6 is glucose $C_6H_{12}O_6$, C1 carbon dioxide CO_2. Mitochondrial outer membrane is omitted.

According to some of newer sources the ATP yield during aerobic respiration is not 36–38, but only about 30–32 ATP molecules / 1 molecule of glucose , because:

- ATP : $NADH+H^+$ and ATP : $FADH_2$ ratios during the oxidative phosphorylation appear to be not 3 and 2, but 2.5 and 1.5 respectively. Unlike in the substrate-level phosphorylation, the stoichiometry here is difficult to establish.
  - ATP synthase produces 1 ATP / 3 H^+. However the exchange of matrix ATP for cytosolic ADP and Pi (antiport with OH^- or symport with H^+) mediated by ATP–ADP translocase and phosphate carrier consumes 1 H^+ / 1 ATP as a result of regeneration of the transmembrane potential changed during this transfer, so the net ratio is 1 ATP : 4 H^+.
  - The mitochondrial electron transport chain proton pump transfers across the inner membrane 10 H^+ / 1 $NADH+H^+$ (4 + 2 + 4) or 6 H^+ / 1 $FADH_2$ (2 + 4).

So the final stoichiometry is

1 $NADH+H^+$: 10 H^+ : 10/4 ATP = 1 $NADH+H^+$: 2.5 ATP

1 $FADH_2$: 6 H^+ : 6/4 ATP = 1 $FADH_2$: 1.5 ATP

- ATP : $NADH+H^+$ coming from glycolysis ratio during the oxidative phosphorylation is
  - 1.5, as for $FADH_2$, if hydrogen atoms ($2H^+$+$2e^-$) are transferred from cytosolic $NADH+H^+$ to mitochondrial FAD by the glycerol phosphate shuttle located in the inner mitochondrial membrane.
  - 2.5 in case of malate-aspartate shuttle transferring hydrogen atoms from cytosolic $NADH+H^+$ to mitochondrial NAD^+

So finally we have, per molecule of glucose

- Substrate-level phosphorylation: 2 ATP from glycolysis + 2 ATP (directly GTP) from Krebs cycle
- Oxidative phosphorylation
  - 2 $NADH+H^+$ from glycolysis: 2 × 1.5 ATP (if glycerol phosphate shuttle transfers hydrogen atoms) or 2 × 2.5 ATP (malate-aspartate shuttle)
  - 2 $NADH+H^+$ from the oxidative decarboxylation of pyruvate and 6 from Krebs cycle: 8 × 2.5 ATP
  - 2 $FADH_2$ from the Krebs cycle: 2 × 1.5 ATP

Altogether this gives 4 + 3 (or 5) + 20 + 3 = 30 (or 32) ATP per molecule of glucose

The total ATP yield in ethanol or lactic acid fermentation is only 2 molecules coming from glycolysis, because pyruvate is not transferred to the mitochondrion and finally oxidized to the carbon dioxide (CO_2), but reduced to ethanol or lactic acid in the cytoplasm.

Fermentation

Without oxygen, pyruvate (pyruvic acid) is not metabolized by cellular respiration but undergoes a process of fermentation. The pyruvate is not transported into the mitochondrion, but remains in the cytoplasm, where it is converted to waste products that may be removed from the cell. This serves the purpose of oxidizing the electron carriers so that they can perform glycolysis again and removing the excess pyruvate. Fermentation oxidizes NADH to NAD+ so it can be re-used in glycolysis. In the absence of oxygen, fermentation prevents the buildup of NADH in the cytoplasm and provides NAD+ for glycolysis. This waste product varies depending on the organism. In skeletal muscles, the waste product is lactic acid. This type of fermentation is called lactic acid fermentation. In strenuous exercise, when energy demands exceed energy supply, the respiratory chain cannot process all of the hydrogen atoms joined by NADH. During anaerobic glycolysis, NAD+ regenerates when pairs of hydrogen combine with pyruvate to form lactate. Lactate formation is catalyzed by lactate dehydrogenase in a reversible reaction. Lactate can also be used as an indirect precursor for liver glycogen. During recovery, when oxygen becomes available, NAD+ attaches to hydrogen from lactate to form ATP. In yeast, the waste products are ethanol and carbon dioxide. This type of fermentation is known as alcoholic or ethanol fermentation. The ATP generated in this process is made by substrate-level phosphorylation, which does not require oxygen.

Fermentation is less efficient at using the energy from glucose: only 2 ATP are produced per glucose, compared to the 38 ATP per glucose nominally produced by aerobic respiration. This is because the waste products of fermentation still contain chemical potential energy that can be released by oxidation. Ethanol, for example, can be burned in an internal combustion engine like gasoline. Glycolytic ATP, however, is created more quickly. For prokaryotes to continue a rapid growth rate when they are shifted from an aerobic environment to an anaerobic environment, they must increase the rate of the glycolytic reactions. For multicellular organisms, during short bursts of strenuous activity, muscle cells use fermentation to supplement the ATP production from the slower aerobic respiration, so fermentation may be used by a cell even before the oxygen levels are depleted, as is the case in sports that do not require athletes to pace themselves, such as sprinting.

Anaerobic Respiration

Cellular respiration is the process by which biological fuels are oxidised in the presence of an inorganic electron acceptor (such as oxygen) to produce large amounts of energy, to drive the bulk production of ATP.

Anaerobic respiration is used by some microorganisms in which neither oxygen (aerobic respiration) nor pyruvate derivatives (fermentation) is the final electron acceptor. Rather, an inorganic acceptor such as sulfate or nitrate is used. Such organisms are typically found in unusual places such as underwater caves or near hydrothermal vents at the bottom of the ocean.

REFERENCES

1. Cellular Respiration (PDF).
2. Bailey, Regina. Cellular Respiration.
3. Porter, R.; Brand, M. (1 September 1995). Mitochondrial proton conductance and H+/O ratio are independent of electron transport rate in isolated hepatocytes.

The Biochemical Journal (Free full text). 310 (Pt 2): 379–382. doi:10.1042/bj3100379. ISSN 0264-6021. PMC 1135905. PMID 7654171.

4. Reece1 Urry2 Cain3 Wasserman4 Minorsky5 Jackson6, Jane1 Lisa2 Michael3 Steven4 Peter5 Robert6 (2010). Campbell Biology Ninth Edition. Pearson Education, Inc. p. 168.
5. Rich, P. R. (2003). The molecular machinery of Keilins respiratory chain. Biochemical Society Transactions. 31 (Pt 6): 1095–1105. doi:10.1042/BST0311095. PMID 14641005.
6. Stryer, Lubert (1995). Biochemistry (fourth ed.). New York – Basingstoke: W. H. Freeman and Company. ISBN 978-0716720096.

CHAPTER 6

Genetic Code

Chapter Contents

The genetic code is a set of instructions for transferring genetic data stored in the form of DNA or RNA into proteins. Proteins are integral to almost all of the biological processes that occur in living things. They are made up of amino acid sequences, and amino acids are produced based on the sequence of the genetic code. This biological method of information storage, then, is among the most important topics in modern biology.

DNA and RNA — the nucleic acids that contain genetic information — are composed of nucleotides, specialized molecules that, in certain orders, code for the production of proteins. Certain combinations of three nucleotides, also known as tri-nucleotide sequences, are called codons. Each codon contains the code for a single amino acid. The nucleotide sequence Adenine-Uracil-Adenine, for example, codes for the amino acid Isoleucine.

INTRODUCTION

The **genetic code** is the set of rules by which information encoded within genetic material (DNA or mRNA sequences) is translated into proteins by living cells. Translation is accomplished by the ribosome, which links amino acids in an order specified by mRNA, using transfer RNA (tRNA) molecules to carry amino acids and to read the mRNA three nucleotides at a time. The genetic code is highly similar among all organisms and can be expressed in a simple table with 64 entries.

The code defines how sequences of nucleotide triplets, called *codons*, specify which amino acid will be added next during protein synthesis. With some exceptions, a three-nucleotide codon in a nucleic acid sequence specifies a single amino acid. Because the vast majority of genes are encoded with exactly the same code (see the RNA codon table), this particular code is often referred to as the canonical or standard genetic code, or simply *the* genetic code, though in fact some variant codes have evolved. For example, protein synthesis in human mitochondria relies on a genetic code that differs from the standard genetic code.

While the "genetic code" determines a protein›s amino acid sequence, other genomic regions determine when and where these proteins are produced according to a multitude of more complex "gene regulatory codes".

DISCOVERY

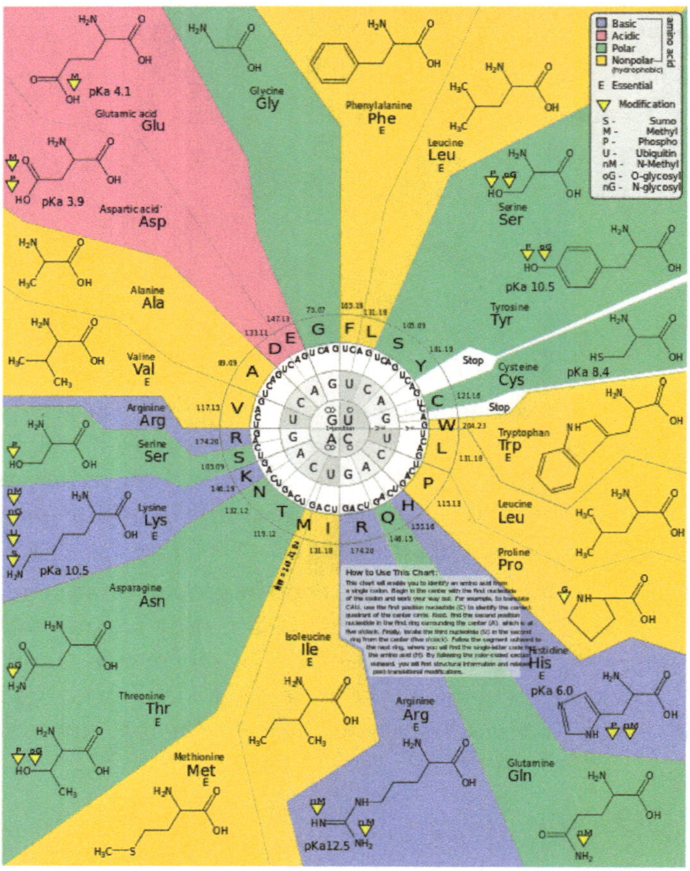

The genetic code.

Serious efforts to understand how proteins are encoded began after the structure of DNA was discovered in 1953. George Gamow postulated that sets of three bases must be employed to encode the 20 standard amino acids used by living cells to build proteins. With four different nucleotides, a code of 2 nucleotides would allow for only a maximum of 4^2 = 16 amino acids. A code of 3 nucleotides could code for a maximum of 4^3 = 64 amino acids.

The Crick, Brenner et al. experiment first demonstrated that codons consist of three DNA bases; Marshall Nirenberg and Heinrich J. Matthaei were the first to elucidate the nature of a codon in 1961 at the National Institutes of Health. They used a cell-free system to translate a poly-uracil RNA sequence (i.e., UUUUU...) and discovered that the polypeptide that they had synthesized consisted of only the amino acid phenylalanine. They thereby deduced that the codon UUU specified the amino acid phenylalanine. This was followed by experiments in Severo Ochoa›s laboratory that demonstrated that the poly-adenine RNA sequence (AAAAA...) coded for the polypeptide poly-lysine and that the poly-cytosine RNA sequence (CCCCC...) coded for the polypeptide poly-proline. Therefore, the codon AAA specified the amino acid lysine, and the codon CCC specified the amino acid proline. Using different copolymers most of the remaining codons were then determined. Subsequent work by Har Gobind Khorana identified the rest of the genetic code. Shortly thereafter, Robert W. Holley determined the structure of transfer RNA (tRNA), the adapter molecule that facilitates the process of translating RNA into protein. This work was based upon earlier studies by Severo Ochoa, who received the Nobel Prize in Physiology or Medicine in 1959 for his work on the enzymology of RNA synthesis.

Extending this work, Nirenberg and Philip Leder revealed the triplet nature of the genetic code and deciphered the codons of the standard genetic code. In these experiments, various combinations of mRNA were passed through a filter that contained ribosomes, the components of cells that translate RNA into protein. Unique triplets promoted the binding of specific tRNAs to the ribosome. Leder and Nirenberg were able to determine the sequences of 54 out of 64 codons in their experiments. In 1968, Khorana, Holley and Nirenberg received the Nobel Prize in Physiology or Medicine for their work.

FEATURES

Reading Frame

A codon is defined by the initial nucleotide from which translation starts and sets the frame for a run of uninterrupted triplets, which is known as an "open reading frame" (ORF). For example, the string GGGAAACCC, if read from the first position, contains the codons GGG, AAA, and CCC; and, if read from the second position, it contains the codons GGA and AAC; if read starting from the third position, GAA and ACC. Every sequence can, thus, be read in its 5' → 3' direction in three reading frames, each of which will produce a different amino acid sequence (in the given example, Gly-Lys-Pro, Gly-Asn, or Glu-Thr, respectively). With double-stranded DNA, there are six possible reading frames, three in the forward orientation on one strand and three reverse on the opposite strand. The actual frame from which a protein sequence is translated is defined by a start codon, usually the first AUG codon in the mRNA sequence.

In eukaryotes, ORFs in exons are often interrupted by introns.

Start and Stop Codons

Translation starts with a chain initiation codon or start codon. Unlike stop codons, the codon alone is not sufficient to begin the process. Nearby sequences such as the Shine-Dalgarno sequence in *E. coli* and initiation factors are also required to start translation. The most common start codon is AUG, which is read as methionine or, in bacteria, as formylmethionine. Alternative start codons depending on the organism include "GUG" or "UUG"; these codons normally represent valine and leucine, respectively, but as start codons they are translated as methionine or formylmethionine.

The three stop codons have been given names: UAG is *amber*, UGA is *opal* (sometimes also called *umber*), and UAA is *ochre*. "Amber" was named by discoverers Richard Epstein and Charles Steinberg after their friend Harris Bernstein, whose last name means "amber" in German. The other two stop codons were named "ochre" and "opal" in order to keep the "color names" theme. Stop codons are also called "termination" or "nonsense" codons. They signal release of the nascent polypeptide from the ribosome because there is no cognate tRNA that has anticodons complementary to these stop signals, and so a release factor binds to the ribosome instead.

Effect of Mutations

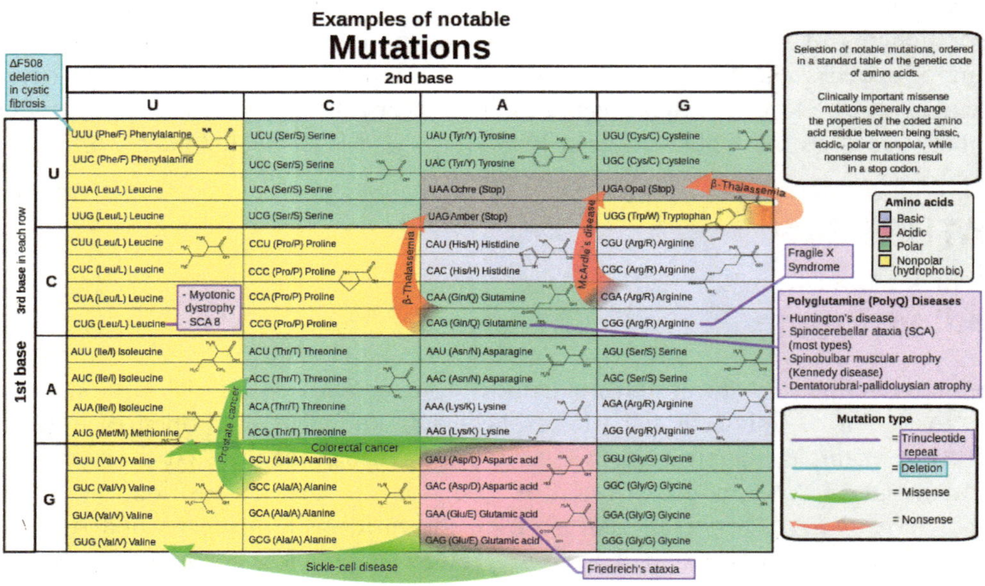

Examples of notable mutations that can occur in humans.

During the process of DNA replication, errors occasionally occur in the polymerization of the second strand. These errors, called mutations, can affect the phenotype of an organism, especially if they occur within the protein coding sequence of a gene. Error rates are usually very low—1 error in every 10–100 million bases—due to the "proofreading" ability of DNA polymerases.

Missense mutations and nonsense mutations are examples of point mutations, which can cause genetic diseases such as sickle-cell disease and thalassemia respectively. Clinically important missense mutations generally change the properties of the coded amino acid residue between being basic, acidic, polar or non-polar, whereas nonsense mutations result in a stop codon.

Mutations that disrupt the reading frame sequence by indels (insertions or deletions) of a non-multiple of 3 nucleotide bases are known as frameshift mutations. These mutations usually result in a completely different translation from the original, and are also very likely to cause a stop codon to be read, which truncates the creation of the protein. These mutations may impair the function of the resulting protein, and are thus rare in *in vivo* protein-coding sequences. One reason inheritance of frameshift mutations is rare is that, if the protein being translated is essential for growth under the selective pressures the organism faces, absence of a functional protein may cause death before the organism is viable. Frameshift mutations may result in severe genetic diseases such as Tay-Sachs disease.

Although most mutations that change protein sequences are harmful or neutral, some mutations have a beneficial effect on an organism. These mutations may enable the mutant organism to withstand particular environmental stresses better than wild type organisms, or reproduce more quickly. In these cases a mutation will tend to become more common in a population through natural selection. Viruses that use RNA as their genetic material have rapid mutation rates, which can be an advantage, since these viruses will evolve constantly and rapidly, and thus evade the defensive responses of e.g. the human immune system. In large populations of asexually reproducing organisms, for example, *E. coli*, multiple beneficial mutations may co-occur. This phenomenon is called clonal interference and causes competition among the mutations.

Degeneracy

Degeneracy is the redundancy of the genetic code. This term was given by Bernfield and Nirenberg. The genetic code has redundancy but no ambiguity (see the codon tables below for the full correlation). For example, although codons GAA and GAG both specify glutamic acid (redundancy), neither of them specifies any other amino acid (no ambiguity). The codons encoding one amino acid may differ in any of their three positions. For example, the amino acid leucine is specified by **YUR** or CU**N** (UUA, UUG, CUU, CUC, CUA, or CUG) codons (difference in the first or third position indicated using IUPAC notation), while the amino acid serine is specified by UC**N** or AG**Y** (UCA, UCG, UCC, UCU, AGU, or AGC) codons (difference in the first, second, or third position).[-117 -] A practical consequence of redundancy is that errors in the third position of the triplet codon cause only a silent mutation or an error that would not affect the protein because the hydrophilicity or hydrophobicity is maintained by equivalent substitution of amino acids; for example, a codon of NUN (where N = any nucleotide) tends to code for hydrophobic amino acids. NCN yields amino acid residues that are small in size and moderate in hydropathy; NAN encodes average size hydrophilic residues. The genetic code is so well-structured for hydropathy that a mathematical analysis (Singular Value Decomposition) of 12 variables (4 nucleotides x 3 positions) yields a remarkable correlation (C = 0.95) for predicting the hydropathy of the encoded amino acid directly from the triplet nucleotide sequence, *without translation.* Note in the table, below, eight amino acids are not affected at all by mutations at the third position of the codon, whereas in the figure above, a mutation at the second position is likely to cause a radical change in the physicochemical properties of the encoded amino acid.

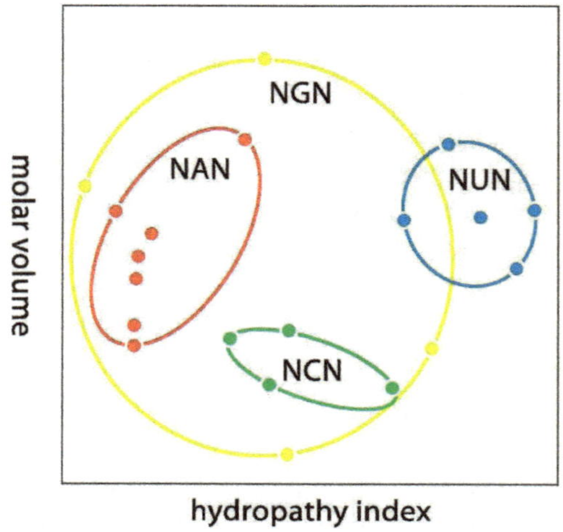

Grouping of codons by amino acid residue molar volume and hydropathy. A more detailed version is available.

Codon Usage Bias

The frequency of codons, also known as codon usage bias, can vary from species to species with functional implications for the control of translation. The following codon usage table is for the human genome.

Human genome codon frequency

Codon	AA	Fraction	Freq ‰	Number	Codon	AA	Fraction	Freq ‰	Number	Codon	AA	Fraction	Freq ‰	Number	Codon	AA	Fraction	Freq ‰	Number
UUU	F	0.46	17.6	714298	UCU	S	0.19	15.2	618711	UAU	Y	0.44	12.2	495699	UGU	C	0.46	10.6	430311
UUC	F	0.54	20.3	824692	UCC	S	0.22	17.7	718892	UAC	Y	0.56	15.3	622407	UGC	C	0.54	12.6	513028
UUA	L	0.08	7.7	311881	UCA	S	0.15	12.2	496448	UAA	*	0.30	1.0	40285	UGA	*	0.47	1.6	63237
UUG	L	0.13	12.9	525688	UCG	S	0.05	4.4	179419	UAG	*	0.24	0.8	32109	UGG	W	1.00	13.2	535595
CUU	L	0.13	13.2	536515	CCU	P	0.29	17.5	713233	CAU	H	0.42	10.9	441711	CGU	R	0.08	4.5	184609
CUC	L	0.20	19.6	796638	CCC	P	0.32	19.8	804620	CAC	H	0.58	15.1	613713	CGC	R	0.18	10.4	423516
CUA	L	0.07	7.2	290751	CCA	P	0.28	16.9	688038	CAA	Q	0.27	12.3	501911	CGA	R	0.11	6.2	250760
CUG	L	0.40	39.6	1611801	CCG	P	0.11	6.9	281570	CAG	Q	0.73	34.2	1391973	CGG	R	0.20	11.4	464485
AUU	I	0.36	16.0	650473	ACU	T	0.25	13.1	533609	AAU	N	0.47	17.0	689701	AGU	S	0.15	12.1	493429
AUC	I	0.47	20.8	846466	ACC	T	0.36	18.9	768147	AAC	N	0.53	19.1	776603	AGC	S	0.24	19.5	791383
AUA	I	0.17	7.5	304565	ACA	T	0.28	15.1	614523	AAA	K	0.43	24.4	993621	AGA	R	0.21	12.2	494682
AUG	M	1.00	22.0	896005	ACG	T	0.11	6.1	246105	AAG	K	0.57	31.9	1295568	AGG	R	0.21	12.0	486463
GUU	V	0.18	11.0	448607	GCU	A	0.27	18.4	750096	GAU	D	0.46	21.8	885429	GGU	G	0.16	10.8	437126
GUC	V	0.24	14.5	588138	GCC	A	0.40	27.7	1127679	GAC	D	0.54	25.1	1020595	GGC	G	0.34	22.2	903565
GUA	V	0.12	7.1	287712	GCA	A	0.23	15.8	643471	GAA	E	0.42	29.0	1177632	GGA	G	0.25	16.5	669873
GUG	V	0.46	28.1	1143534	GCG	A	0.11	7.4	299495	GAG	E	0.58	39.6	1609975	GGG	G	0.25	16.5	669768

Variation

While slight variations on the standard code had been predicted earlier, none were discovered until 1979, when researchers studying human mitochondrial genes discovered they used an alternative code. Many slight variants have been discovered since then, including various alternative mitochondrial codes, and small variants such as translation of the codon UGA as tryptophan in *Mycoplasma* species, and translation of CUG as a serine rather than a leucine in yeasts of the "CTG clade" (*Candida albicans* is member of this group). Because viruses must use the same genetic code as their hosts, modifications to the standard genetic code could interfere with the synthesis or functioning of viral proteins. However, some viruses (such as totiviruses) have adapted to the genetic code modification of the host. In bacteria and archaea, GUG and UUG are common start codons, but in rare cases, certain proteins may use alternative start codons not normally used by that species.

In certain proteins, non-standard amino acids are substituted for standard stop codons, depending on associated signal sequences in the messenger RNA. For example, UGA can code for selenocysteine and UAG can code for pyrrolysine. Selenocysteine is now viewed as the 21st amino acid, and pyrrolysine is viewed as the 22nd. Unlike selenocysteine, pyrrolysine encoded UAG is translated with the participation of a dedicated aminoacyl-tRNA synthetase. Both selenocysteine and pyrrolysine may be present in the same organism. Although the genetic code is normally fixed in an organism, the achaeal prokaryote *Acetohalobium arabaticum* can expand its genetic code from 20 to 21 amino acids (by including pyrrolysine) under different conditions of growth.

Despite these differences, all known naturally occurring codes are very similar to each other, and the coding mechanism is the same for all organisms: three-base codons, tRNA, ribosomes, reading the code in the same direction and translating the code three letters at a time into sequences of amino acids.

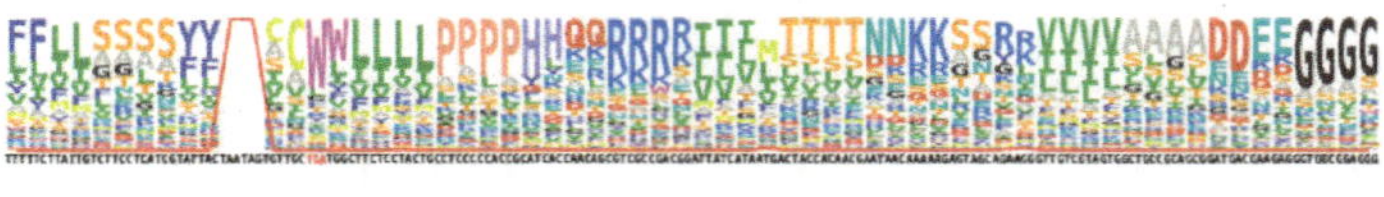

Genetic code logo of the *Globobulimina pseudospinescens* mitochondrial genome. The logo shows the 64 codons from left to right, predicted alternatives in red (relative to the standard genetic code). Red line: stop codons. The height of each amino acid in the stack shows how often it is aligned to the codon in homologous protein domains. The stack height indicates the support for the prediction.

Variant genetic codes used by an organism can be inferred by identifying highly conserved genes encoded in that genome, and comparing its codon usage to the amino acids in homologous proteins of other organisms. For example, the program FACIL infers a genetic code by searching which amino acids in homologous protein domains are most often aligned to every codon. The resulting amino acid probabilities for each codon are displayed in a genetic code logo, that also shows the support for a stop codon.

RNA CODON TABLE

nonpolar | polar | basic | acidic | (stop codon)

Standard genetic code									
1st base	**2nd base**								**3rd base**
	U		**C**		**A**		**G**		
U	UUU	(Phe/F) Phenylalanine	UCU	(Ser/S) Serine	UAU	(Tyr/Y) Tyrosine	UGU	(Cys/C) Cysteine	**U**
	UUC		UCC		UAC		UGC		**C**
	UUA	(Leu/L) Leucine	UCA		UAA	Stop (*Ochre*)	UGA	Stop (*Opal*)	**A**
	UUG		UCG		UAG	Stop (*Amber*)	UGG	(Trp/W) Tryptophan	**G**
C	CUU		CCU	(Pro/P) Proline	CAU	(His/H) Histidine	CGU	(Arg/R) Arginine	**U**
	CUC		CCC		CAC		CGC		**C**
	CUA		CCA		CAA	(Gln/Q) Glutamine	CGA		**A**
	CUG		CCG		CAG		CGG		**G**
A	AUU	(Ile/I) Isoleucine	ACU	(Thr/T) Threonine	AAU	(Asn/N) Asparagine	AGU	(Ser/S) Serine	**U**
	AUC		ACC		AAC		AGC		**C**
	AUA		ACA		AAA	(Lys/K) Lysine	AGA	(Arg/R) Arginine	**A**
	AUG[A]	(Met/M) Methionine	ACG		AAG		AGG		**G**
G	GUU	(Val/V) Valine	GCU	(Ala/A) Alanine	GAU	(Asp/D) Aspartic acid	GGU	(Gly/G) Glycine	**U**
	GUC		GCC		GAC		GGC		**C**
	GUA		GCA		GAA	(Glu/E) Glutamic acid	GGA		**A**
	GUG		GCG		GAG		GGG		**G**

[A] The codon AUG both codes for methionine and serves as an initiation site: the first AUG in an mRNA›s coding region is where translation into protein begins.

Inverse table (compressed using IUPAC notation)					
Amino acid	**Codons**	**Compressed**	**Amino acid**	**Codons**	**Compressed**
Ala/A	GCU, GCC, GCA, GCG	GCN	**Leu/L**	UUA, UUG, CUU, CUC, CUA, CUG	YUR, CUN
Arg/R	CGU, CGC, CGA, CGG, AGA, AGG	CGN, MGR	**Lys/K**	AAA, AAG	AAR
Asn/N	AAU, AAC	AAY	**Met/M**	AUG	
Asp/D	GAU, GAC	GAY	**Phe/F**	UUU, UUC	UUY
Cys/C	UGU, UGC	UGY	**Pro/P**	CCU, CCC, CCA, CCG	CCN
Gln/Q	CAA, CAG	CAR	**Ser/S**	UCU, UCC, UCA, UCG, AGU, AGC	UCN, AGY
Glu/E	GAA, GAG	GAR	**Thr/T**	ACU, ACC, ACA, ACG	ACN
Gly/G	GGU, GGC, GGA, GGG	GGN	**Trp/W**	UGG	
His/H	CAU, CAC	CAY	**Tyr/Y**	UAU, UAC	UAY
Ile/I	AUU, AUC, AUA	AUH	**Val/V**	GUU, GUC, GUA, GUG	GUN
START	AUG		**STOP**	UAA, UGA, UAG	UAR, URA

DNA CODON TABLE

The DNA codon table is essentially identical to that for RNA, but with U replaced by T.

Origin

The origin of the genetic code is a part of the question of the origin of life. Under the main hypothesis for the origin of life, the RNA world hypothesis, any model for the emergence of genetic code is intimately related to a model of the transfer from ribozymes (RNA enzymes) to proteins as the principal enzymes in cells. In line with the RNA world hypothesis, transfer RNA molecules appear to have evolved before modern aminoacyl-tRNA synthetases, so the latter cannot be part of the explanation of its patterns.

A consideration of a hypothetical random genetic code further motivates a biochemical or evolutionary model for the origin of the genetic code. If amino acids were randomly assigned to triplet codons, there would be 1.5×10^{84} possible genetic codes to choose from. This number is found by calculating how many ways there are to place 21 items (20 amino acids plus one stop) in 64 bins, wherein each item is used at least once. In fact, the distribution of codon assignments in the genetic code is nonrandom. In particular, the genetic code clusters certain amino acid assignments. For example, amino acids that share the same biosynthetic pathway tend to have the same first base in their codons. This could be an evolutionary relic of early simpler genetic code with fewer amino acids, that later diverged to code for a larger set of amino acids. It could also reflect steric and chemical properties that had another effect on the codon during its evolution. Amino acids with similar physical properties also tend to have similar codons, reducing the problems caused by point mutations and mistranslations.

Given the non-random genetic triplet coding scheme, it has been suggested that a tenable hypothesis for the origin of genetic code should address multiple aspects of the codon table such as absence of codons for D-amino acids, secondary codon patterns for some amino acids, confinement of synonymous positions to third position, a limited set of only 20 amino acids instead of a number closer to 64, and the relation of stop codon patterns to amino acid coding patterns.

There are three main ideas for the origin of the genetic code, and many models belong to either one of them or to a combination thereof:

- **"Frozen accident"**: the genetic code has been randomly created. For example, early tRNA-like ribozymes may have had different affinities for amino acids, with codons emerging from another part of the ribozyme which exhibited random variability. Once enough peptides were coded for, any major random change in the genetic code would have been lethal, hence it is "frozen".
- **Stereochemical affinity**: the genetic code is a result of a high affinity between each amino acid and its codon or anti-codon; the latter option implies that pre-tRNA molecules matched their corresponding amino acids by this affinity. Later during evolution, this matching has been gradually replaced with the one performed today by aminoacyl-tRNA synthetases.
- **Optimality**: the genetic code continued to evolve after its initial creation, so

that the current code reflects adaptation that maximizes some fitness function, usually some kind of error minimization.

Hypotheses for the origin of the genetic code have addressed a variety of scenarios:

- **Chemical principles** govern specific RNA interaction with amino acids. Experiments with aptamers showed that some amino acids have a selective chemical affinity for the base triplets that code for them. Recent experiments show that of the 8 amino acids tested, 6 show some RNA triplet-amino acid association.
- **Biosynthetic expansion**. The standard modern genetic code grew from a simpler earlier code through a process of "biosynthetic expansion". Here the idea is that primordial life "discovered" new amino acids (for example, as by-products of metabolism) and later incorporated some of these into the machinery of genetic coding. Although much circumstantial evidence has been found to suggest that fewer different amino acids were used in the past than today, precise and detailed hypotheses about which amino acids entered the code in what order have proved far more controversial.
- **Natural selection** has led to codon assignments of the genetic code that minimize the effects of mutations. A recent hypothesis suggests that the triplet code was derived from codes that used longer than triplet codons (such as quadruplet codons). Longer than triplet decoding would have higher degree of codon redundancy and would be more error resistant than the triplet decoding. This feature could allow accurate decoding in the absence of highly complex translational machinery such as the ribosome and before cells began making ribosomes.
- **Information channels:** Information-theoretic approaches model the process of translating the genetic code into corresponding amino acids as an error-prone information channel. The inherent noise (that is, the error) in the channel poses the organism with a fundamental question: how can a genetic code be constructed to withstand the effect of noisewhile accurately and efficiently translating information? These "rate-distortion" models suggest that the genetic code originated as a result of the interplay of the three conflicting evolutionary forces: the needs for diverse amino-acids, for error-tolerance and for minimal cost of resources. The code emerges at a coding transition when the mapping of codons to amino-acids becomes nonrandom. The emergence of the code is governed by the topology defined by the probable errors and is related to the map coloring problem.
- **Game theory:** Models based on signaling games combine elements of game theory, natural selection and information channels. Such models have been used to suggest that the first polypeptides were likely short and had some use other than enzymatic function. Game theoretic models have also suggested that the organization of RNA strings into cells may have been necessary to prevent "deceptive" use of the genetic code, i.e. preventing the ancient equivalent of viruses from overwhelming the RNA world.

- **Stop codons:** Codons for translational stops are also an interesting aspect to the problem of the origin of the genetic code. As an example for addressing stop codon evolution, it has been suggested that the stop codons are such that they are most likely to terminate translation early in the case of a frame shift error. In contrast, some stereochemical molecular models explain the origin of stop codons as "unassignable".

EXPANDED GENETIC CODES (SYNTHETIC BIOLOGY)

Since 2001, 40 non-natural amino acids have been added into protein by creating a unique codon (recoding) and a corresponding transfer-RNA:aminoacyl – tRNA-synthetase pair to encode it with diverse physicochemical and biological properties in order to be used as a tool to exploring protein structure and function or to create novel or enhanced proteins.

H. Murakami and M. Sisido have extended some codons to have four and five bases. Steven A. Benner constructed a functional 65th (*in vivo*) codon.

CODON DEGENERACY

Degeneracy of codons is the redundancy of the genetic code, exhibited as the multiplicity of three-base pair codon combinations that specify an amino acid. The degeneracy of the genetic code is what accounts for the existence of synonymous mutations.[:Chp 15]

Degeneracy of the genetic code was identified by Lagerkvist. For instance, codons GAA and GAG both specify glutamic acid and exhibit redundancy; but, neither specifies any other amino acid and thus are not ambiguous or demonstrate no ambiguity.

The codons encoding one amino acid may differ in any of their three positions; however, more often than not, this difference is in the second or third position. For instance, the amino acid glutamic acid is specified by GAA and GAG codons (difference in the third position); the amino acid leucine is specified by UUA, UUG, CUU, CUC, CUA, CUG codons (difference in the first or third position); and the amino acid serine is specified by UCA, UCG, UCC, UCU, AGU, AGC (difference in the first, second, or third position).[-]

Degeneracy results because there are more codons than encodable amino acids. For example, if there were two bases per codon, then only 16 amino acids could be coded for (4^2=16). Because at least 21 codes are required (20 amino acids plus stop) and the next largest number of bases is three, then 4^3 gives 64 possible codons, meaning that some degeneracy must exist.[-]

Implications

These properties of the genetic code make it more fault-tolerant for point mutations. For example, in theory, fourfold degenerate codons can tolerate any point mutation at the third position, although codon usage bias restricts this in practice in many organisms; twofold degenerate codons can tolerate one out of the three possible point mutations at the third position. Since transition mutations (purine to purine or pyrimidine to pyrimidine mutations) are more likely than transversion (purine to pyrimidine or vice versa) mutations, the equivalence of purines or that of pyrimidines at twofold degenerate sites adds a further fault-tolerance.

A practical consequence of redundancy is that some errors in the genetic code cause only a silent mutation or an error that would not affect the protein because the hydrophilicity or hydrophobicity is maintained by equivalent substitution of amino acids; for example, a codon of NUN (where N = any nucleotide) tends to code for hydrophobic amino acids. NCN yields amino acid residues that are small in size and moderate in hydropathy; NAN encodes average size hydrophilic residues. These tendencies may result from the shared ancestry of the aminoacyl tRNA synthetases related to these codons.

These variable codes for amino acids are allowed because of modified bases in the first base of the anticodon of the tRNA, and the base-pair formed is called a wobble base pair. The modified bases include inosine and the Non-Watson-Crick U-G basepair.

Terminology

A position of a codon is said to be a *n*-fold degenerate site if only *n* of four possible nucleotides (A, C, G, T) at this position specify the same amino acid. A nucleotide substitution at a fourfold degenerate site is referred to as a synonymous nucleotide substitution,⁻ whereas nucleotide substitutions in which the substitution involves the change of a purine to a pyrimidine, or vice versa, are non-synonymous transversion substitutions.⁻

A position of a codon is said to be a non-degenerate site if any mutation at this position results in amino acid substitution. There is only one threefold degenerate site where changing to three of the four nucleotides may have no effect on the amino acid (depending on what it is changed to), while changing to the fourth possible nucleotide always results in an amino acid substitution. This is the third position of an isoleucine codon: AUU, AUC, or AUA all encode isoleucine, but AUG encodes methionine. In computation, this position is often treated as a twofold degenerate site

There are three amino acids encoded by six different codons: serine, leucine, and arginine. Only two amino acids are specified by a single codon. One of these is the amino-acid methionine, specified by the codon AUG, which also specifies the start of translation; the other is tryptophan, specified by the codon UGG.

Inverse table (compressed using IUPAC notation)

Amino acid	Codons	Compressed	Amino acid	Codons	Compressed
Ala/A	GCU, GCC, GCA, GCG	GCN	**Leu/L**	UUA, UUG, CUU, CUC, CUA, CUG	YUR, CUN
Arg/R	CGU, CGC, CGA, CGG, AGA, AGG	CGN, MGR	**Lys/K**	AAA, AAG	AAR
Asn/N	AAU, AAC	AAY	**Met/M**	AUG	
Asp/D	GAU, GAC	GAY	**Phe/F**	UUU, UUC	UUY
Cys/C	UGU, UGC	UGY	**Pro/P**	CCU, CCC, CCA, CCG	CCN
Gln/Q	CAA, CAG	CAR	**Ser/S**	UCU, UCC, UCA, UCG, AGU, AGC	UCN, AGY
Glu/E	GAA, GAG	GAR	**Thr/T**	ACU, ACC, ACA, ACG	ACN
Gly/G	GGU, GGC, GGA, GGG	GGN	**Trp/W**	UGG	
His/H	CAU, CAC	CAY	**Tyr/Y**	UAU, UAC	UAY
Ile/I	AUU, AUC, AUA	AUH	**Val/V**	GUU, GUC, GUA, GUG	GUN
START	AUG		**STOP**	UAA, UGA, UAG	UAR, URA

DNA CODON TABLE

The genetic code is traditionally represented as an RNA codon table because, when proteins are made in a cell by ribosomes, it is mRNA that directs protein synthesis. The mRNA sequence is determined by the sequence of genomic DNA. With the rise of computational biology and genomics, most genes are now discovered at the DNA level, so a **DNA codon table** is becoming increasingly useful. The DNA codons in such tables occur on the sense DNA strand and are arranged in a 5› → 3› direction.

nonpolar	polar	basic	acidic	(stop codon)

Standard genetic code

1st base	2nd base: T		C		A		G		3rd base
T	TTT	(Phe/F) Phenylalanine	TCT	(Ser/S) Serine	TAT	(Tyr/Y) Tyrosine	TGT	(Cys/C) Cysteine	**T**
	TTC		TCC		TAC		TGC		**C**
	TTA	(Leu/L) Leucine	TCA		TAA	Stop (*Ochre*)	TGA	Stop (*Opal*)	**A**
	TTG		TCG		TAG	Stop (*Amber*)	TGG	(Trp/W) Tryptophan	**G**
C	CTT		CCT	(Pro/P) Proline	CAT	(His/H) Histidine	CGT	(Arg/R) Arginine	**T**
	CTC		CCC		CAC		CGC		**C**
	CTA		CCA		CAA	(Gln/Q) Glutamine	CGA		**A**
	CTG		CCG		CAG		CGG		**G**
A	ATT	(Ile/I) Isoleucine	ACT	(Thr/T) Threonine	AAT	(Asn/N) Asparagine	AGT	(Ser/S) Serine	**T**
	ATC		ACC		AAC		AGC		**C**
	ATA		ACA		AAA	(Lys/K) Lysine	AGA	(Arg/R) Arginine	**A**
	ATG[A]	(Met/M) Methionine	ACG		AAG		AGG		**G**

G	GTT	(Val/V) Valine	GCT	(Ala/A) Alanine	GAT	(Asp/D) Aspartic acid	GGT	(Gly/G) Glycine	T
	GTC		GCC		GAC		GGC		C
	GTA		GCA		GAA	(Glu/E) Glutamic acid	GGA		A
	GTG		GCG		GAG		GGG		G

[A] The codon ATG both codes for methionine and serves as an initiation site: the first ATG in an mRNA›s coding region is where translation into protein begins.

The historical basis for designating the stop codons as amber, ochre and opal is described in an autobiography by Sydney Brenner and in an historical article by Bob Edgar.

Inverse table (compressed using IUPAC notation)

Amino acid	Codons	Compressed	Amino acid	Codons	Compressed
Ala/A	GCT, GCC, GCA, GCG	GCN	**Leu/L**	TTA, TTG, CTT, CTC, CTA, CTG	YTR, CTN
Arg/R	CGT, CGC, CGA, CGG, AGA, AGG	CGN, MGR	**Lys/K**	AAA, AAG	AAR
Asn/N	AAT, AAC	AAY	**Met/M**	ATG	
Asp/D	GAT, GAC	GAY	**Phe/F**	TTT, TTC	TTY
Cys/C	TGT, TGC	TGY	**Pro/P**	CCT, CCC, CCA, CCG	CCN
Gln/Q	CAA, CAG	CAR	**Ser/S**	TCT, TCC, TCA, TCG, AGT, AGC	TCN, AGY
Glu/E	GAA, GAG	GAR	**Thr/T**	ACT, ACC, ACA, ACG	ACN
Gly/G	GGT, GGC, GGA, GGG	GGN	**Trp/W**	TGG	
His/H	CAT, CAC	CAY	**Tyr/Y**	TAT, TAC	TAY
Ile/I	ATT, ATC, ATA	ATH	**Val/V**	GTT, GTC, GTA, GTG	GTN
START	ATG		**STOP**	TAA, TGA, TAG	TAR, TRA

LIST OF GENETIC CODES

While there is a lot of commonality, different parts of the tree of life use slightly different genetic codes.

Notably the mitochondrial codes vary.

When translating from genome to protein, the use of the correct genetic code is essential. Other mechanisms also play a part in protein biosynthesis, such as post-transcriptional modification.

- Translation table 1: The standard code
- Translation table 2: The vertebrate mitochondrial code
- Translation table 3: The yeast mitochondrial code
- Translation table 4: The mold, protozoan, and coelenterate mitochondrial code and the mycoplasma/spiroplasma code
- Translation table 5: The invertebrate mitochondrial code
- Translation table 6: The ciliate, dasycladacean and hexamita nuclear code
- Translation table 7: Kinetoplast code: now merged into translation table 4
- Translation table 8: merged to table 1; all plant chloroplast differences due to RNA edit

- Translation table 9: The echinoderm and flatworm mitochondrial code
- Translation table 10: The euplotid nuclear code
- Translation table 11: The bacterial, archaeal and plant plastid code
- Translation table 12: The alternative yeast nuclear code
- Translation table 13: The ascidian mitochondrial code
- Translation table 14: The alternative flatworm mitochondrial code
- Translation table 15: Blepharisma nuclear code
- Translation table 16: Chlorophycean mitochondrial code
- Translation table 21: Trematode mitochondrial code
- Translation table 22: Scenedesmus obliquus mitochondrial code
- Translation table 23: Thraustochytrium mitochondrial code
- Translation table 24: Pterobranchia mitochondrial code
- Translation table 25: Candidate division SR1 and gracilibacteria code
- Translation table 26: Pachysolen tannophilus nuclear code

REFERENCES

1. The Nobel Prize in Physiology or Medicine 1959 (Press release). The Royal Swedish Academy of Science. 1959. Retrieved 2010-02-27. The Nobel Prize in Physiology or Medicine 1959 was awarded jointly to Severo Ochoa and Arthur Kornberg ‹for their discovery of the mechanisms in the biological synthesis of ribonucleic acid and deoxyribonucleic acid›.
2. The Nobel Prize in Physiology or Medicine 1968 (Press release). The Royal Swedish Academy of Science. 1968. Retrieved 2010-02-27. The Nobel Prize in Physiology or Medicine 1968 was awarded jointly to Robert W. Holley, Har Gobind Khorana and Marshall W. Nirenberg ‹for their interpretation of the genetic code and its function in protein synthesis›.
3. (Boillée 2006, p. 39)
4. Freeland SJ, Wu T, Keulmann N (Oct 2003).The case for an error minimizing standard genetic code. Origins of Life and Evolution of the Biosphere. 33 (4–5): 457–77. doi:10.1023/A5771327614. PMID 14604186.
5. Yarus M, Widmann JJ, Knight R (Nov 2009).RNA-amino acid binding: a stereochemical era for the genetic code. Journal of Molecular Evolution. 69 (5): 406–29. doi:10.1007/s00239-009-9270-1. PMID 19795157.
6. Amirnovin R (May 1997).An analysis of the metabolic theory of the origin of the genetic code. Journal of Molecular Evolution. 44 (5): 473–6. doi:10.1007/PL00006170. PMID 9115171.
7. Baranov PV, Venin M, Provan G (2009). Gemmell NJ, ed.Codon size reduction as the origin of the triplet genetic code. PLOS ONE. 4 (5): e5708. Bibcode9PLoSO...4.5708B. doi:10.1371/journal.pone.0005708. PMC 2682656. PMID 19479032.

8. Barrell BG, Bankier AT, Drouin J (1979).A different genetic code in human mitochondria. Nature. 282 (5735): 189–194. doi:10.1038/282189a0. ()

9. Boillée S, Vande Velde C, Cleveland DW (Oct 2006).ALS: a disease of motor neurons and their nonneuronal neighbors. Neuron. 52 (1): 39–59. doi:10.1016/j.neuron.2006.09.018. PMID 17016.

10. Bridges KR (2002).Malaria and the Red Cell. Harvard.

11. Brooks DJ, Fresco JR, Lesk AM, Singh M (Oct 2002).Evolution of amino acid frequencies in proteins over deep time: inferred order of introduction of amino acids into the genetic code. Molecular Biology and Evolution. 19 (10): 1645–55. doi:10.1093/oxfordjournals.molbev.a003988. PMID 12270892.

12. Butler G, Rasmussen MD, Lin MF, et al. (Jun 2009).Evolution of pathogenicity and sexual reproduction in eight Candida genomes. Nature. 459 (7247): 657–62. Bibcode9Natur.459..657B. doi:10.1038/nature08064. PMC 2834264. PMID 19465905.

13. Chang JC, Kan YW (Jun 1979).beta 0 thalassemia, a nonsense mutation in man. Proceedings of the National Academy of Sciences of the United States of America. 76 (6): 2886–9. Bibcode9PNAS...76.2886C. doi:10.1073/pnas.76.6.2886. PMC 383714. PMID 88735.

14. Crick F (1988).Chapter 8: The genetic code. What mad pursuit: a personal view of scientific discovery. New York: Basic Books. pp. 89–101. ISBN 0-465-09138-5.

15. Crick FH (Dec 1968).The origin of the genetic code. Journal of Molecular Evolution. 38 (3): 367–79. doi:10.1016/0022-2836(68)90392-6. PMID 4887876.

16. Crick FH, Orgel LE (1973).Directed panspermia. Icarus. 19 (3): 341–6, 344. Bibcode3Icar...19..341C. doi:10.1016/0019-1035(73)90110-3. It is a little surprising that organisms with somewhat different codes do not coexist. (Further discussion)

17. Crow JF (1993).How much do we know about spontaneous human mutation rates?. Environmental and Molecular Mutagenesis. 21 (2): 122–9. doi:10.1002/em.2850210205. PMID 8444142.

18. de Visser JA, Rozen DE (Apr 2006).Clonal interference and the periodic selection of new beneficial mutations in Escherichia coli. Genetics. 172 (4): 2093–100. doi:10.1534/genetics.105.052373. PMC 1456385. PMID 16489229.

19. Di Giulio M (Oct 1989).The extension reached by the minimization of the polarity distances during the evolution of the genetic code. Journal of Molecular Evolution. 29 (4): 288–93. doi:10.1007/BF02103616. PMID 2514270.

20. Drake JW, Holland JJ (Nov 1999).Mutation rates among RNA viruses. Proceedings of the National Academy of Sciences of the United States of America. 96 (24): 13910–3. Bibcode9PNAS...9613910D. doi:10.1073/pnas.96.24.13910. PMC 24164. PMID 10570172.

21. Dutilh BE, Jurgelenaite R, Szklarczyk R, van Hijum SA, Harhangi HR, Schmid M, de Wild B, Françoijs KJ, Stunnenberg HG, Strous M, Jetten MS, Op den Camp HJ, Huynen MA (Jul 2011).FACIL: Fast and Accurate Genetic Code Inference

and Logo. Bioinformatics. 27 (14): 1929–33. doi:10.1093/bioinformatics/btr316. PMID 21653513.

22. Edgar B (Oct 2004).The genome of bacteriophage T4: an archeological dig. Genetics. 168 (2): 575–82. PMC 1448817. PMID 15514035.
23. Elzanowski A, Ostell J (2008-04-07).The Genetic Codes. National Center for Biotechnology Information (NCBI). Retrieved 2010-03-10.
24. Erives A (Aug 2011).A model of proto-anti-codon RNA enzymes requiring L-amino acid homochirality. Journal of Molecular Evolution. 73 (1–2): 10–22. doi:10.1007/s00239-011-9453-4. PMC 3223571. PMID 21779963.
25. Fitzpatrick DA, Logue ME, Stajich JE, Butler G (1 January 2006).A fungal phylogeny based on 42 complete genomes derived from supertree and combined gene analysis. BMC Evolutionary Biology. 6: 99. doi:10.1186/1471-2148-6-99. PMC 1679813. PMID 17121679.
26. Freeland SJ, Hurst LD (Sep 1998).The genetic code is one in a million. Journal of Molecular Evolution. 47 (3): 238–48. doi:10.1007/PL00006381. PMID 9732450.
27. Freeland SJ, Knight RD, Landweber LF, Hurst LD (Apr 2000).Early fixation of an optimal genetic code. Molecular Biology and Evolution. 17 (4): 511–18. doi:10.1093/oxfordjournals.molbev.a026331. PMID 10742043.
28. Freisinger E, Grollman AP, Miller H, Kisker C (Apr 2004).Lesion (in)tolerance reveals insights into DNA replication fidelity. The EMBO Journal. 23 (7): 1494–505. doi:10.1038/sj.emboj.7600158. PMC 391067. PMID 15057282.
29. Füllen G, Youvan DC (1994).Genetic Algorithms and Recursive Ensemble Mutagenesis in Protein Engineering. Complexity International 1.
30. Gardner RS, Wahba AJ, Basilio C, Miller RS, Lengyel P, Speyer JF (Dec 1962).Synthetic polynucleotides and the amino acid code. VII. Proceedings of the National Academy of Sciences of the United States of America. 48 (12): 2087–94. Bibcode2PNAS...48.2087G. doi:10.1073/pnas.48.12.2087. PMC 221128. PMID 13946552.
31. Griffiths AJ, Miller JH, Suzuki DT, Lewontin RC, et al., eds. (2000).Spontaneous mutations. An Introduction to Genetic Analysis (7th ed.). New York: W. H. Freeman. ISBN 0-7167-3520-2.
32. Holland J, Spindler K, Horodyski F, Grabau E, Nichol S, VandePol S (Mar 1982).Rapid evolution of RNA genomes. Science. 215 (4540): 1577–85. Bibcode2Sci...215.1577H. doi:10.1126/science.7041255. PMID 7041255.
33. Hopfield JJ (1978).Origin of the genetic code: a testable hypothesis based on tRNA structure, sequence, and kinetic proofreading.. PNAS. 75: 4334–4338. doi:10.1073/pnas.75.9.4334. PMC 336109. PMID 279919.
34. http://www.kazusa.or.jp/codon/cgi-bin/showcodon.cgi?species=9606&aa=1&style=N
35. Isbrandt D, Hopwood JJ, von Figura K, Peters C (1996).Two novel frameshift mutations causing premature stop codons in a patient with the severe form

of Maroteaux-Lamy syndrome. Human Mutation. 7 (4): 361–3. doi:10.1002/(SICI)1098-1004(1996)7:4<361::AID-HUMU12>3.0.CO;2-0. PMID 8723688.

36. Itzkovitz S, Alon U (2007).The genetic code is nearly optimal for allowing additional information within protein-coding sequences. Genome Research. 17 (4): 405–412. doi:10.1101/gr.5987307.

37. Jee J, Sundstrom A, Massey SE, Mishra B (Nov 2013).What can information-asymmetric games tell us about the context of Crick›s ‹frozen accident›?. Journal of the Royal Society, Interface / the Royal Society. 10 (88): 20130614. doi:10.1098/rsif.2013.0614. PMC 3785830. PMID 23985735.

38. Jukes TH, Osawa S (Dec 1990).The genetic code in mitochondria and chloroplasts. Experientia. 46 (11–12): 1117–26. doi:10.1007/BF01936921. PMID 2253709.

39. Knight RD, Freeland SJ, Landweber LF (Jun 1999).Selection, history and chemistry: the three faces of the genetic code. Trends in Biochemical Sciences. 24 (6): 241–7. doi:10.1016/S0968-0004(99)01392-4. PMID 10366854.

40. Knight RD, Landweber LF (Sep 1998).Rhyme or reason: RNA-arginine interactions and the genetic code. Chemistry & Biology. 5 (9): R215–20. doi:10.1016/S1074-5521(98)90001-1. PMID 9751648.

41. Krzycki JA (Dec 2005).The direct genetic encoding of pyrrolysine. Current Opinion in Microbiology. 8 (6): 706–12. doi:10.1016/j.mib.2005.10.009. PMID 16256420.

42. Lewis R (2005). Human Genetics: Concepts and Applications (6th ed.). Boston, Mass: McGraw Hill. pp. 227–228. ISBN 0-07-111156-5.

43. Maloy S (2003-11-29).How nonsense mutations got their names. Microbial Genetics Course. San Diego State University. Retrieved 2010-03-10.

44. Mulligan PK, King RC, Stansfield WD (2006). A dictionary of genetics. Oxford [Oxfordshire]: Oxford University Press. p. 608. ISBN 0-19-530761-5.

45. Nakamoto T (March 2009).Evolution and the universality of the mechanism of initiation of protein synthesis. Gene. 432 (1–2): 1–6. doi:10.1016/j.gene.2008.11.001. PMID 19056476.

46. Nirenberg M, Leder P, Bernfield M, Brimacombe R, Trupin J, Rottman F, O›Neal C (May 1965).RNA codewords and protein synthesis, VII. On the general nature of the RNA code. Proceedings of the National Academy of Sciences of the United States of America. 53 (5): 1161–8. Bibcode5PNAS...53.1161N. doi:10.1073/pnas.53.5.1161. PMC 301388. PMID 5330357.

47. Nirenberg MW, Matthaei JH (Oct 1961).The dependence of cell-free protein synthesis in E. coli upon naturally occurring or synthetic polyribonucleotides. Proceedings of the National Academy of Sciences of the United States of America. 47 (10): 1588–602. Bibcode1PNAS...47.1588N. doi:10.1073/pnas.47.10.1588. PMC 223178. PMID 14479932.

48. Prat L, Heinemann IU, Aerni HR, Rinehart J, O›Donoghue P, Söll D (Dec 2012). Carbon source-dependent expansion of the genetic code in bacteria. Proceedings of the National Academy of Sciences of the United States of America. 109

(51): 21070–5. Bibcode2PNAS..10921070P. doi:10.1073/pnas.1218613110. PMC 3529041. PMID 23185002.

49. References for the image are found in Wikimedia Commons page at: Commons:File:Notable mutations.svg#References.

50. Ribas de Pouplana L, Turner RJ, Steer BA, Schimmel P (Sep 1998).Genetic code origins: tRNAs older than their synthetases?. Proceedings of the National Academy of Sciences of the United States of America. 95 (19): 11295–300. Bibcode8PNAS...9511295D. doi:10.1073/pnas.95.19.11295. PMC 21636. PMID 9736730.

51. Ronneberg TA, Landweber LF, Freeland SJ (Dec 2000).Testing a biosynthetic theory of the genetic code: fact or artifact?. Proceedings of the National Academy of Sciences of the United States of America. 97 (25): 13690–5. Bibcode0PNAS...9713690R. doi:10.1073/pnas.250403097. PMC 17637. PMID 11087835.

52. Santos MA, Tuite MF (May 1995).The CUG codon is decoded in vivo as serine and not leucine in Candida albicans. Nucleic Acids Research. 23 (9): 1481–6. doi:10.1093/nar/23.9.1481. PMC 306886. PMID 7784200.

53. Sawyer SA, Parsch J, Zhang Z, Hartl DL (Apr 2007).Prevalence of positive selection among nearly neutral amino acid replacements in Drosophila. Proceedings of the National Academy of Sciences of the United States of America. 104 (16): 6504–10. Bibcode7PNAS..104.6504S. doi:10.1073/pnas.0701572104. PMC 1871816. PMID 17409186.

54. Sella G, Ardell DH (Sep 2006).The coevolution of genes and genetic codes: Crick›s frozen accident revisited. Journal of Molecular Evolution. 63 (3): 297–313. doi:10.1007/s00239-004-0176-7. PMID 16838217.

55. Sengupta S, Higgs PG (2015).Pathways of genetic code evolution in ancient and modern organisms. Journal of Molecular Evolution. 80: 229–243. doi:10.1007/s00239-015-9686-8.

56. Simon M (2005). Emergent computation: emphasizing bioinformatics. New York: AIP Press/Springer Science+Business Media. pp. 105–106. ISBN 0-387-22046-1.

57. Sonneborn TM (1965). Bryson V, Vogel H, eds. Evolving genes and proteins. New York: Academic Press. pp. 377–397.

58. Taylor DJ, Ballinger MJ, Bowman SM, Bruenn JA (2013).Virus-host co-evolution under a modified nuclear genetic code. PeerJ. 1: e50. doi:10.7717/peerj.50. PMC 3628385. PMID 23638388.

59. Taylor FJ, Coates D (1989).The code within the codons. Bio Systems. 22 (3): 177–87. doi:10.1016/0303-2647(89)90059-2. PMID 2650752.

60. Tlusty T (Feb 2008).Rate-distortion scenario for the emergence and evolution of noisy molecular codes. Physical Review Letters. 100 (4): 048101. arXiv7.4149. Bibcode8PhRvL.100d8101T. doi:10.1103/PhysRevLett.100.048101. PMID 18352335.

61. Tlusty T (Nov 2007).A model for the emergence of the genetic code as a

transition in a noisy information channel. Journal of Theoretical Biology. 249 (2): 331–42. doi:10.1016/j.jtbi.2007.07.029. PMID 17826800.

62. Tlusty T (Sep 2010).A colorful origin for the genetic code: information theory, statistical mechanics and the emergence of molecular codes. Physics of Life Reviews. 7 (3): 362–76. arXiv7.3906. Bibcode0PhLRv...7..362T. doi:10.1016/j.plrev.2010.06.002. PMID 20558115.

63. Touriol C, Bornes S, Bonnal S, Audigier S, Prats H, Prats AC, Vagner S (2003). Generation of protein isoform diversity by alternative initiation of translation at non-AUG codons. Biology of the Cell / Under the Auspices of the European Cell Biology Organization. 95 (3–4): 169–78. doi:10.1016/S0248-4900(03)00033-9. PMID 12867081.

64. Turanov AA, Lobanov AV, Fomenko DE, Morrison HG, Sogin ML, Klobutcher LA, Hatfield DL, Gladyshev VN (Jan 2009).Genetic code supports targeted insertion of two amino acids by one codon. Science. 323 (5911): 259–61. doi:10.1126/science.1164748. PMC 3088105. PMID 19131629.

65. Wahba AJ, Gardner RS, Basilio C, Miller RS, Speyer JF, Lengyel P (Jan 1963).Synthetic polynucleotides and the amino acid code. VIII. Proceedings of the National Academy of Sciences of the United States of America. 49 (1): 116–22. Bibcode3PNAS...49..116W. doi:10.1073/pnas.49.1.116. PMC 300638. PMID 13998282.

66. Wang Q, Parrish AR, Wang L (Mar 2009).Expanding the genetic code for biological studies. Chemistry & Biology. 16 (3): 323–36. doi:10.1016/j.chembiol.2009.03.001. PMC 2696486. PMID 19318213.

67. Watson JD, Baker TA, Bell SP, Gann A, Levine M, Oosick R (2008). Molecular Biology of the Gene. San Francisco: Pearson/Benjamin Cummings. ISBN 0-8053-9592-X.

68. Witzany, G (2016) Crucial steps to life: From chemical reactions to code using agents. Biosystems 140: 49–57. doi: 10.1016/j.biosystems.2015.12.007. PMID 26723230

69. Wong JT (Feb 1980).Role of minimization of chemical distances between amino acids in the evolution of the genetic code. Proceedings of the National Academy of Sciences of the United States of America. 77 (2): 1083–6. Bibcode0PNAS...77.1083W. doi:10.1073/pnas.77.2.1083. PMC 348428. PMID 6928661.

70. Xie J, Schultz PG (Dec 2005).Adding amino acids to the genetic repertoire. Current Opinion in Chemical Biology. 9 (6): 548–54. doi:10.1016/j.cbpa.2005.10.011. PMID 16260173.

71. Yang et al. (1990) in Michel-Beyerle, M. E., ed. Reaction centers of photosynthetic bacteria: Feldafing-II-Meeting 6. Berlin: Springer-Verlag. pp. 209–18. ISBN 3-540-53420-2.

72. Yarus M (2010). Life from an RNA World: The Ancestor Within. Cambridge: Harvard University Press. p. 163. ISBN 0-674-05075-4.

73. Zhang Y, Baranov PV, Atkins JF, Gladyshev VN (May 2005).Pyrrolysine and

selenocysteine use dissimilar decoding strategies. The Journal of Biological Chemistry. 280 (21): 20740–51. doi:10.1074/jbc.M501458200. PMID 15788401.

CHAPTER 7

Peptide Synthesis

Chapter Contents

- **Introduction**
- **Chemistry**
- **Liquid-Phase Synthesis**
- **Solid-Phase Synthesis**
- **Solid Supports**
- **Protecting Groups**
- **Activating Groups**
- **Regioselective Disulfide Bond Formation**
- **Synthesizing Long Peptides**
- **Microwave-Assisted Peptide Synthesis**
- **Cyclic Peptides**
- **Fluorenylmethyloxycarbonyl Chloride**
- **Amino Acid Synthesis**

Peptides are organic molecules in which multiple amino acids are linked by peptide bonds. Each amino acid has a different side chain. All amino acids are comprised of an amino group, which is NH2, and a carboxylate group, which is COOH. When these groups react, they create a peptide bond. When carried out chemically outside of the cell, the peptide is known as a synthetic peptide.

INTRODUCTION

In organic chemistry, peptide synthesis is the production of peptides, which are organic compounds in which multiple amino acids are linked via amide bonds, also known as peptide bonds. The biological process of producing long peptides (proteins) is known as protein biosynthesis.

CHEMISTRY

Peptides are synthesized by coupling the carboxyl group of one amino acid to the amino group of another amino acid molecule. Due to the possibility of unintended reactions, protecting groups are usually necessary. Chemical peptide synthesis most commonly starts at the carboxyl end of the peptide, and proceeds toward the amino-terminus. This is the opposite direction of protein biosynthesis.

LIQUID PHASE SYNTHESIS

Liquid-phase peptide synthesis is a classical approach to peptide synthesis. It has been replaced in most labs by solid-phase synthesis (see below). However, it retains usefulness in large-scale production of peptides for industrial purposes.

SOLID PHASE SYNTHESIS

Solid-phase peptide synthesis (SPPS), pioneered by Robert Bruce Merrifield, caused a paradigm shift within the peptide synthesis community, and it is now the standard method for synthesizing peptides and proteins in the lab. SPPS allows for the synthesis of natural peptides which are difficult to express in bacteria, the incorporation of unnatural amino acids, peptide/protein backbone modification, and the synthesis of D-proteins, which consist of D-amino acids.

Small porous beads are treated with functional units (‹linkers›) on which peptide chains can be built. The peptide will remain covalently attached to the bead until cleaved from it by a reagent such as anhydrous hydrogen fluoride or trifluoroacetic acid. The peptide is thus ‹immobilized› on the solid-phase and can be retained during a filtration process while liquid-phase reagents and by-products of synthesis are flushed away.

The general principle of SPPS is one of repeated cycles of deprotection-wash-coupling-wash. The free N-terminal amine of a solid-phase attached peptide is coupled (see below) to a single N-protected amino acid unit. This unit is then deprotected, revealing a new N-terminal amine to which a further amino acid may be attached. The superiority of this technique partially lies in the ability to perform wash cycles after each reaction, removing excess reagent with all of the growing peptide of interest remaining covalently attached to the insoluble resin.

The overwhelmingly important consideration is to generate extremely high yield in each step. For example, if each coupling step were to have 99% yield, a 26-amino acid peptide would be synthesized in 77% final yield (assuming 100% yield in each deprotection); if each step were 95%, it would be synthesized in 25% yield. Thus each amino acid is added in major excess (2~10x) and coupling amino acids together is highly optimized by a series of well-characterized agents.

There are two majorly used forms of SPPS – *Fmoc* and *Boc*. Unlike ribosome protein synthesis, solid-phase peptide synthesis proceeds in a C-terminal to N-terminal fashion. The N-termini of amino acid monomers is protected by either of these two groups and added onto a deprotected amino acid chain. Automated synthesizers are available for both techniques, though many research groups continue to perform SPPS manually.

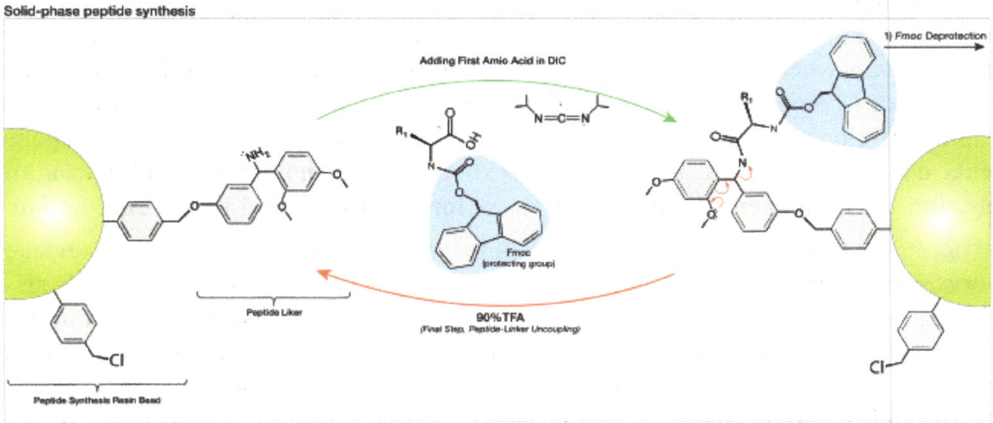

Solid-phase peptide synthesis on a Rink amide resin, using Fmoc-α-amine-protected amino acids.

SPPS is limited by yields, and typically peptides and proteins in the range of 70 amino acids are pushing the limits of synthetic accessibility. Synthetic difficulty also is sequence dependent; typically amyloid peptides and proteins are difficult to make. Longer lengths can be accessed by using native chemical ligation to couple two peptides together with quantitative yields.

Since its introduction over 40 years ago, SPPS has been significantly optimized. First, the resins themselves have been optimized. Furthermore, the 'linkers' between the C-terminal amino acid and polystyrene resin have improved attachment and cleavage to the point of mostly quantitative yields. The evolution of side chain protecting groups has limited the frequency of unwanted side reactions. In addition, the evolution of new activating groups on the carboxyl group of the incoming amino acid have improved coupling and decreased epimerization. Finally, the process itself has been optimized. In Merrifield's initial report, the deprotection of the α-amino group resulted in the formation of a peptide-resin salt, which required neutralization with base prior to coupling. The time between neutralization of the amino group and coupling of the next amino acid allowed for aggregation of peptides, primarily through the formation of secondary structures, and adversely affected coupling. The Kent group reported that concomitant neutralization of the α-amino group and coupling of the next amino acid led to improved coupling. Each of these improvements has helped SPPS become the robust technique that it is today.

SOLID SUPPORTS

The name solid support implies that reactions are carried out on the surface of the support, but this is not the case. Reactions also occur within these particles, and thus the term "solid support" better describes the insolubility of the polymer. The physical properties of the solid support, and the applications to which it can be utilized, vary with the material from which the support is constructed, the amount of cross-linking, as well as the linker and handle being used. Most scientists in the field believe that supports should have the minimum amount of cross-linking to confer stability. This should result in a well-solvated system where solid-phase peptide synthesis can be carried out. Nonetheless, the characteristics of an efficient solid support include:It must be physically stable and permit the rapid filtration of liquids, such as excess reagents, it must be inert to all reagents and solvents used during SPPS, it must swell extensively in the solvents used to allow for penetration of the reagents, and tt must allow for the attachment of the first amino acid.

There are three primary types of solid supports: gel-type supports, surface-type supports, and composites. Gel-type supports are highly solvated polymers with an equal distribution of functional groups. This type of support is the most common, and includes polystyrene (styrene cross-linked with 1–2% divinylbenzene), polyacrylamide (hydrophilic alternative to polystyrene), polyethylene glycol (PEG) (PEG-polystyrene (PEG-PS) is more stable than polystyrene and spaces the site of synthesis from the polymer backbone), and PEG-based supports composed of a PEG-polypropylene glycol network or PEG with polyamide or polystyrene. Surface-type supports: Many materials have been developed for surface functionalization, including controlled pore glass, cellulose fibers, and highly cross-linked polystyrene. Composites are gel-type polymers supported by rigid matrices.

Polystyrene Resin

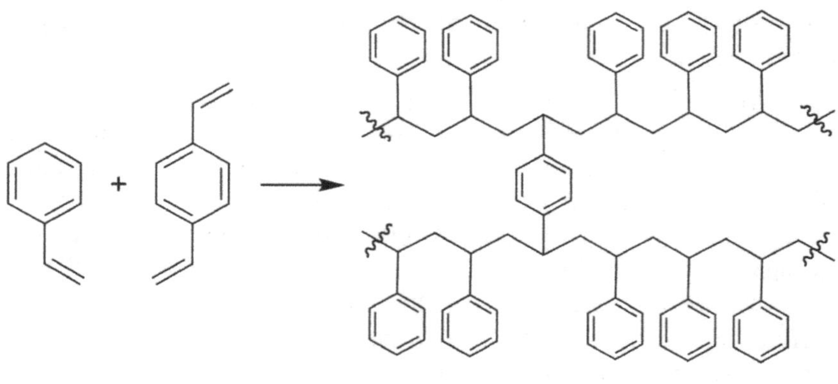

Polystyrene cross-linked with divinylbenzene. This is the most common solid support used in SPPS, and was the support pioneered by R. Bruce Merrifield.

Polystyrene resin is a versatile resin and it is quite useful in multi-well, automated peptide synthesis, due to its minimal swelling in dichloromethane. The initial support used by R. Bruce Merrifield was polysytrene cross-linked with 2% divinylbenzene. This support is sometimes referred to as the ‹Merrifield resin.› This resin produces a hydrophobic bead that is solvated by a nonpolar solvent such as dichloromethane or dimethylformamide. Since then, new resins have been developed that have the advantages of chemical inertness, and enhanced swelling or rigidity (a property of mechanical strength). For instance, highly cross-linked (50%) polystyrene has been developed that possesses the features of increased mechanical stability, better filtration of reagents and solvents, and rapid reaction kinetics.

Polystyrene resins are also available as PEG hybrids. An example of this type of resin is the Tentagel resin. The base resin is polystyrene onto which is attached long chains (MW ca. 3000 Da) of polyethylene glycol (PEG; also known as polyethylene oxide). Synthesis is carried out on the distal end of the PEG spacer making it suited for long and difficult peptides. In addition, it is also attractive for the synthesis of combinatorial Peptide libraries and on resin screening experiments. It does not expand much during synthesis, making it a preferred resin for robotic peptide synthesis.

Polyamide Resin

PEG-based Resin

Improvements to solid supports used for peptide synthesis enhance their ability to withstand the repeated use of TFA during the deprotection step of SPPS. Furthermore, different resins allow for different functional groups at the C-terminus. The oxymethyl phenylacetamidomethyl (PAM) resin results in the conventional C-terminal carboxylic acid. On the other hand, the paramethylbenzhydrylamine (pMBHA) resin yields a C-terminal amide, which is useful in mimicking the interior of a protein.

Along with the development of Fmoc SPPS, different resins have also been created to be removed by TFA. Similar to the Boc strategy, two primary resins are used, based on whether a C-terminal carboxylic acid or amide is desired. The Wang resin was, as of 1996 the most commonly used resin for peptides with C-terminal carboxylic acids. If a C-terminal amide is desired, the Rink amide resin is used.

PROTECTING GROUPS

Amino acids have reactive α-carboxylic acid and α-amine groups that allow for their linking into polymers, but that also complicate the aim coupling specific pairs of amino acids, in precise order. In addition, many amino acids have reactive side chain functional groups, which can also react in a variety of ways, including with free α-carboxylic and α-amino groups during peptide synthesis (given the very reactive reagents present), “side-reactions” that would negatively influence yield and purity. Chemical groups have been developed to facilitate the synthesis of peptides with precise amino acid sequences, with minimal side reactions, groups that block or “protect” all functional groups present in amino acids except that pair whose coupling is desired. These protecting groups, while very many in practice, can be described in three groups: α-carboxylic acid (C-terminal) protecting groups, α-amino (N-terminal) protecting groups, and side chain protecting groups.

C-terminal Protecting Groups

Protecting groups of the carboxylic acid are the least used given the direction and methods applied in solid-supported peptide synthesis, but are covered first because to the brevity of the topic. These protecting groups are mostly used in liquid-phase synthesis, and there is some redundancy in the chemistry with respect to groups used to protect carboxylates in side chains (see below).

N-terminal Protecting Groups

Protected amino acids being added in a given step of peptide synthesis are added in excess to ensure maximal yields during each synthesis step. Without N-terminal protection of the added amino acid, its self-coupling (polymerization) would compete with the desired peptide synthesis, resulting in low yield of even failure of the desired peptide synthesis. N-terminal protection requires an additional step of removing the protecting group in each peptide synthesis cycle, a deprotection step, prior to the next coupling step.

As of this date, two protecting groups, *tert*-butyloxycarbonyl (*t*-Boc) and 9H-fluoren-9-ylmethoxycarbonyl (Fmoc) are most commonly used to protect the α-amine group of the "incoming" (newly added) amino acid in a solid-phase peptide synthesis cycle.

t-Boc and Fmoc protecting groups

Tert-butyloxycarbonyl (t-Boc) protection

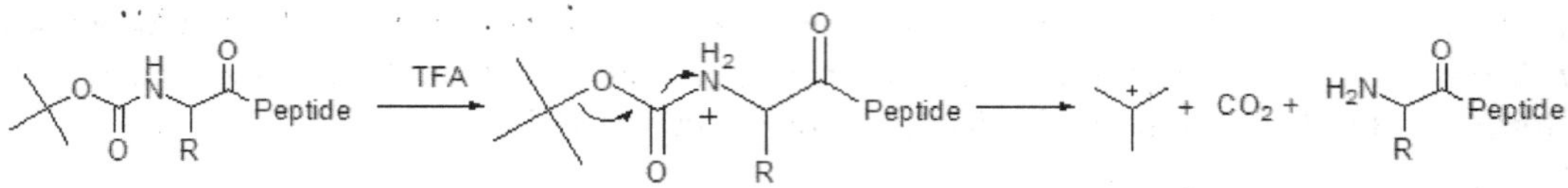

Boc cleavage.

The original method for the synthesis of proteins relied on *tert*-butyloxycarbonyl (or more simply "Boc") to temporarily protect the α-amino group. In this method, the Boc group is covalently bound to the amino group to suppress its nucleophilicity. The C-terminal amino acid is covalently linked to the resin through a linker. Next, the Boc group is removed with acid, such as trifluoroacetic acid (TFA). This forms a positively charged amino group (in the presence of excess TFA; note image on the right illustrates neutral amino group), which is neutralized (via in-situ or non-in-situ methods) and coupled to the incoming activated amino acid. Reactions are driven to completion by the use of excess (2- to 4-fold) activated amino acid. After each deprotection and coupling step, a wash with dimethylformamide (DMF) is performed to remove excess reagents, allowing (by year 2000 for high yields (~99%) during each cycle.

t-Boc protecting strategies retain usefulness in reducing peptide aggregation during synthesis. *t*-Boc groups can be added to amino acids with *t*-Boc anhydride and a suitable base. Some researchers prefer Boc SPPS for complex syntheses. In addition, when synthesizing nonnatural peptide analogs, which are base-sensitive (such as depsipeptides), the *t*-Boc protecting group is necessary, because Fmoc SPPS uses a base to deprotect the α-amino group.

Permanent side-chain protecting groups are typically benzyl or benzyl-based groups. Final removal of the peptide from the linkage occurs simultaneously with side-chain deprotection with anhydrous hydrogen fluoride via hydrolytic cleavage. The final product is a fluoride salt which is relatively easy to solubilize. Importantly, scavengers such as cresol are added to the HF in order to prevent reactive *t*-butyl cations from generating undesired products. In fact, the use of harsh hydrogen fluoride may degrade some peptides, which was the premise for the development of a milder, base-labile method of SPPS—namely, the Fmoc method.

9H-fluoren-9-Ylmethoxycarbonyl (fmoc) Protection

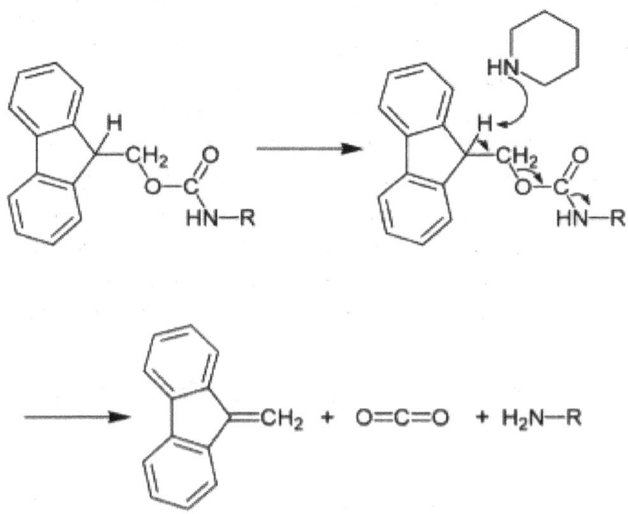

Cleavage of the amine-protecting Fmoc group. Treatment of the Fmoc-protected amino acid, abbreviated by "R," with piperidine, resulting in proton abstraction from the methine group of the fluorenyl ring system, which results in cleavage of that ring system as dibenzofulvene, and release of the amino acid as a carbamate, which decomposes to carbon dioxide (CO_2) and the amino acid moiety with free amine group. The gentleness of the deprotection is believed to lie in the acidity of the fluorenyl proton, resulting from stabilization of the resulting aromatic anion. Absent a scavenger (e.g., such as a thiol), the dibenzofulvene product can react with nucleophiles such as the piperidine (which is in large excess), or even the released amine. See Jones (1992).

The capacity for anhydrous hydrogen fluoride to degrade proteins during the final cleavage conditions led to a new α-amino protecting group based on 9-fluorenylmethyloxycarbonyl (Fmoc). The Fmoc method allows for a milder deprotection scheme. This method utilizes a base, usually piperidine (20–50%) in DMF in order to remove the Fmoc group to expose the α-amino group for reaction with an incoming activated amino acid. Unlike the acid used to deprotect the α-amino group in Boc methods, Fmoc SPPS uses a base, and thus the exposed amine is neutral. Therefore, no neutralization of the peptide-resin is required, but the lack of electrostatic repulsions between the peptides can lead to increased aggregation. Because the liberated fluorenyl group is a chromophore, deprotection by Fmoc can be monitored by UV absorbance of the runoff, a strategy which is employed in automated synthesizers.

The advantage of Fmoc is that it is cleaved under very mild basic conditions (e.g. piperidine), but stable under acidic conditions, although this has not always held true in certain synthetic sequences. This allows mild acid-labile protecting groups that are stable under basic conditions, such as Boc and benzyl groups, to be used on the side-chains of amino acid residues of the target peptide. This orthogonal protecting group strategy is common in organic synthesis. Fmoc is preferred over BOC due to ease of cleavage; however it is less atom-economical, as the fluorenyl group is much larger than the tert-butyl group. Accordingly, prices for Fmoc amino acids were high until the large-scale piloting of one of the first synthesized peptide drugs, enfuvirtide, began in the 1990s, when market demand adjusted the relative prices of the two sets of amino acids.

Semipermanent side chain protecting groups are t-butyl-based, and final cleavage of the protein from the resin and removal of permanent protecting groups is performed with TFA in the presence of scavengers. Water and triisopropylsilane (TIPS) present in a 1:1 ratio are often used as scavengers. Thus, the Fmoc method is orthogonal in two directions: deprotection of any α-amino group, deprotection of side groups and final cleavage from the resin occur by independent mechanisms. The resulting final product is a TFA salt, which is more difficult to solubilize than the fluoride salts generated in Boc SPPS. This method is thus milder than the Boc method because the deprotection/cleavage-from-resin steps occur with different conditions rather than with different reaction rates.

Comparison of *t*-Boc and Fmoc solid-phase Peptide Synthesis

Both the Fmoc and Boc methods offer advantages and disadvantages. The selection of one technique over another is thus made on a case-by-case basis.

	Boc	**Fmoc**
Requires special equipment	Yes	No
Cost of reagents	Lower	Higher
Solubility of peptides	Higher	Lower
Purity of hydrophobic peptides	High	May be lower
Problems with aggregation	Less frequently	More frequently
Synthesis time	~20 min/amino acid	~20–60 min/amino acid
Cleavage from resin	HF	TFA
Safety	Potentially dangerous	Relatively safe
Orthogonal	No	Yes

Boc SPPS uses special equipment to handle the final cleavage and deprotection step, which requires anhydrous hydrogen fluoride. Because the final cleavage of the peptide with Fmoc SPPS uses TFA, this special equipment is not necessary. The solubility of peptides generated by Boc SPPS is generally higher than those generated with the Fmoc method, because fluoride salts are higher in solubility than TFA salts. Next, problems with aggregation are generally more of an issue with Fmoc SPPS, primarily because the removal of a Boc group with TFA yields a positively charged α-amino group, whereas the removal of an Fmoc group yields a neutral α-amino group. The steric hindrance of the positively charged α-amino group limits the formation of secondary structure on the resin.Finally, the Fmoc method is considered orthogonal, since α-amino group deprotection is with base, while final cleavage from the resin is with acid. The Boc method utilizes acid for both deprotection and cleavage from the resin. Hence, both methods possess advantages and disadvantages for their application in specific situations, and several factors must be considered to decide between the methods.

Other Protecting Groups

Benzyloxy-Carbonyl

The (Z) group is another carbamate-type amine protecting group, first used by Max Bergmann in the synthesis of oligopeptides. It is removed under harsh conditions using HBr in acetic acid, or milder conditions of catalytic hydrogenation. While it has been used periodically for α-amine protection in peptide synthesis, of this date, it is almost exclusively used for side chain protection.

Alloc and Miscellaneous Groups

The allyloxycarbonyl (alloc) protecting group is sometimes used to protect an amino group (or carboxylic acid or alcohol group) when an orthogonal deprotection scheme is required. It is also sometimes used when conducting on-resin cyclic peptide formation, where the peptide is linked to the resin by a side-chain functional group. The Alloc group can be removed using tetrakis(triphenylphosphine)palladium(0).

For special applications like synthetic steps involving protein microarrays, protecting groups sometimes termed "lithographic" are used, which are amenable to photochemistry at a particular wavelength of light, and so which can be removed during lithographic types of operations.

Side Chain Protecting Groups

Amino acid side chains represent a broad range of functional groups and are sites of nonspecific reactivity during peptide synthesis. Because of this, many different protecting groups are required that are usually based on the benzyl (Bzl) or tert-butyl (tBu) group. The specific protecting groups used during the synthesis of a given peptide vary depending on the peptide sequence and the type of N-terminal protection used (see next paragraph). Side chain protecting groups are known as permanent or semipermanent protecting groups, because they can withstand the multiple cycles of chemical treatment during synthesis and are only removed during treatment with strong acids after peptide synthesis is completed.

Because N-terminal deprotection occurs repeatedly during peptide synthesis, protecting schemes are established such that different types of side chain protecting groups (e.g., Bzl, tBu, etc.) are matched to either Boc or Fmoc, respectively, for ultimate deprotection that is optimized. Because multiple protecting groups are normally used during peptide synthesis of peptides greater in length than oligomers, care must be taken such that all side chain protecting groups are compatible, so that when deprotection of individual protecting groups is required (e.g., to selectively modify the side chain of one amino acid of a synthetic peptide), the one deprotection step does not affect other side chains. Protecting schemes are therefore developed in each particular case of a peptide synthesis to assign protecting groups to each amino acid residue.

ACTIVATING GROUPS

For coupling the peptides the carboxyl group is usually activated. This is important for speeding up the reaction. There are two main types of activating groups: carbodiimides and triazolols. However the use of pentafluorophenyl esters (FDPP,PFPOH) and BOP-Cl are useful for cyclising peptides.

Carbodiimides

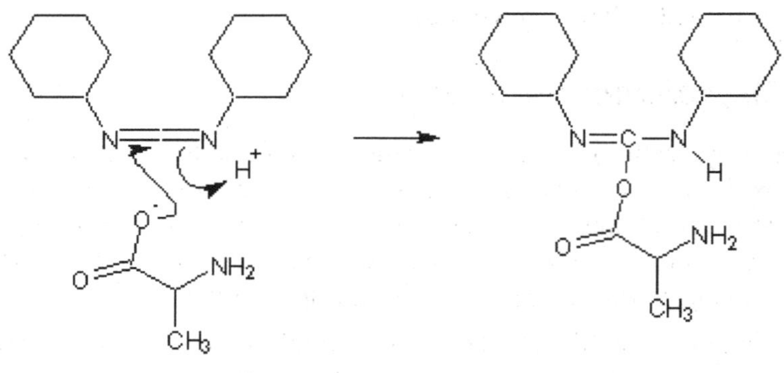

Alanine attaching to DCC.

These activating agents were first developed. Most common are dicyclohexylcarbodiimide (DCC) and diisopropylcarbodiimide (DIC). Reaction with a carboxylic acid yields a highly reactive O-acylisourea. During artificial protein synthesis (such as Fmoc solid-state synthesizers), the C-terminus is often used as the attachment site on which the amino acid monomers are added. To enhance the electrophilicity of carboxylate group, the negatively charged oxygen must first be "activated" into a better leaving group. DCC is used for this purpose. The negatively charged oxygen will act as a nucleophile, attacking the central carbon in DCC. DCC is temporarily attached to the former carboxylate group (which is now an ester group), making nucleophilic attack by an amino group (on the attaching amino acid) to the former C-terminus (carbonyl group) more efficient. The problem with carbodiimides is that they are too reactive and that they can therefore cause racemization of the amino acid.

Triazoles

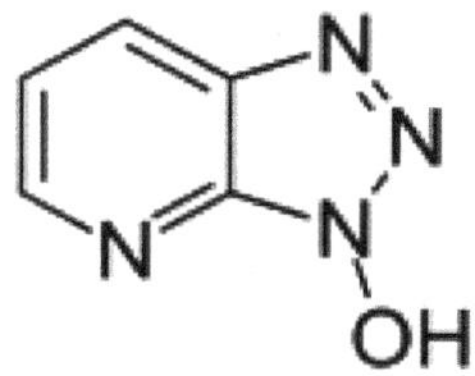

HOBt

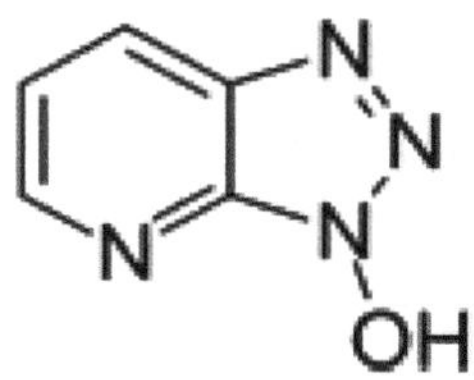

HOAt

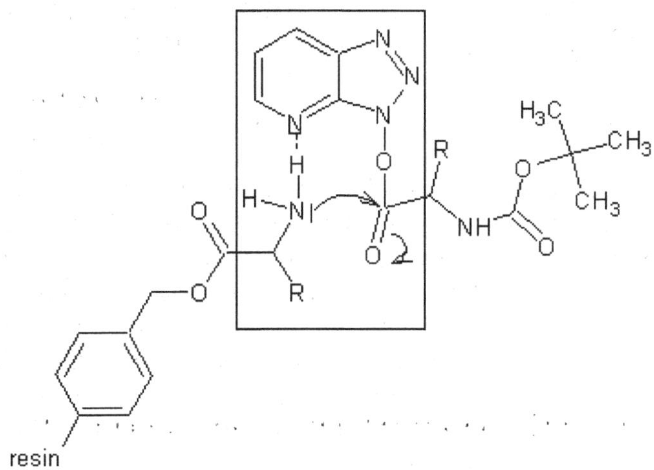

Neighbouring group effect of HOAt.

To solve the problem of racemization, triazoles were introduced. The most important ones are 1-hydroxy-benzotriazole (HOBt) and 1-hydroxy-7-aza-benzotriazole (HOAt), though others have also been developed. These substances can react with the O-acylurea to form an active ester which is less reactive and less in danger of racemization. HOAt is especially favourable because of a neighbouring group effect. As of this date, HOBt has been removed from many chemical vendor catalogues; although almost always found as a hydrate, HOBt may be explosive when allowed to fully dehydrate and shipment by air or sea is heavily restricted. Alternatives to HOBt and HOAt have been introduced. One of the most promising and inexpensive is ethyl 2-cyano-2-(hydroxyimino)acetate (trade name Oxyma Pure), which is not explosive and has a reactivity of that in between HOBt and HOAt.

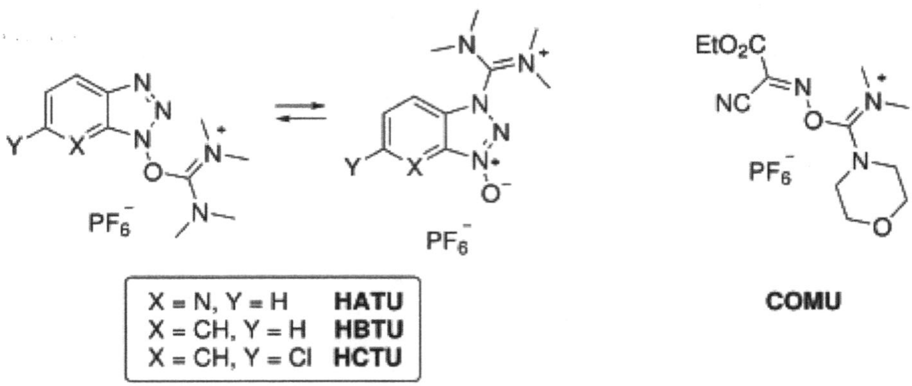

Uronium-based peptide coupling reagents.

Newer developments omit the carbodiimides totally: the active ester is introduced as a uronium or phosphonium salt of a non-nucleophilic anion (tetrafluoroborate or hexafluorophosphate): HBTU, HATU, HCTU, TBTU, PyBOP. Two uronium types of the coupling additive of Oxyma Pure is also available as COMU or TOTU reagent.

REGIOSELECTIVE DISULFIDE BOND FORMATION

The formation of multiple native disulfides remains one of the primary challenges of native peptide synthesis by solid-phase methods. Random chain combination typically results in several products with nonnative disulfide bonds. Stepwise formation of disulfide bonds is typically the preferred method, and performed with thiol protecting groups. Different thiol protecting groups provide multiple dimensions of orthogonal protection. These orthogonally protected cysteines are incorporated during the solid-phase synthesis of the peptide. Successive removal of these groups, to allow for selective exposure of free thiol groups, leads to disulfide formation in a stepwise manner. The order of removal of the groups must be considered so that only one group is removed at a time. Using this method, Kiso and coworkers reported the first total synthesis of insulin in 1993.

Thiol protecting groups used in peptide synthesis requiring later regioselective disulfide bond formation must possess multiple characteristics. First, they must be reversible with conditions that do not affect the unprotected side chains. Second, the protecting group must be able to withstand the conditions of solid-phase synthesis. Third, the removal of the thiol protecting group must be such that it leaves intact other thiol protecting groups, if orthogonal protection is desired. That is, the removal of PG A should not affect PG B. Some of the thiol protecting groups commonly used include the acetamidomethyl (Acm), tert-butyl (But), 3-nitro-2-pyridine sulfenyl (NPYS), 2-pyridine-sulfenyl (Pyr), and triphenylmethyl (Trt) groups. Importantly, the NPYS group can replace the Acm PG to yield an activated thiol.

Important to the discussion of disulfide bond formation is the order in which disulfides are formed. The synthesis insulin by Kiso and coworkers is illustrative of the logic and methods for regioselective disulfide bond formation.In this work, the A-chain of insulin was prepared with following protecting groups in place on its cysteines: CysA6(But), CysA7(Acm), and CysA11(But), leaving CysA20 unprotected. Synthesis of the B-chain was performed with the following protecting groups in place CysB7(Acm) and CysB19(Pyr). The first disulfide bond, CysA20–CysB19, was formed by mixing the two chains in 8 M urea, pH 8 (RT) for 50 min, while the second disulfide bond, CysA7–CysB7, was formed by treatment with iodine in aqueous acetic acid to remove the Acm groups. The third disulfide, the intramolecular CysA6–CysA11, was formed after the removal of the But groups by methyltrichlorosilane with diphenyl sulfoxide in TFA. Importantly, formation of the first disulfide in 8 M urea, pH 8 does not affect the other protecting groups, namely Acm and But groups. Likewise, formation of the second disulfide bond with iodine in aqueous acetic acid does not affect the But groups. From a logical standpoint, the order in which the thiol groups are exposed to form disulfides should be of little consequence, since the other cysteines are protected; however, it is observed, practically, that the order in which disulfides are formed can have a significant effect on yields.

SYNTHESIZING LONG PEPTIDES

Stepwise elongation, in which the amino acids are connected step-by-step in turn, is ideal for small peptides containing between 2 and 100 amino acid residues. Another method is fragment condensation, in which peptide fragments are coupled. Although the former can elongate the peptide chain without racemization, the yield drops if only it is used in the creation of long or highly polar peptides. Fragment condensation is better than stepwise elongation for synthesizing sophisticated long peptides, but its use must be restricted in order to protect against racemization. Fragment condensation is also undesirable since the coupled fragment must be in gross excess, which may be a limitation depending on the length of the fragment.

A new development for producing longer peptide chains is chemical ligation: unprotected peptide chains react chemoselectively in aqueous solution. A first kinetically controlled product rearranges to form the amide bond. The most common form of native chemical ligation uses a peptide thioester that reacts with a terminal cysteine residue. Other methods applicable for covalently linking polypeptides in aqueous solution include the use of split inteins, spontaneous isopeptide bond formation and sortase ligation.

In order to optimize synthesis of long peptides, Zealand Pharma (located in Denmark in Medicon Valley) invented a method for converting a difficult peptide sequence into an easy peptide sequence. The new technology, called SIP-technology, uses "structure-inducing probes" (SIP) to facilitate the synthesis of long peptides. The SIP-technology is a small pre-sequence peptide sequence (e.g. Lysine (Lysn); Glutamic Acid (Glun);

(LysGlu)n) that is incorporated at the C-terminus of subsequent resin bound peptide to induce an alpha-helix-like structure in the peptide. The SIP technology constrains the parent peptide into a more ordered conformation using intramolecular hydrogen bonds. This allows the peptide structure to stabilize, and the utilized hydrogen bonds reduce the likelihood of aggregation and degradation by enzymes. In this way, the SIP technology is designed to optimize peptide synthesis, increase biological half-life, improve peptide stability and inhibit enzymatic degradation without altering pharmacological activity or profile of action.

MICROWAVE-ASSISTED PEPTIDE SYNTHESIS

Although microwave irradiation has been around since the late 1940s, it was not until 1986 that microwave energy was used in organic chemistry. During the end of the 1980s and 1990s, microwave energy was an obvious source for completing chemical reactions in minutes that would otherwise take several hours to days. Through several technical improvements at the end of the 1990s and beginning of the 2000s, microwave synthesizers have been designed to provide both low and high energy pockets of microwave energy so that the temperature of the reaction mixture could be controlled. The microwave energy used in peptide synthesis is of a single frequency providing maximum penetration depth of the sample which is in contrast to conventional kitchen microwaves.

In peptide synthesis, microwave irradiation has been used to complete long peptide sequences with high degrees of yield and low degrees of racemization. Microwave irradiation during the coupling of amino acids to a growing polypeptide chain is catalyzed not only by the increase in temperature but also by the alternating electric field of the microwave. This is because the polar *N*-terminal amine group and peptide backbone continuously try to align with the alternating electric field, thus helping prevent aggregation and increasing access to the solid phase reaction matrix. This increases yields of the final peptide products. There is however no clear evidence that microwave is better than simple heating and some peptide laboratories regard microwave just as a convenient method for rapid heating of the peptidyl resin. Heating to above 50–55 degrees Celsius also prevents aggregation and accelerates the coupling.

Despite the main advantages of microwave irradiation of peptide synthesis, the main disadvantage is the racemization which may occur with the coupling of cysteine and histidine. A typical coupling reaction with these amino acids are performed at lower temperatures than the other 18 natural amino acids. A number of peptides do not survive microwave synthesis or heating in general. One of the more serious side effects is dehydration (loss of water) which for certain peptides can be almost quantitative like pancreatic polypeptide (PP). This side effect is also seen by simple heating without the use of microwave.

CYCLIC PEPTIDES

On Resin Cyclization

Peptides can be cyclized on a solid support. A variety of cylization reagents can be used such as HBTU/HOBt/DIEA, PyBop/DIEA, PyClock/DIEA. Head-to-tail peptides can be made on the solid support. The deprotection of the C-terminus at some suitable point allows on-resin cyclization by amide bond formation with the deprotected N-terminus. Once cyclization has taken place, the peptide is cleaved from resin by acidolysis and purified. The strategy for the solid-phase synthesis of cyclic peptides in not limited to attachment through Asp, Glu or Lys side chains. Cysteine has a very reactive sulfhydryl group on its side chain. A disulfide bridge is created when a sulfur atom from one Cysteine forms a single covalent bond with another sulfur atom from a second cysteine in a different part of the protein. These bridges help to stabilize proteins, especially those secreted from cells. Some researchers use modified cysteines using S-acetomidomethyl (Acm) to block the formation of the disulfide bond but preserve the cysteine and the protein's original primary structure.

Off-resin Cyclization

Off-resin cyclization is a solid-phase synthesis of key intermediates, followed by the key cyclization in solution phase, the final deprotection of any masked side chains is also carried out in solution phase. This has the disadvantages that the efficiencies of solid-phase synthesis are lost in the solution phase steps, that purification from by-products, reagents and unconverted material is required, and that undesired oligomers can be formed if macrocycle formation is involved.

FLUORENYLMETHYLOXYCARBONYL CHLORIDE

Fluorenylmethyloxycarbonyl chloride (FMOC-Cl) is a chloroformate ester. It is used to introduce FMOC group as the FMOC carbamate.

Preparation

This compound may be prepared by reacting 9-fluorenylmethanol with phosgene:

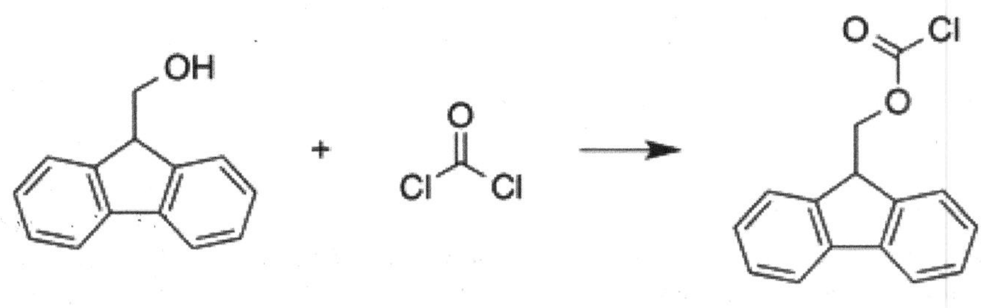

Reactions

The FMOC carbamate is often used as a protecting group for amines. The FMOC group can be introduced by reacting the amine with FMOC-Cl, e.g.:

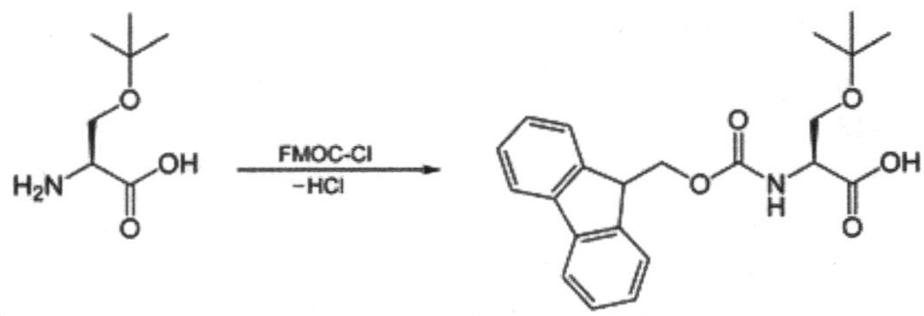

The other common method for introducing the FMOC group is through 9-fluorenylmethyl succinimidyl carbonate (FMOC-OSu), which may itself be obtained by the reaction of FMOC-Cl with the dicyclohexylammonium salt of *N*-hydroxysuccinimide.

It may be cleaved by bases, typically a solution of piperidine:

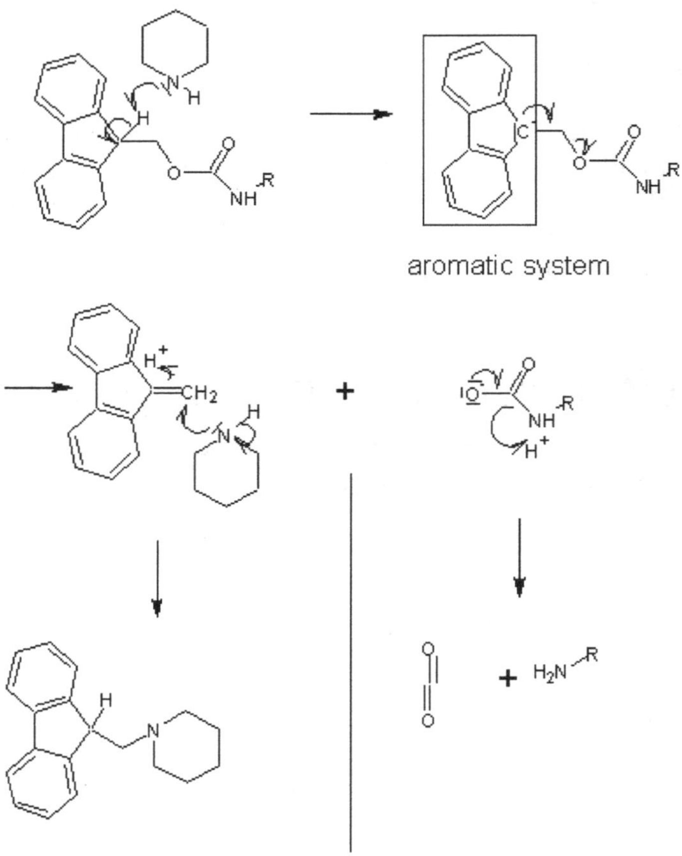

FMOC protection has found significant use in solid phase peptide synthesis because its removal with piperidine solution does not disturb the acid labile linker between the peptide and the resin.

Because the fluorenyl group is highly fluorescent, certain UV-inactive compounds may be reacted to give the FMOC derivatives, suitable for analysis by reversed phase HPLC. Analytical uses of FMOC-Cl that do not use chromatography may be limited by the requirement that excess FMOC-Cl be removed before an analysis of fluorescence.

Amine Protection - Fluorenylmethyloxycarbonyl (Fmoc)

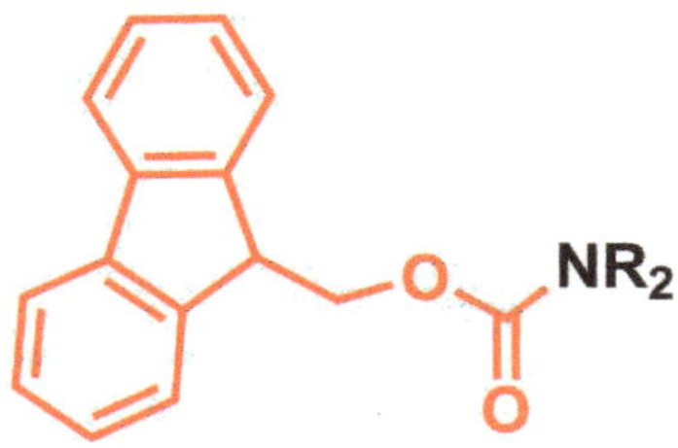

Fluorenylmethyloxycarbonyl (**Fmoc**) group is used as a protecting group for amines in organic synthesis.

Common Amine Protection Methods

- Fluorenylmethyloxycarbonyl chloride or 9-fluorenylmethyloxycarbonyl azide (itself made by reacting FMOC-Cl with sodium azide), sodium bicarbonate and aqueous dioxane

Common Amine Deprotection Methods

- 20% Piperidine in dimethylformamide (Fmoc Group has an approximate half life of 6 seconds in this solution)
- Tetra-n-butylammonium fluoride in the presence of dimethylformamide

AMINO ACID SYNTHESIS

Amino acid synthesis is the set of biochemical processes (metabolic pathways) by which the various amino acids are produced from other compounds. The substrates for these processes are various compounds in the organism's diet or growth media. Not all organisms are able to synthesise all amino acids. Humans are excellent example of this, since humans can only synthesise 11 of the 20 standard amino acids (aka non-essential amino acid), and in time of accelerated growth, histidine, can be considered an essential amino acid.

A fundamental problem for biological systems is to obtain nitrogen in an easily usable form. This problem is solved by certain microorganisms capable of reducing the inert N≡N molecule (nitrogen gas) to two molecules of ammonia in one of the most remarkable reactions in biochemistry. Ammonia is the source of nitrogen for all the amino acids. The carbon backbones come from the glycolytic pathway, the pentose phosphate pathway, or the citric acid cycle.

In amino acid production, one encounters an important problem in biosynthesis, namely stereochemical control. Because all amino acids except glycine are chiral, biosynthetic pathways must generate the correct isomer with high fidelity. In each of the 19 pathways for the generation of chiral amino acids, the stereochemistry at the α-carbon atom is established by a transamination reaction that involves pyridoxal phosphate. Almost all the transaminases that catalyze these reactions descend from a common ancestor, illustrating once again that effective solutions to biochemical problems are retained throughout evolution.

Biosynthetic pathways are often highly regulated such that building-blocks are synthesized only when supplies are low. Very often, a high concentration of the final product of a pathway inhibits the activity of enzymes that function early in the pathway. Often present are allosteric enzymes capable of sensing and responding to concentrations of regulatory species. These enzymes are similar in functional properties to aspartate transcarbamoylase and its regulators. Feedback and allosteric mechanisms ensure that all twenty amino acids are maintained in sufficient amounts for protein synthesis and other processes.

Nitrogen Fixation

Microorganisms use ATP and reduced ferredoxin, a powerful reductant, to reduce atmospheric nitrogen (N_2) to ammonia (NH_3). An iron-molybdenum cluster in nitrogenase deftly catalyzes the fixation of N_2, a very inert molecule. Higher organisms consume the fixed nitrogen to synthesize amino acids, nucleotides, and other nitrogen-containing biomolecules. The major points of entry of ammonia into metabolism are glutamine or glutamate.

Transamination

Most amino acids are synthesized from α-ketoacids, and later transaminated from another amino acid, usually glutamate. The enzyme involved in this reaction is an aminotransferase.

α-ketoacid + glutamate ⇄ amino acid + α-ketoglutarate

Glutamate itself is formed by amination of α-ketoglutarate:

α-ketoglutarate + NH^{+4} ⇄ glutamate

From Intermediates of the Citric Acid Cycle and Other Pathways

Of the basic set of twenty amino acids (not counting selenocysteine), there are eight that human beings cannot synthesize. In addition, the amino acids arginine, cysteine, glycine, glutamine, histidine, proline, serine, and tyrosine are considered **conditionally essential**, meaning they are not normally required in the diet, but must be supplied exogenously to specific populations that do not synthesize it in adequate amounts. For example, enough arginine is synthesized by the urea cycle to meet the needs of an adult but perhaps not those of a growing child. Amino acids that must be obtained from the diet are called essential amino acids. Nonessential amino acids are produced in the body. The pathways for the synthesis of nonessential amino acids are quite simple. Glutamate dehydrogenase catalyzes the reductive amination of α-ketoglutarate to glutamate. A transamination reaction takes place in the synthesis of most amino acids. At this step, the chirality of the amino acid is established. Alanine and aspartate are synthesized by the transamination of pyruvate and oxaloacetate, respectively. Glutamine is synthesized from NH4+ and glutamate, and asparagine is synthesized similarly. Proline and arginine are derived from glutamate. Serine, formed from 3-phosphoglycerate, is the precursor of glycine and cysteine. Tyrosine is synthesized by the hydroxylation of phenylalanine, an essential amino acid. The pathways for the biosynthesis of essential amino acids are much more complex than those for the nonessential ones. Activated Tetrahydrofolate, a carrier of one-carbon units, plays an important role in the metabolism of amino acids and nucleotides. This coenzyme carries one-carbon units at three oxidation states, which are interconvertible: most reduced—methyl; intermediate—methylene; and most oxidized—formyl, formimino, and methenyl. The major donor of activated methyl groups is S-adenosylmethionine, which is synthesized by the transfer of an adenosyl group from ATP to the sulfur atom of methionine. S-Adenosylhomocysteine is formed when the activated methyl group is transferred to an acceptor. It is hydrolyzed to adenosine and homocysteine, the latter of which is then methylated to methionine to complete the activated methyl cycle.

Cortisol inhibits protein synthesis.

REGULATION BY FEEDBACK INHIBITION

Most of the pathways of amino acid biosynthesis are regulated by feedback inhibition, in which the committed step is allosterically inhibited by the final product. Branched pathways require extensive interaction among the branches that includes both negative and positive regulation. The regulation of glutamine synthetase from *E. coli* is a striking demonstration of cumulative feedback inhibition and of control by a cascade of reversible covalent modifications.

α-Ketoglutarates

The α-ketoglutarate family of amino acid synthesis (synthesis of glutamate, glutamine, proline and arginine) begins with α-ketoglutarate, an intermediate in the Citric Acid Cycle. The concentration of α-ketoglutarate is dependent on the activity and metabolism within the cell along with the regulation of enzymatic activity. In *E. coli* citrate synthase, the enzyme involved in the condensation reaction initiating the Citric Acid Cycle is strongly inhibited by α-ketoglutarate feedback inhibition and can be inhibited by DPNH as well high concentrations of ATP. This is one of the initial regulations of the α-ketoglutarate family of amino acid synthesis.

The regulation of the synthesis of glutamate from α-ketoglutarate is subject to regulatory control of the Citric Acid Cycle as well as mass action dependent on the concentrations of reactants involved due to the reversible nature of the transamination and glutamate dehydrogenase reactions.

The conversion of glutamate to glutamine is regulated by glutamine synthetase (GS) and is a highly significant step in nitrogen metabolism. This enzyme is regulated by at least four different mechanisms: 1. Repression and depression due to nitrogen levels; 2. Activation and inactivation due to enzymatic forms (taut and relaxed); 3. Cumulative feedback inhibition through end product metabolites; and 4. Alterations of the enzyme due to adenylation and deadenylation. In rich nitrogenous media or growth conditions containing high quantities of ammonia there is a low level of GS, whereas in limiting quantities of ammonia the specific activity of the enzyme is 20-fold higher. The confirmation of the enzyme plays a role in regulation depending on if GS is in the taut or relaxed form. The taut form of GS is fully active but, the removal of manganese converts the enzyme to the relaxed state. The specific conformational state occurs based on the binding of specific divalent cations and is also related to adenylation. The feedback inhibition of GS is due to a cumulative feedback due to several metabolites including L-tryptophan, L-histidine, AMP, CTP, glucosamine-6-phosphate and carbamyl phosphate, alanine, and glycine. An excess of any one product does not individually inhibit the enzyme but a combination or accumulation of all the end products have a strong inhibitory effect on the synthesis of glutamine. Glutamine synthase activity is also inhibited via adenylation. The adenylation activity is catalyzed by the bifunctional adenylyltransferase/adenylyl removal (AT/AR) enzyme. Glutamine and a regulatory protein called PII act together to stimulate adenylation.

The regulation of proline biosynthesis can be dependent on the initial controlling step through negative feedback inhibition. In *E. coli*, proline allosterically inhibits Glutamate 5-kinase which catalyzes the reaction from L-glutamate to an unstable intermediate L-γ-Glutamyl phosphate.

Arginine synthesis also utilizes negative feedback as well as repression through a repressor encoded by the gene *argR*. The gene product of *argR*, ArgR an aporepressor, and arginine as a corepressor affect the operon of arginine biosynthesis. The degree of repression is determined by the concentrations of the repressor protein and corepressor level.

Erythrose 4-Phosphate and Phosphoenolpyruvate

Phenylalanine, tyrosine, and tryptophan are known as the aromatic amino acids. The synthesis of all three share a common beginning to their pathways; the formation of chorismate from phosphoenolpyruvate (PEP) and erythrose 4- phosphate (E4P). The first step, condensation of 3-deoxy-D-arabino-heptulosonic acid 7-phosphate (DAHP) from PEP/E4P, uses three isoenzymes AroF, AroG, and AroH. Each one of these has its synthesis regulated from tyrosine, phenylalanine, and tryptophan, respectively. These isoenzymes all have the ability to help regulate synthesis of DAHP by the method of feedback inhibition. This acts in the cell by monitoring the concentrations of each of the three aromatic amino acids. When there is too much of any one of them, that one will allosterically control the DAHP synthetase by "turning it off". With the first step of the common pathway shut off, synthesis of the three amino acids can not proceed. The rest of the enzymes in the common pathway (conversion of DAHP to chorismate) appear to be synthesized constitutively, except for shikimate kinase which can be inhibited by shikimate through linear mixed-type inhibition. If too much shikimate has been produced then it can bind to shikimate kinase to stop further production.

Besides the regulations described above, each amino acids terminal pathway can be regulated. These terminal pathways progress from chorismate to the final end product, either tyrosine, phenylalanine, or tryptophan. Each one of these pathways is regulated in a similar fashion to the common pathway; with feedback inhibition on the first committed step of the pathway.

Tyrosine and phenylalanine share the same initial step in their terminal pathways, chorismate converted to prephenate which is converted to an amino acid-specific intermediate. This process is mediated by a phenylalanine (PheA) or tyrosine (TyrA) specific chorismate mutase-prephenate dehydrogenase. The reason for the amino acid-specific enzymes is because PheA uses a simple dehydrogenase to convert prephenate to phenylpyruvate, while TyrA uses a NAD-dependent dehydrogenase to make 4-hydroxylphenylpyruvate. Both PheA and TyrA are feedback inhibited by their respective amino acids. Tyrosine can also be inhibited at the transcriptional level by the TyrR repressor. TyrR binds to the TyrR boxes on the operon near the promoter of the gene that it wants to repress.

In the terminal-tryptophan synthesis pathway, the initial step converts chorismate to anthranilate using anthranilate synthase. This enzyme requires either ammonia or glutamine as the amino group donor. Anthranilate synthase is regulated by the gene products of trpE and trpD. trpE encodes the first subunit, which binds to chorismate and moves the amino group from the donor to chorismate. trpD encodes the second subunit, which is simply used to bind glutamine and use it as the amino group donor so that the amine group can transfer to the chorismate. Anthranilate synthase is also regulated by feedback inhibition. The finished product of tryptophan, once produced in great enough quantities, is able to act as the co-repressor to the TrpR repressor which represses expression of the trp operon.

Oxaloacetate and Aspartate

The oxaloacetate/aspartate family of amino acids is composed of lysine, asparagine, methionine, threonine, and isoleucine. Aspartate can be converted into lysine, asparagine, methionine and threonine. Threonine also gives rise to isoleucine. All of these amino acids contain different mechanisms for their regulation, some being more complex than others. All the enzymes in this biosynthetic pathway are subject to regulation via feedback inhibition and/or repression at the genetic level. As is typical in highly branched metabolic pathways, there is additional regulation at each branch point of the pathway. This type of regulatory scheme allows control over the total flux of the aspartate pathway in addition to the total flux of individual amino acids. The aspartate pathway uses L-aspartic acid as the precursor for the biosynthesis of one fourth of the building block amino acids. Without this pathway, protein synthesis would not be possible.

Aspartate

The enzyme aspartokinase, which catalyzes the phosphorylation of aspartate and initiates its conversion into other amino acids, can be broken up into 3 isozymes, AK-I, II and III. AK-I is feed-back inhibited by threonine, while AK-II and III are inhibited by lysine. As a sidenote, AK-III catalyzes the phosphorylation of aspartic acid that is the commitment step in this biosynthetic pathway. The higher the concentration of threonine or lysine, the more aspartate kinase becomes downregulated.

Lysine

Lysine is synthesized from aspartate via the diaminopimelate (DAP) pathway. The initial two stages of the DAP pathway are catalyzed by aspartokinase and aspartate semialdehyde dehydrogenase and play a key role in the biosynthesis of lysine, threonine and methionine. There are two bifunctional aspartokinase/homoserine dehydrogenases, ThrA and MetL, in addition to a monofunctional aspartokinase, LysC. Transcription of aspartokinase genes is regulated by concentrations of the subsequently produced amino acids, lysine, threonine and methionine. The higher these amino acids concentrations, the less the gene is transcribed. ThrA and LysC are also feed-back inhibited by threonine and lysine. Finally, DAP decarboxylase LysA mediates the last step of the lysine synthesis and is common for all studied bacterial species. The formation of aspartate kinase (AK), which catalyzes the phosphorylation of aspartate and initiates its conversion into other amino acids, is also inhibited by both lysine and threonine, which prevents the formation of the amino acids derived from aspartate. Additionally, high lysine concentrations inhibit the activity of dihydrodipicolinate synthase (DHPS). So, in addition to inhibiting the first enzyme of the aspartate families biosynthetic pathway, lysine also inhibits the activity of the first enzyme after the branch point, i.e. the enzyme that is specific for lysine's own synthesis.

Asparagine

There are two different asparagine synthetases found in bacterial species. These two synthetases, which are both referred to as the AsnC protein, are coded for by two genes: AsnA and AsnB. AsnC is autogenously regulated, which is where the product of a structural gene regulates the expression of the operon in which the genes reside. The stimulating effect of AsnC on AsnA transcription is downregulated by asparagine. However, the autoregulation of AsnC is not affected by asparagine.

Methionine

Methionine synthesis is under tight regulation. The repressor protein MetJ, in cooperation with the corepressor protein S-adenosyl-methionine, mediates the repression of methionine's biosynthetic pathway. Recently, a new regulator focus, MetR has been identified. The MetR protein is required for MetE and MetH gene expression and functions as a transactivator of transcription for these genes. MetR transcriptional activity is regulated by homocystein, which is the metabolic precursor of methionine. It is also known that vitamin B12 can repress MetE gene expression, which is mediated by the MetH holoenzyme.

Threonine

The biosynthesis of threonine is regulated via allosteric regulation of its precursor, homoserine, by structurally altering the enzyme homoserine dehydrogenase. This reaction occurs at a key branch point in the pathway, with the substrate homoserine serving as the precursor for the biosynthesis of lysine, methionine, threonin and isoleucine. High levels of threonine result in low levels of homoserine synthesis. The synthesis of aspartate kinase (AK), which catalyzes the phosphorylation of aspartate and initiates its conversion into other amino acids, is feed-back inhibited by lysine, isoleucine, and threonine, which prevents the synthesis of the amino acids derived from aspartate. So, in addition to inhibiting the first enzyme of the aspartate families biosynthetic pathway, threonine also inhibits the activity of the first enzyme after the branch point, i.e. the enzyme that is specific for threonine's own synthesis.

Isoleucine

The enzymes threonine deaminase, dihydroxy acid dehydrase and transaminase are controlled by end-product regulation. I.e. the presence of isoleucine will downregulate the formation of all three enzymes, resulting in the downregulation of threonine biosynthesis. High concentrations of isoleucine also result in the downregulation of aspartate's conversion into the aspartyl-phosphate intermediate, hence halting further biosynthesis of lysine, methionine, threonine, and isoleucine.

Ribose 5-phosphates

The synthesis of histidine in *E. coli* is a complex pathway involving 10 reactions and 10 enzymes. Synthesis begins with 5-phosphoribosyl-pyrophosphate (PRPP) and finishes with histidine and occurs through the reactions of the following enzymes:

HisG-> HisE/HisI-> HisA-> HisH-> HisF-> HisB-> HisC-> HisB-> HisD (HisE/I and HisB are both bifunctional enzymes)

All of the enzymes are coded for on the his operon. This operon has a distinct block of the leader sequence, called block 1:

Met-Thr-Arg-Val-Gln-Phe-Lys-His-His-His-His-His-His-His-Pro-Asp

This leader sequence is very important for the regulation of histidine in "E. coli". The *his* operon operates under a system of coordinated regulation where all the gene products will be repressed or depressed equally. The main factor in the repression or derepression of histidine synthesis is the concentration of histidine charged tRNAs. The regulation of histidine is actually quite simple considering the complexity of its biosynthesis pathway and, it closely resembles regulation of tryptophan. In this system the full leader sequence has 4 blocks of complementary strands that can form hairpin loops structures. Block one, shown above, is the key to regulation. When histidine charged tRNA levels are low in the cell the ribosome will stall at the string of His residues in block 1. This stalling of the ribosome will allow complementary strands 2 and 3 to form a hairpin loop. The loop formed by strands 2 and 3 forms an anti-terminator and translation of the *his* genes will continue and histidine will be produced. However when histidine charged tRNA levels are high the ribosome will not stall at block 1, this will not allow strands 2 and 3 to form a hairpin. Instead strands 3 and 4 will form a hairpin loop further downstream of the ribosome. The hairpin loop formed by strands 3 and 4 is a terminating loop, when the ribosome comes into contact with the loop, it will be "knocked off" the transcript. When the ribosome is removed the *his* genes will not be translated and histidine will not be produced by the cell.

3-Phosphoglycerates

Serine

Serine is the first amino acid in this family to be produced; it is then modified to produce both glycine and cysteine (and many other biologically important molecules). Serine is formed from 3-phosphoglycerate in the following pathway:

3-phosphoglycerate-> phosphohydroxyl-pyruvate-> phosphoserine-> serine

The conversion from 3-phosphoglycerate to phosphohydroxyl-pyruvate is achieved by the enzyme phosphoglycerate dehydrogenase. This enzyme is the key regulatory step in this pathway. Phosphoglycerate dehydrogenase is regulated by the concentration of serine in the cell. At high concentrations this enzyme will be inactive and serine will not be produced. At low concentrations of serine the enzyme will be fully active and serine will be produced by the bacterium. Since serine is the first amino acid produced in this family both glycine and cysteine will be regulated by the available concentration of serine in the cell.

Glycine

Glycine is synthesized from serine using the enzyme serine hydromethyltransferase (SHMT), which is coded by the gene *glyA*. The enzyme effectively removes a hydroxyl group from serine and replaces it with a methyl group to yield glycine. This reaction is the only way *E. coli* can produce glycine. The regulation of *glyA* is very complex and is known to incorporate serine, glycine, methionine, purines, thymine, and folates however, the full mechanism has yet to be elucidated. The methionine gene product MetR and the methionine intermediate homocysteine are known to positively regulate glyA. Homocysteine is a coactivator of *glyA* and must act in concert with MetR. On the other hand, PurR, a protein which plays a role in purine synthesis and S-adeno-sylmethionine are known to down regulate *glyA*. PurR binds directly to the control region of *glyA* and effectively turns the gene off so that glycine will not be produced by the bacterium.

Cysteine

Cysteine is a very important molecule for a bacterium's survival. This amino acid harbors a sulfur atom and can actively participate in disulfide bond formation. The genes required for the synthesis of cysteine are coded for on the *cys* regulon. The integration of sulfur into the molecule is positively regulated by CysB. CysB is the main focus of cysteine regulation. Effective inducers of this regulon are N-acetyl-serine (NAS) and very small amounts of reduced sulfur. CysB functions by binding to DNA half sites on the *cys* regulon. These half sites differ in quantity and arrangement depending on the promoter of interest. There is however one half site that is conserved. It lies just upstream of the -35 site of the promoter. There are also multiple accessory sites depending on the promoter. In the absence of the inducer, NAS, CysB will bind the DNA and cover many of the accessory half sites. Without the accessory half sites the regulon cannot be transcribed and cysteine will not be produced. It is believed that the presence of NAS causes CysB to undergo a conformational change. This conformational change allows CysB to bind properly to all the half sites and causes the recruitment of the RNA polymerase. The RNA polymerase will then transcribe the *cys* regulon and cysteine will be produced.

Further regulation is required for this pathway, however. CysB can actually down regulate its own transcription by binding to its own DNA sequence and blocking the RNA polymerase. In this case NAS will act to disallow the binding of CysB to its own DNA sequence. OAS is a precursor of NAS, cysteine itself can inhibit CysE which functions to create OAS. Without the necessary OAS, NAS will not be produced and cysteine will not be produced. There are two other negative regulators of cysteine. These are the molecules sulfide and thiosulfate, they act to bind to CysB and they compete with NAS for the binding of CysB.

Pyruvates

Pyruvate is the end result of glycolysis and can feed into both the TCA cycle and fermentation processes. Reactions beginning with either one or two molecules of pyruvate cause the synthesis of alanine, valine, and leucine. Feedback inhibition of final products is the main method of inhibition, and, in *E. coli*, the *ilvEDA* operon also plays a part in this regulation.

Alanine

Alanine is produced by the transamination of one molecule of pyruvate using two alternate steps: 1) conversion of glutamate to α-ketoglutarate using a glutamate-alanine transaminase, and 2) conversion of valine to α-ketoisovalerate via Transaminase C.

Not much is known about the regulation of alanine synthesis. The only definite method is the bacterium's ability to repress Transaminase C activity by either valine or leucine (see ***ilvEDA* operon**). Other than that, alanine biosynthesis does not seem to be regulated.

Valine

Valine is produced by a four-enzyme pathway. It begins with the reaction of two pyruvate molecules catalyzed by Acetohydroxy acid synthase yielding α-acetolactate. Step two is the NADPH+ + H+ - dependent reduction of α-acetolactate and migration of the methane groups to produce α, β-dihydroxyisovalerate. This is catalyzed by Acetohydroxy isomeroreductase. The third reaction is the dehydration reaction of α, β-dihydroxyisovalerate catalyzed by Dihydroxy acid dehydrase resulting in α-ketoisovalerate. Finally, a transamination catalyzed either by an alanine-valine transaminase or a glutamate-valine transaminase results in valine.

Valine performs feedback inhibition to inhibit the Acetohydroxy acid synthase used to combine the first two pyruvate molecules.

Leucine

The leucine synthesis pathway diverges from the valine pathway beginning with α-ketoisovalerate. α-Isopropylmalate synthase reacts with this substrate and Acetyl CoA to produce α-isopropylmalate. An isomerase then isomerizes α-isopropylmalate to β-isopropylmalate. The third step is the NAD+-dependent oxidation of β-isopropylmalate via the action of a dehydrogenase to yield α-ketoisocaproate. Finally is the transamination via the action of a glutamate-leucine transaminase to result in leucine.

Leucine, like valine, regulates the first step of its pathway by inhibiting the action of the α-Isopropylmalate synthase.Because leucine is synthesized by a diversion from the valine synthetic pathway, the feedback inhibition of valine on its pathway also can inhibit the synthesis of leucine.

ilvEDA operon

The genes that encode both the Dihydroxy acid dehydrase used in the creation of α-ketoisovalerate and Transaminase E, as well as other enzymes are encoded on the ilvEDA operon. This operon is bound and inactivated by valine, leucine, and isoleucine. (Isoleucine is not a direct derivative of pyruvate, but is produced by the use of many of the same enzymes used to produce valine and, indirectly, leucine.) When one of these amino acids is limited, the gene furthest from the amino-acid binding site of this operon can be transcribed. When a second of these amino acids is limited, the next-closest gene to the binding site can be transcribed, and so forth.

Amino acids as precursors to other biomolecules

Amino acids are precursors of a variety of biomolecules. Glutathione (γ-Glu-Cys-Gly) serves as a sulfhydryl buffer and detoxifying agent. Glutathione peroxidase, a selenoenzyme, catalyzes the reduction of hydrogen peroxide and organic peroxides by glutathione. Nitric oxide, a short-lived messenger, is formed from arginine. Porphyrins are synthesized from glycine and succinyl CoA, which condense to give δ-aminolevulinate. Two molecules of this intermediate become linked to form porphobilinogen. Four molecules of porphobilinogen combine to form a linear tetrapyrrole, which cyclizes to uroporphyrinogen III. Oxidation and side-chain modifications lead to the synthesis of protoporphyrin IX, which acquires an iron atom to form heme.

REFERENCES

1. Akaji, K.; Fujino, K.; Tatsumi, T.; Kiso, Y. (1993). "Total synthesis of human insulin by regioselective disulfide formation using the silyl chloride-sulfoxide method". Journal of the American Chemical Society. 115 (24): 11384–11392. doi:10.1021/ja00077a043.
2. Albericio, F. (2000). Solid-Phase Synthesis: A Practical Guide (1 ed.). Boca Raton: CRC Press. p. 848. ISBN 0824703596.
3. Aranko AS, Wlodawer A, Iwaï H (2014). "Nature's recipe for splitting inteins". Prot Eng Des Sel. 27: 263–71. doi:10.1093/protein/gzu028. PMC 4133565. PMID 25096198.
4. Bergmann, Max & Zervas, Leonidas (1932). "Über ein allgemeines Verfahren der Peptid-Synthese". Berichte der deutschen chemischen Gesellschaft. 65 (7): 1192–1201. doi:10.1002/cber.19320650722.
5. Feinberg, R. S.; Merrifield, R. B. (1974). "Zinc chloride-catalyzed chloromethylation of resins for solid phase peptide synthesis". Tetrahedron. 30 (17): 3209–3212. doi:10.1016/S0040-4020(01)97575-1.
6. Haridas V, Sadanandan S, Dheepthi NU (2014). "Sortase-based bio-organic strategies for macromolecular synthesis". Chembiochem. 15: 1857–67. doi:10.1002/cbic.201402013. PMID 25111709.
7. Hermkens, P. H. H.; Ottenheijm, H. C. J.; Rees, D. C. (1997). "Solid-phase organic reactions II: A review of the literature Nov 95 – Nov 96". Tetrahedron. 53 (16): 5643–5678. doi:10.1016/S0040-4020(97)00279-2.
8. Jones, J. (1992). Amino Acid and Peptide Synthesis. Oxford, UK: Oxford University Press
9. K. C. Nicolaou; Natarajan, Swaminathan; Li, Hui; Jain, Nareshkumar F.; Hughes, Robert; Solomon, Michael E.; Ramanjulu, Joshi M.; Boddy, Christopher N. C.; Takayanagi, Masaru (1998). "Total Synthesis of Vancomycin Aglycon – Part 1: Synthesis of Amino Acids 4–7 and Construction of the AB-COD Ring Skeleton". Angew. Chem. Int. Ed. 37 (19): 2708–2714. doi:10.1002/(SICI)1521-3773(19981016)37:19<2708::AID-ANIE2708>3.0.CO;2-E.
10. Kapusta, D. R.; Thorkildsen, C; Kenigs, VA; Meier, E; Vinge, MM; Quist, C; Petersen, JS (2005). "Pharmacodynamic Characterization of ZP120 (Ac-RYYRWKKKKKKK-NH2), a Novel, Functionally Selective Nociceptin/Orphanin FQ Peptide Receptor Partial Agonist with Sodium-Potassium-Sparing Aquaretic Activity". Journal of Pharmacology and Experimental Therapeutics. 314 (2): 652–60. doi:10.1124/jpet.105.083436. PMID 15855355.
11. L. A. Carpino (1993). "1-Hydroxy-7-azabenzotriazole. An efficient peptide coupling additive". J. Am. Chem. Soc. 115 (10): 4397–4398. doi:10.1021/ja00063a082.

12. Matsueda, G. R. a. S., J.M. (1981). "A p-methylbenzylhydrlamine resin for improved solid-phase synthesis of peptide amides". Peptides. 2 (1): 45–50. doi:10.1016/S0196-9781(81)80010-1. PMID 7243625.

13. Mitchell, A. R. K., S.B.H.; Engelhard, M.; Merrifield, R.B. (1978). "A new synthetic route to tert-butyloxycarbonylaminoacyl-4-(oxymethyl) phenylacetamidomethyl-resin, an improved support for solid-phase peptide synthesis". J. Org. Chem. 43 (13): 2845–2852. doi:10.1021/jo00408a022.

14. Nilsson BL, Soellner MB, Raines RT (2005). "Chemical Synthesis of Proteins". Annu. Rev. Biophys. Biomol. Struct. 34: 91–118. doi:10.1146/annurev.biophys.34.040204.144700. PMC 2845543. PMID 15869385.

15. Ottl, J.; Battistuta, R.; Pieper, M.; Tschesche, H.; Bode, W.; Kuhn, K.; Moroder, L. (1996). "Design and synthesis of heterotrimeric collagen peptides with a built-in cystine-knot. Models for collagen catabolism by matrix-metalloproteases". FEBS Lett. 398 (1): 31–36. doi:10.1016/S0014-5793(96)01212-4. PMID 8946948.

16. Palasek, Stacey A.; Cox, Zachary J.; and Collins, Jonathan M. (2007). "Limiting racemization and aspartimide formation in microwave-enhanced Fmoc solid phase peptide synthesis". Journal of Peptide Science. 13 (3): 143–148. doi:10.1002/psc.804. PMID 17121420.

17. Peter Scott (13 October 2009). Linker Strategies in Solid-Phase Organic Synthesis. John Wiley & Sons. pp. 135–137. ISBN 978-0-470-74905-0.

18. R. B. Merrifield (1963). "Solid Phase Peptide Synthesis. I. The Synthesis of a Tetrapeptide". J. Am. Chem. Soc. 85 (14): 2149–2154. doi:10.1021/ja00897a025.

19. R. Baker; J. L. Castro (1989). "The total synthesis of (+)-macbecin I". Chem. Commun. (6): 378–381. doi:10.1039/C39890000378.

20. Reddington SC, Howarth M (2015). "Secrets of a covalent interaction for biomaterials and biotechnology: SpyTag and SpyCatcher". Curr Op Chem Biol. 29: 94–9. doi:10.1016/j.cbpa.2015.10.002. PMID 26517567.

21. Rizzi A, Rizzi D, Marzola G, et al. (October 2002). "Pharmacological characterization of the novel nociceptin/orphanin FQ receptor ligand, ZP120: in vitro and in vivo studies in mice". Br. J. Pharmacol. 137 (3): 369–74. doi:10.1038/sj.bjp.0704894. PMC 1573505. PMID 12237257.

22. Schmidt; Joullié, Madeleine M. (1998). "Synthetic studies of 14-membered cyclopeptide alkaloids". Tetrahedron Lett. 39 (40): 7211–7214. doi:10.1016/S0040-4039(98)01589-5.

23. Schnolzer, M. A., P.; Jones, A.; Alewood, D.; Kent, S.B.H. (2007). "In Situ Neutralization in Boc-chemistry Solid Phase Peptide Synthesis". Int. J. Peptide Res. Therap. 13 (1–2): 31–44. doi:10.1007/s10989-006-9059-7.

24. Sieber, P. (1987). "A new acid-labile anchor group for the solid-phase synthesis of C-terminal peptide amides by the Fmoc method". Tetrahedron Lett. 28: 2107–10. doi:10.1016/S0040-4039(00)96055-6.

25. Sieber, P.; Kamber, B.; Hartmann, A.; Jöhl, A.; Riniker, B.; Rittel, W. (1977). "Total synthesis of human insulin. IV. Description of the final steps (author's

transl)". Helvetica Chimica Acta. 60 (1): 27–37. doi:10.1002/hlca.19770600105. PMID 838597.

26. This may be because the formation of the CysA20–CysB19 disulfide may place the thiol group of CysB7 in close proximity with both CysA6 and CysA7, leading to multiple disulfide products

27. Wang, S.-S. (1973). "p-alkoxybenzyl alcohol resin and p-alkoxybenzyloxycarbonylhydrazide resin for solid phase synthesis of protected peptide fragments.". J. Am. Chem. Soc. 95 (4): 1328–33. doi:10.1021/ja00785a052. PMID 4687686.

28. Zhang, J.-W.; Wu, Cui Rong; Liu, Wen; Zhang, Jing Wen (1991). "Disulfide bond formation in peptides by dimethyl sulfoxide. Scope and applications". J. Am. Chem. Soc. 113 (17): 6657–6662. doi:10.1021/ja00017a044.

CHAPTER 8

Essential of Human Nutrition/Amino acids

Chapter Contents

- **Amino Acids**
- **Glucogenic**
- **Ketogenic**
- **Urea**
- **Essential Amino Acid**
- **Complete Proteins in Non-Human Animals**
- **Interchangeability**
- **Effects of Deficiency**
- **Protein (Nutrient)**

Nutrition can be defined as food or nourishment needed to keep an organism growing, healthy and viable. It also refers to the process of providing or receiving food or other life-supporting substances. The study of nutrition covers the types of food needed to keep an organism thriving and the means by which the organism derives nourishment by the digestive process. Every living thing needs proper nutrition to survive. For human needs, nutrition can be as basic as gruel or as complex as a five-star meal.

AMINO ACIDS

Amino acids are the monomers of proteins and are an essential part of human growth, development, and health. There are a total of twenty amino acids, with Asparagine being the first to be discovered in 1806. Amino acids are all composed of a carboxyl group, an amino group, and a hydrogen atom bonded to the same carbon atom-the alpha carbon (Basic Structure, 2003). They differ from one another in their side chains, or the R groups bonded to the alpha carbon. The R groups of the different amino acids can differ in size and structure, as well as electric charge (acidic or basic), which influences the solubility of the amino acids in water (Nelson and Cox, 2013).

There twenty amino acids that are generally found in proteins, and they are: Glycine, Alanine, Valine, Isoleucine, Leucine, Proline, Methionine, Phenylalanine, Tyrosine, Tryptophan, Serine, Cysteine, Threonine, Asparagine, Glutamine, Aspartic acid, Glutamic acid, Histidine, Lysine, and Arginine. Proteins are broken down using hydrolysis reactions in which a water molecule is added to the protein, and this results in individual amino acids being formed. Proteins are synthesized using dehydration reactions (condensation reaction), in which a molecule of water is removed and a peptide bond forms between the amino acids. When two amino acids are joined together, the resulting molecule is called a dipeptide. When three are joined together, the molecule is called a tripeptide (Whitney and Rolfes, 2015). As a chain of many amino acids forms and grows, the chain is called a polypeptide.

The human body needs and uses the different amino acids to make proteins to help the body: 1) Metabolize food, 2) Repair torn or damaged body tissues, 3) Grow, and 4) Perform other important body functions (Amino acids, 2013).

The twenty amino acids are separated into three groups: 1) Essential amino acids, 2) Nonessential amino acids, and 3) Conditional Amino Acids. Essential amino acids are the amino acids that the body cannot synthesize by itself or cannot make in adequate quantities. Instead it must get these amino acids through food obtained in the diet. There are a total of nine essential amino acids. These are: Valine, Isoleucine, Leucine, Threonine, Histidine, Lysine, Phenylalanine, and Tryptophan. The nonessential amino acids are those that the body can synthesize by itself and make in large enough quantities. There are 11 nonessential amino acids and they can be supplied by food in the diet but it is not a requirement. Nonessential amino acids can be produces as long as there is a supply of Nitrogen to produce the amino group of the amino acid and pieces of fat or carbohydrates to form the rest of the structure. Conditional amino acids are amino acids that are usually nonessential but become essential during times of stress, illness, or other special circumstances. One such illness is Phenylketonuria, an inherited disease in which the nonessential amino acid tyrosine becomes essential because the body cannot convert phenylalanine into tyrosine (Whitney and Rolfes, 2015).

There are several foods that one should eat to obtain all essential amino acids. These foods include: beans, chicken, lean meat, fish, nuts and seeds, peanut butter, tofu, lentils and many others (Protein in diet, 2013).

According to the Merriam-Webster dictionary, an amino acid is defined as "an amphoteric organic acid containing the amino group NH2." In simpler terms, amino acids are the building blocks of proteins. All amino acids are composed of an amino group (NH2), an acid group (COOH), a hydrogen atom, a central carbon atom, and a side group. The side group is what distinguishes all the different amino acids from each other.

There are 20 amino acids. Of the 20 amino acids, 11 are nonessential, meaning that they can be produced and synthesized by the body. The remaining nine are essential, which means that they must be obtained from food. The essential amino acids are either not produced at all by the body or are not produced in sufficient amounts. Some amino acids are conditionally essential, meaning that they are normally nonessential, but must be obtained from the diet under special circumstances (Whitney & Rolfes, 2015).

In order to be used in the metabolic pathway, amino acids must undergo deamination. Deamination means they lose their nitrogen-containing amino group, and the only thing left is the carbon skeleton. After this process, they are able to enter the TCA cycle (Whitney & Rolfes, 2015).

The structure of a basic amino acid consists of a central carbon (C), an amino group (NH2), am atom of hydrogen (H), and an acid group (CHO2). Unlike carbohydrates or lipids, amino acids have a varying side group, or R-group, which occupies the remaining bond on the carbon and differentiates the twenty amino acids from each other. This R-group can be rather simple, being a hydrogen atom on the amino acid glycine, or rather complex as it is on the amino acid phenylalanine which has a multi carbon-hydrogen R-group (Whitney/Rolfes, 2013).

Overall there are two types of amino acids regarding human nutrition, essential and nonessential. Nonessential amino acids are ones that the human body can produce by itself using bodily nitrogen and excess carbs and lipids for the remaining carbon, hydrogen, and oxygen pieces of the amino acid. There are eleven nonessential amino acids and they include alanine, arginine, asparagine, aspartic acid, cysteine, glutamic acid, glutamine, glycine, proline, serine, and tyrosine. Most proteins usually contain nonessential amino acids but it is not a requirement for our diet. On the other hand, essential amino acids are required in the human diet as they cannot be synthesized by the body. There are nine essential amino acids including histidine, isoleucine, leucine, lysine, methionine, phenylalanine, threonine, tryptophan, and valine. It is not necessarily vital to eat essential and nonessential proteins at every meal but it is important to balance their intake throughout the day (National Library of Medicine, 2015). There are special cases though in which one must include a nonessential amino acid into their diet for specific reasons, making this amino acid conditionally essential. For people with a disease known as phenylketonuria for example, they must include the nonessential amino acid tyrosine in their diet as tyrosine is made from phenylalanine, and if there is a complication in absorbing phenylalanine, than tyrosine has become conditionally essential for that person (Whitney/ Rolfes, 2013). Initially in a newborn only five of the nonessential amino acids are actually nonessential while the rest are conditionally essential until the body develops enough so that it can create the remaining nonessential amino acids in an efficient manner.

A protein is made by amino acids being linked together during a condensation reaction forming a dipeptide, tripeptide, or a polypeptide. The type of the amino acids and the order in which they sequence is vital as this directly determines the shape and function of the resulting protein (Australian Nutrient Reference Values, 2014). The general sequence of the amino acids in the amino acid chain determines what's called its primary structure. The weak electrical charges with that polypeptide then determine the way one part of the chain interacts with another, creating its secondary structure. The unique side group on each amino acid and the way this side group interacts with the surrounding area determines the polypeptide's tertiary structure. Then, if this polypeptide's function requires that it binds with one or more other polypeptide then that creates a multiple polypeptide structure, or a quaternary structure.

GLUCOGENIC

Amino acids can be classified on the basis of essentiality, polarity, hydrophobia and their fate within the body once consumed. Specifically, amino acids can be separated into two groups according to the futures of their carbon fragments following deamination. If a carbon fragment later becomes a component of glucose, the amino acid to which it belongs is called a glucogenic amino acid (Whitney, 2002, p.183). Specifically, if an amino acid becomes a pyruvate or a pyruvate-associated molecule within the Krebs Cycle, it is considered glucogenic. The production of glucose from glucogenic amino acids through a process called gluconeogenesis (closely associated with the Krebs cycle) occurs in the liver. In the first step of this two-step process, glucogenic amino acids are converted to alpha keto acids. In the second, alpha keto acids become glucose (Schutz, 2011). There are thirteen known glucogenic amino acids in the human body. Some examples of glucogenic amino acids in humans are glycine (used in some pharmaceuticals and metal finishing), serine (important in biosynthesis of purine and pyrimidines), valine, and histidine (precursor for histamine and carnosine synthesis). There are also some amino acids which can be considered both glucogenic and ketogenic, including tyrosine (important role in photosynthesis and signal transduction processes), tryptophan (essential amino acid important in protein biosynthesis) and phenylalanine (used in norepinephrine and epinephrine synthesis).

A glucogenic amino acid is one that can be converted to pyruvate and can provide glucose. Thus, proteins are a good source of glucose when carbohydrates are not available. According to King (2015), "all amino acids except lysine and leucine are at least partly glucogenic." Amino acids that are made into glucose go through a process known as glucogenesis. Glucogenesis occurs mainly in the liver, but also in the kidneys under certain circumstances, such as starvation. When amino acids are not used to make glucose, they are used instead as an energy source for other body cells (Walker & Rolfes, 2015).

KETOGENIC

If the carbon fragment within an amino acid later becomes a component of ketone bodies, fats or sterols rather than glucose as in glucogenic amino acids, the amino acid is ketogenic. However, there are also some ketogenic amino acids that can also be considered glucogenic depending on the fate of their carbon fragment (such as tyrosine, phenylalanine and tryptophan). By definition, ketogenic amino acids are those that can be degraded directly into acetyl CoA which is the precursor to ketone bodies (Noguchi, 2010). Only two known amino acids are exclusively ketogenic in the human body: leucine and lysine. Leucine is used in formation of sterols in muscle and adipose tissue whereas lysine is closely correlated to serotonin function. There are five amino acids known in the human body which are both ketogenic and glucogenic, including isoleucine (involved in gluconeogenesis and Acetyl CoA), phenylalanine, tryptophan, tyrosine and threonine (precursor to glycine). While there are no disease specifically associated with any of the ketogenic amino acids, there is some evidence which indicates that ketogenic essential amino acid replacement diets can decrease the effects of a liver ailment known as hepatic steatosis in mice (Xu, 2013).

Ketogenic amino acids are those that make acetyl CoA, but cannot make glucose. King (2015) states that "lysine and leucine are the only amino acids that are solely ketogenic." Ketogenic amino acids are converted into ketone bodies. Ketone bodies are acidic compounds and are produced by the liver when carbohydrates are not available and fats do not completely break down. Ketone bodies are normally produced and used in small enough amounts that provide the brain cells with fuel. Keto acids are compounds that contain a carbonyl group. When there are too many keto acids in the body, blood pH drops, signaling that the body's chemistry is not in balance. This is known as ketosis. Ketosis also causes a loss of appetite, which may be beneficial when food is unavailable. Once a person is able to eat again, appetite returns and the body leaves ketosis (Whitney & Rolfes, 2015).

UREA

Proteins from diet can be broken down in the liver or in muscle through several processes. These proteins are broken down into amino acids and those amino acids have to further dispose of their amino groups. This process can occur through transamination which is the removal of the amino group. This allows the resulting parts of the amino acid to be utilized for energy. However, these amino acids must be removed from the body because a build up of amino groups could be a potential toxin for body. Even in small amounts amino groups could be fatal towards an individual. Essentially, urea is created when proteins are broken down. The process by which the urea is safely removed from the body is called the Urea Cycle (also referred to as the ornithine cycle. The Urea cycle occurs in the liver and is the main method in removing excess nitrogen from the body. In addition, the Urea cycle works in unity with the citric acid cycle as well. This is accomplished through the exchanging different intermediates and substances needed for each reaction. Urea is typically removed from the body by way of blood. Urea travels through the body from the liver to the kidney. There the kidney filters out the Urea from blood and it excreted out of the body in urine. However, there are tests that can be performed to see the blood urea nitrogen (Chemistry).This test is very important to see if an individual's liver and kidney are healthy and functioning. If a person's blood nitrogen level is higher than normal it could mean that the liver or kidney are not functioning properly (Webmd) . Doctors will be able to tell if individual has disease in her kidney through these tests. Some of these diseases could be either acute kidney failure or end stage renal disease (Webmd). Urea is the main end product of nitrogen metabolism. Urea was first discovered by German chemist Friedrich Wohler in 1828 while he was trying to make ammonium cyanate from from silver cyanide and ammonium chloride. However, by mistake he ended up making Urea. Organically, Urea is a carbamide which a compound that is made up of two amino groups that are linked by a carbonyl (Boswick). Some of the main qualities of Urea is that it does not smell, has no color, and is water soluble. The reason behind urea being soluble is that in water it can get displaced into ammonium ion and bicarbonate ion. The water solubility is why urea is excreted in urine because it is the most efficient process. Urea is also utilized outside the body as well. For example, Urea is one main components of fertilizer. In addition, Urea can be synthetically made to be utilized for plastic, glue, detergent, or even pesticides (Boswick). This illustrates that Urea could have many potential uses not just used in the body.

Ammonia is a highly toxic substance to humans. If not excreted from the body, its accumulation can lead to liver damage, and even death (Ophardt, 2003). Ammonia is cleared from the body via urea. Urea is made in the liver and is excreted in the kidneys as urine. Urea is the main excretion method of unused nitrogen. The more protein a person consumes, the more urea is produced. In order to keep urea in solution, water must also be consumed. Thus, a person who eats a lot of protein must also drink a lot of water. This will help to dilute and excrete urea. If a person on a high-protein diet doesn't drink enough water, they may become dehydrated. Without extra water, the body uses its stored water to get rid of urea. This is why it is common to see water loss in those who eat a lot of protein. Losing water makes high-protein diets seem effective, but actually has no value to losing body fat (Whitney & Rolfes, 2015).

ESSENTIAL AMINO ACID

An **essential amino acid**, or **indispensable amino acid**, is an amino acid that cannot be synthesized *de novo* (from scratch) by the organism, and thus must be supplied in its diet. The nine amino acids humans cannot synthesize are phenylalanine, valine, threonine, tryptophan, methionine, leucine, isoleucine, lysine, and histidine (i.e., F V T W M L I K H).

Six other amino acids are considered **conditionally essential** in the human diet, meaning their synthesis can be limited under special pathophysiological conditions, such as prematurity in the infant or individuals in severe catabolic distress. These six are arginine, cysteine, glycine, glutamine, proline, and tyrosine (i.e. R C G Q P Y). Five amino acids are **dispensable** in humans, meaning they can be synthesized in the body. These five are alanine, aspartic acid, asparagine, glutamic acid and serine (i.e., A D N E S).

Essentiality in Humans

Essential	Non-Essential
Histidine (H)	Alanine (A)
Isoleucine (I)	Arginine* (R)
Leucine (L)	Aspartic acid (D)
Lysine (K)	Cysteine* (C)
Methionine (M)	Glutamic acid (E)
Phenylalanine (F)	Glutamine* (Q)
Threonine (T)	Glycine* (G)
Tryptophan (W)	Proline* (P)
Valine (V)	Serine* (S)
	Tyrosine* (Y)
	Asparagine* (N)
	Selenocysteine (U)
	Pyrrolysine** (O)

(*) Essential only in certain cases.

(**) Pyrrolysine, sometimes considered "the 22nd amino acid", is not used by humans.

Eukaryotes can synthesize some of the amino acids from other substrates. Consequently, only a subset of the amino acids used in protein synthesis are essential nutrients.

Minimum Daily Intake

Estimating the daily requirement for the indispensable amino acids has proven to be difficult; these numbers have undergone considerable revision over the last 20 years. The following table lists the WHO recommended daily amounts currently in use for essential amino acids in **adult humans**, together with their standard one-letter abbreviations. Food sources are identified based on the USDA National Nutrient Database Release.

Amino acid(s)	mg per kg body weight	mg per 70 kg	mg per 100 kg
H Histidine	10	700	1000
I Isoleucine	20	1400	2000
L Leucine	39	2730	3900
K Lysine	30	2100	3000
M Methionine + **C** Cysteine	10.4 + 4.1 (15 total)	1050	1500
F Phenylalanine + **Y** Tyrosine	25 (total)	1750	2500
T Threonine	15	1050	1500
W Tryptophan	4	280	400
V Valine	26	1820	2600

The recommended daily intakes for children aged three years and older is 10% to 20% higher than adult levels and those for infants can be as much as 150% higher in the first year of life. Cysteine (or sulphur-containing amino acids), tyrosine (or aromatic amino acids), and arginine are always required by infants and growing children.

Relative Amino Acid Composition of Protein Sources

Various attempts have been made to express the "quality" or "value" of various kinds of protein. Measures include the biological value, net protein utilization, protein efficiency ratio, protein digestibility-corrected amino acid score and complete proteins concept. These concepts are important in the livestock industry, because the relative lack of one or more of the essential amino acids in animal feeds would have a limiting effect on growth and thus on feed conversion ratio. Thus, various feedstuffs may be fed in combination to increase net protein utilization, or a supplement of an individual amino acid (methionine, lysine, threonine, or tryptophan) can be added to the feed.

Although proteins from plant sources tend to have a relatively lower concentrations of protein by mass in comparison to protein from eggs or milk, they are nevertheless "complete" in that they contain at least trace amounts of all of the amino acids that are essential in human nutrition. Eating various plant foods in combination can provide a protein of higher biological value.Certain native combinations of foods, such as corn and beans, soybeans and rice, or red beans and rice, contain the essential amino acids necessary for humans in adequate amounts.

Additionally, certain types of algae and marine phytoplankton predate the division between animal and plant life on the planet; they have both chlorophyll as do plants, and also all the essential amino acids, as do animal proteins.

Protein Per Calorie

It can be shown that common vegetable sources contain adequate protein, often more protein per Calorie than the standard reference, whole raw egg, while other plant sources, particularly fruits contain less. For example, while 100 g of raw broccoli only provides 28 kcal and 3 g of protein, it has over 100 mg of protein per kcal. An egg contains five times as many calories (143 kcal) but only four times as much protein, roughly 90 mg of protein per kcal. However, a carrot has only 23 mg protein per kcal or twice the minimum recommendation, a banana meets the minimum, and an apple is below recommendation. It is recommended that adult humans obtain 10–35% of their calories as protein, or roughly 11–39 mg of protein per kcal per day (22–78 g for 2000 kcal). The US FDA daily reference value of 50 g protein per 2000 kcal is 25 mg/kcal per day.

Source	protein (g)	Calories (kcal)	protein/Calorie (mg / kcal)	L (mg)	T (mg)	W (mg)	M+C (mg)
Apples, raw (100 g)	0.26	52	**5**	12	6	1	2
Minimum daily reference	22	2000	**11**				
Bananas, raw (100 g)	1	89	**12**	500	28	9	17
Carrot, raw (100 g)	1	41	**23**	101	191	12	103
US FDA daily / WHO (70 kg)	50	2000	**25**	2730	1050	280	1050
Upper daily reference	78	2000	**39**				
Peanut, valencia, raw (100 g)	48	570	**84**	1,627	859	244	630
Soybeans, dry (100 g)	40	451	**88**	2634	1719	575	1172
Egg, whole, raw (100 g)	13	143	**91**	912	556	167	652
Broccoli, raw (100 g)	3	28	**107**	141	91	29	54
Soy Sauce, typical (100 g)	11	60	**175**	729	403	182	576
Beef, grass-fed, lean (100 g)	23	117	**197**				

COMPLETE PROTEINS IN NON-HUMAN ANIMALS

Scientists had known since the early 20th century that rats could not survive on a diet whose only protein source was zein, which comes from maize (corn), but recovered if they were fed casein from cow's milk. This led William Cumming Rose to the discovery of the essential amino acid threonine. Through manipulation of rodent diets, Rose was able to show that ten amino acids are essential for rats: lysine, tryptophan, histidine, phenylalanine, leucine, isoleucine, methionine, valine, and arginine, in addition to threonine. Rose›s later work showed that eight amino acids are essential for adult human beings, with histidine also being essential for infants. Longer term studies established histidine as also essential for adult humans.

INTERCHANGEABILITY

The distinction between essential and non-essential amino acids is somewhat unclear, as some amino acids can be produced from others. The sulfur-containing amino acids, methionine and homocysteine, can be converted into each other but neither can be synthesized *de novo* in humans. Likewise, cysteine can be made from homocysteine but cannot be synthesized on its own. So, for convenience, sulfur-containing amino acids are sometimes considered a single pool of nutritionally equivalent amino acids as are the aromatic amino acid pair, phenylalanine and tyrosine. Likewise arginine, ornithine, and citrulline, which are interconvertible by the urea cycle, are considered a single group.

EFFECTS OF DEFICIENCY

If one of the nonessential amino acids is less than needed for an individual the utilization of other amino acids will be hindered and thus protein synthesis will be less than what it usually is, even in the presence of adequate total nitrogen intake.

Protein deficiency has been shown to affect all of the body's organs and many of its systems, including the brain and brain function of infants and young children; the immune system, thus elevating risk of infection; gut mucosal function and permeability, which affects absorption and vulnerability to systemic disease; and kidney function. The physical signs of protein deficiency include edema, failure to thrive in infants and children, poor musculature, dull skin, and thin and fragile hair. Biochemical changes reflecting protein deficiency include low serum albumin and low serum transferrin.

The amino acids that are essential in the human diet were established in a series of experiments led by William Cumming Rose. The experiments involved elemental diets to healthy male graduate students. These diets consisted of cornstarch, sucrose, butterfat without protein, corn oil, inorganic salts, the known vitamins, a large brown "candy" made of liver extract flavored with peppermint oil (to supply any unknown vitamins), and mixtures of highly purified individual amino acids. The main outcome measure was nitrogen balance. Rose noted that the symptoms of nervousness, exhaustion, and dizziness were encountered to a greater or lesser extent whenever human subjects were deprived of an essential amino acid.

Essential amino acid deficiency should be distinguished from protein-energy malnutrition, which can manifest as marasmus or kwashiorkor. Kwashiorkor was once attributed to pure protein deficiency in individuals who were consuming enough calories ("sugar baby syndrome"). However, this theory has been challenged by the finding that there is no difference in the diets of children developing marasmus as opposed to kwashiorkor. Still, for instance in Dietary Reference Intakes (DRI) maintained by the USDA, lack of one or more of the essential amino acids is described as protein-energy malnutrition.

PROTEIN (NUTRIENT)

Proteins are essential nutrients for the human body. They are one of the building blocks of body tissue, and can also serve as a fuel source. As a fuel, proteins provide as much energy density as carbohydrates: 4 kcal (17 kJ) per gram; in contrast, lipids provide 9 kcal (37 kJ) per gram. The most important aspect and defining characteristic of protein from a nutritional standpoint is its amino acid composition.

Proteins are polymer chains made of amino acids linked together by peptide bonds. During human digestion, proteins are broken down in the stomach to smaller polypeptide chains via hydrochloric acid and protease actions. This is crucial for the synthesis of the essential amino acids that cannot be biosynthesized by the body.

There are nine essential amino acids which humans must obtain from their diet in order to prevent protein-energy malnutrition and resulting death. They are phenylalanine, valine, threonine, tryptophan, methionine, leucine, isoleucine, lysine, and histidine. There are five dispensable amino acids which humans are able to synthesize in the body. These five are alanine, aspartic acid, asparagine, glutamic acid and serine. There are six conditionally essential amino acids whose synthesis can be limited under special pathophysiological conditions, such as prematurity in the infant or individuals in severe catabolic distress. These six are arginine, cysteine, glycine, glutamine, proline and tyrosine.

Humans need the essential amino acids in certain ratios. Some protein sources contain amino acids in a more or less ‹complete› sense. This has given rise to various ranking systems for protein sources, as described in the article.

Dietary sources of protein include both animals and plants: meats, dairy products, fish and eggs as well as grains, legumes and nuts. Vegetarians and vegans can get enough essential amino acids by eating a variety of plant proteins. It is commonly believed that athletes should consume a higher-than-normal protein intake to maintain optimal physical performance.

Protein Functions in Body

Protein is a nutrient needed by the human body for growth and maintenance. Aside from water, proteins are the most abundant kind of molecules in the body. Protein can be found in all cells of the body and is the major structural component of all cells in the body, especially muscle. This also includes body organs, hair and skin. Proteins are also used in membranes, such as glycoproteins. When broken down into amino acids, they are used as precursors to nucleic acid, co-enzymes, hormones, immune response, cellular repair, and other molecules essential for life. Additionally, protein is needed to form blood cells.

Protein Function in Exercise

Proteins are believed to increase performance in terms of athletics. Amino acids, the building blocks of proteins, are used for building muscle tissue and repairing damaged tissues. Protein is only used as anaerobic fuel when carbohydrates are low, or as aerobic fuel when lipid resources are also low.

Sources

Protein can be found in a wide range of food. The best combination of protein sources depends on the region of the world, access, cost, amino acid types and nutrition balance, as well as acquired tastes. Some foods are high in certain amino acids, but their digestibility and the anti-nutritional factors present in these foods make them of limited value in human nutrition. Therefore, one must consider digestibility and secondary nutrition profile such as calories, cholesterol, vitamins and essential mineral density of the protein source. On a worldwide basis, plant protein foods contribute over 60 percent of the per capita supply of protein, on average. In North America, animal-derived foods contribute about 70 percent of protein sources.

Meat, products from milk, eggs, soy, and fish are sources of complete protein.

Whole grains and cereals are another source of proteins. However, these tend to be limiting in the amino acid lysine or threonine, which are available in other vegetarian sources and meats. Examples of food staples and cereal sources of protein, each with a concentration greater than 7 percent, are (in no particular order) buckwheat, oats, rye, millet, maize (corn), rice, wheat, sorghum, amaranth, and quinoa.

Vegetarian sources of proteins include legumes, nuts, seeds and fruits. Legumes, some of which are called pulses in certain parts of the world, have higher concentrations of amino acids and are more complete sources of protein than whole grains and cereals. Examples of vegetarian foods with protein concentrations greater than 7 percent include soybeans, lentils, kidney beans, white beans, mung beans, chickpeas, cowpeas, lima beans, pigeon peas, lupines, wing beans, almonds, Brazil nuts, cashews, pecans, walnuts, cotton seeds, pumpkin seeds, hemp seeds, sesame seeds, and sunflower seeds.

Food staples that are poor sources of protein include roots and tubers such as yams, cassava and sweet potato. Plantains, another major staple, are also a poor source of essential amino acids. Fruits, while rich in other essential nutrients, are another poor source of amino acids. The protein content in roots, tubers and fruits is between 0 and 2 percent. Food staples with low protein content must be complemented with foods with complete, quality protein content for a healthy life, particularly in children for proper development.

A good source of protein is often a combination of various foods, because different foods are rich in different amino acids. A good source of dietary protein meets two requirements:

- The requirement for the nutritionally indispensable amino acids (histidine, isoleucine, leucine, lysine, methionine, phenylalanine, threonine, tryptophan, and valine) under all conditions and for conditionally indispensable amino acids (cystine, tyrosine, taurine, glycine, arginine, glutamine, proline) under specific physiological and pathological conditions

- The requirement for nonspecific nitrogen for the synthesis of the nutritionally dispensable amino acids (aspartic acid, asparagine, glutamic acid, alanine, serine) and other physiologically important nitrogen-containing compounds such as nucleic acids, creatine, and porphyrins.

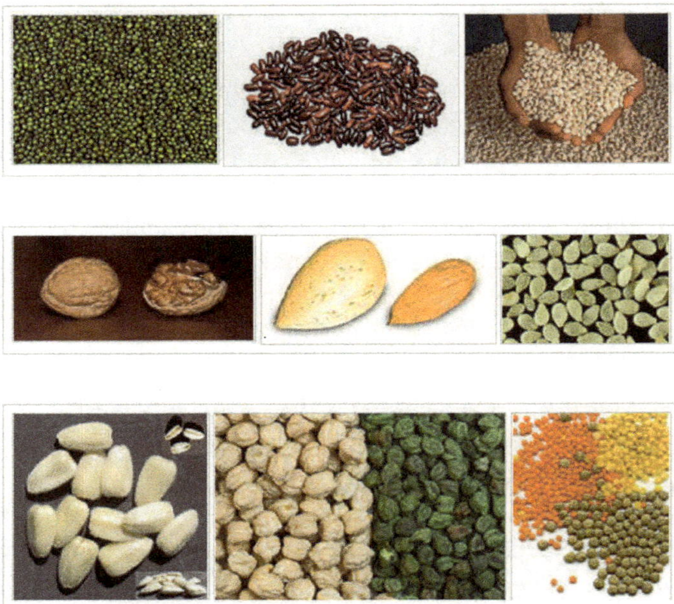

Plant sources of protein.

Healthy people eating a balanced diet rarely need protein supplements. Except for a few amino acids, most are readily available in human diet. The limiting amino acids are lysine, threonine, tryptophan and sulfur-containing amino acids.

The table below presents the most important food groups as protein sources, from a worldwide perspective. It also lists their respective performance as source of the commonly limiting amino acids, in milligrams of limiting amino acid per gram of total protein in the food source. The table reiterates the need for a balanced mix of foods to ensure adequate amino acid source.

Food source	Lysine	Threonine	Tryptophan	Sulfur-containing amino acids
Legumes	64	38	12	25
Cereals and whole grains	31	32	12	37
Nuts and seeds	45	36	**17**	**46**
Fruits	45	29	11	27

Animal	**85**	**44**	12	38
Protein source with highest density of respective amino acid.				
Protein source with lowest density of respective amino acid.				

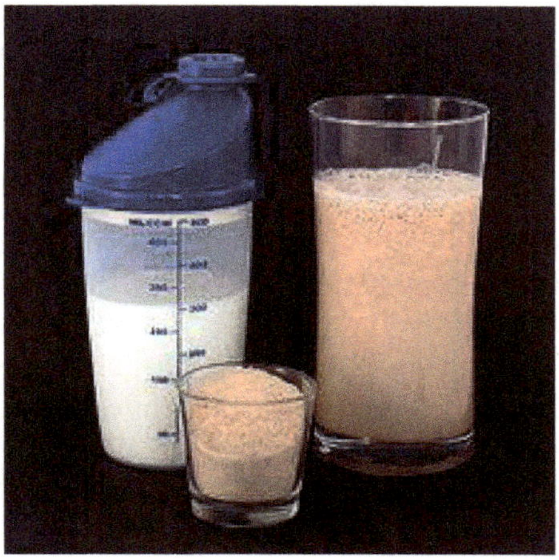

Protein milkshakes, made from protein powder (center) and milk (left), are a common bodybuilding supplement.

Protein powders – such as casein, whey, egg, rice and soy – are processed and manufactured sources of protein. These protein powders may provide an additional source of protein for bodybuilders. The type of protein is important in terms of its influence on protein metabolic response and possibly on the muscle's exercise performance. The different physical and/or chemical properties within the various types of protein may affect the rate of protein digestion. As a result, the amino acid availability and the accumulation of tissue protein is altered because of the various protein metabolic responses.

Protein Quality

The most important aspect and defining characteristic of protein from a nutritional standpoint is its amino acid composition. There are multiple systems which rate proteins by their usefulness to an organism based on their relative percentage of amino acids and, in some systems, the digestibility of the protein source. They include biological value, net protein utilization, and PDCAAS (Protein Digestibility Corrected Amino Acids Score). Also see complete protein, nitrogen balance and protein combining. The PDCAAS was developed by the FDA as an improvement over the Protein efficiency ratio (PER) method. The PDCAAS rating is a fairly recent evaluation method; it was adopted by the US Food and Drug Administration (FDA) and the Food and Agricultural Organization of the United Nations/World Health Organization (FAO/WHO) in 1993 as "the preferred 'best'" method to determine protein quality. These organizations have suggested that other methods for evaluating the quality of protein are inferior.

Digestion

Most proteins are decomposed to single amino acids by digestion in the gastro-intestinal tract.

Digestion typically begins in the stomach when pepsinogen is converted to pepsin by the action of hydrochloric acid, and continued by trypsin and chymotrypsin in the small intestine. Before the absorption in the small intestine, most proteins are already reduced to single amino acid or peptides of several amino acids. Most peptides longer than four amino acids are not absorbed. Absorption into the intestinal absorptive cells is not the end. There, most of the peptides are broken into single amino acids.

Absorption of the amino acids and their derivatives into which dietary protein is degraded is done by the gastrointestinal tract. The absorption rates of individual amino acids are highly dependent on the protein source; for example, the digestibilities of many amino acids in humans, the difference between soy and milk proteins and between individual milk proteins, beta-lactoglobulin and casein. For milk proteins, about 50% of the ingested protein is absorbed between the stomach and the jejunum and 90% is absorbed by the time the digested food reaches the ileum. Biological value (BV) is a measure of the proportion of absorbed protein from a food which becomes incorporated into the proteins of the organism›s body.

Newborn

Newborns of mammals are exceptional in protein digestion and assimilation in that they can absorb intact proteins at the small intestine. This enables passive immunity from milk.

Dietary Requirements

An education campaign launched by the United States Department of Agriculture about 100 years ago, on cottage cheese as a lower-cost protein substitute for meat.

Considerable debate has taken place regarding issues surrounding protein intake requirements. The amount of protein required in a person›s diet is determined in large part by overall energy intake, the body›s need for nitrogen and essential amino acids, body weight and composition, rate of growth in the individual, physical activity level, individual›s energy and carbohydrate intake, as well as the presence of illness or injury. Physical activity and exertion as well as enhanced muscular mass increase the need for protein. Requirements are also greater during childhood for growth and development, during pregnancy or when breast-feeding in order to nourish a baby, or when the body needs to recover from malnutrition or trauma or after an operation.

If not enough energy is taken in through diet, as in the process of starvation, the body will use protein from the muscle mass to meet its energy needs, leading to muscle wasting over time. If the individual does not consume adequate protein in nutrition, then muscle will also waste as more vital cellular processes (e.g. respiration enzymes, blood cells) recycle muscle protein for their own requirements.

According to US & Canadian Dietary Reference Intake guidelines, women aged 19–70 need to consume 46 grams of protein per day, while men aged 19–70 need to consume 56 grams of protein per day to avoid a deficiency. The generally accepted daily protein dietary allowance, measured as intake per kilogram of body weight, is 0.8 g/kg. However, this recommendation is based on structural requirements, but disregards use of protein for energy metabolism. This requirement is for a normal sedentary person.

Active People

Several studies have concluded that active people and athletes may require elevated protein intake (compared to 0.8 g/kg) due to increase in muscle mass and sweat losses, as well as need for body repair and energy source. Suggested amounts vary between 1.6 g/kg and 1.8 g/kg, while a proposed *maximum* daily protein intake would be approximately 25% of energy requirements i.e. approximately 2 to 2.5 g/kg. However, many questions still remain to be resolved.

In addition, some have suggested that athletes using restricted-calorie diets for weight loss should further increase their protein consumption, possibly to 1.8–2.0 g/kg, in order to avoid loss of lean muscle mass.

Aerobic Exercise Protein Needs

Endurance athletes differ from strength-building athletes in that endurance athletes do not build as much muscle mass from training as strength-building athletes do. Research suggests that individuals performing endurance activity require more protein intake than sedentary individuals so that muscles broken down during endurance workouts can be repaired. Although the protein requirement for athletes still remains controversial (for instance see Lamont, Nutrition Research Reviews, pages 142 - 149, 2012), research does show that endurance athletes can benefit from increasing protein intake because the type of exercise endurance athletes participate in still alters the protein metabolism pathway. The overall protein requirement increases because of amino acid oxidation in endurance-trained athletes. Endurance athletes who exercise over a long period (2–5 hours per training session) use protein as a source of 5–10% of their total energy expended. Therefore, a slight increase in protein intake may be beneficial to endurance athletes by replacing the protein lost in energy expenditure and protein lost in repairing muscles. Some scientists suggest that endurance athletes may increase daily protein intake to a maximum of 1.2–1.4 g per kg body weight.

Anaerobic Exercise Protein Needs

Research also indicates that individuals performing strength-training activity require more protein than sedentary individuals. Strength-training athletes may increase their daily protein intake to a maximum of 1.4–1.8 g per kg body weight to enhance muscle protein synthesis, or to make up for the loss of amino acid oxidation during exercise. Many athletes maintain a high-protein diet as part of their training, and so protein deficiency is less likely among this group than among non-athletes. In fact, some athletes who specialize in anaerobic sports (e.g., weightlifting) assume a very high level of protein intake is necessary, and may over-consume. Research indicates that many athletes consume more protein than they need even without the use of protein supplements.

Special Populations

Phenylketonuria

Individuals with phenylketonuria (PKU) must keep their intake of phenylalanine extremely low to prevent a mental disability and other metabolic complications.

Maple Syrup Urine Disease

Maple syrup urine disease is associated with genetic anomalies in the metabolism of branched-chain amino acids (BCAAs). They have high blood levels of BCAAs and must severely restrict their intake of BCAAs in order to prevent mental retardation and death.

Excess Consumption

Research indicates that a high protein diet is carcinogenic, and that the cancer risk is somewhat decreased if it's non-animal protein. When a high dietary protein intake is consumed, there is an increase in urea excretion, which suggests that amino acid oxidation is increased.High levels of protein intake increase the activity of branched-chain ketoacid dehydrogenase.As a result, oxidation is facilitated, and the amino group of the amino acid is excreted to the liver. This process suggests that excess protein consumption results in protein oxidation and that the protein is excreted. The body is unable to store excess protein. Protein is digested into amino acids, which enter the bloodstream. Excess amino acids are converted to other usable molecules by the liver in a process called deamination. Deamination converts nitrogen from the amino acid into ammonia, which is converted by the liver into urea in the urea cycle. Excretion of urea is performed by the kidneys. These organs can normally cope with any extra workload, but, if kidney disease occurs, a decrease in protein will often be prescribed. When there is excess protein intake, amino acids can be converted to glucose or ketones, in addition to being oxidized for fuel. When food protein intake is periodically high or low, the body tries to keep protein levels at an equilibrium by using the "labile protein reserve", which serves as a short-term protein store to be used for emergencies or daily variations in protein intake. However, that reserve is not utilized as longer-term storage for future needs.

Many researchers have also found that excessive intake of protein increases calcium excretion in urine. It has been thought that this occurs to maintain the pH imbalance from the oxidation of sulfur amino acids. Also, it is inconclusive whether bone resorption contributes to bone loss and osteoporosis. However, it is also found that a regular intake of calcium would be able to stabilize this loss.

Another issue arising from over-consumption of protein is a higher risk of kidney stone formation from calcium in the renal circulatory system. It has been found that high animal protein intake in healthy individuals increases the probability of forming kidney stones by 250 percent.

An epidemiological study from 2006 has found no relationship between total protein intake and blood pressure; it did, however, find an inverse relationship between vegetable protein intake and blood pressure.

Saying they eat too much protein, the *2015–2020 Dietary Guidelines for Americans* asked men and teenage boys to increase their consumption of vegetables or other underconsumed foods.

Testing in Foods

The classic assays for protein concentration in food are the Kjeldahl method and the Dumas method. These tests determine the total nitrogen in a sample. The only major component of most food which contains nitrogen is protein (fat, carbohydrate and dietary fibre do not contain nitrogen). If the amount of nitrogen is multiplied by a factor depending on the kinds of protein expected in the food the total protein can be determined. This value is known as the "crude protein" content. On food labels the protein is given by the nitrogen multiplied by 6.25, because the average nitrogen content of proteins is about 16%. The Kjeldahl test is typically used because it is the method the AOAC International has adopted and is therefore used by many food standards agencies around the world, though the Dumas method is also approved by some standards organizations.

Accidental contamination and intentional adulteration of protein meals with non-protein nitrogen sources that inflate crude protein content measurements have been known to occur in the food industry for decades. To ensure food quality, purchasers of protein meals routinely conduct quality control tests designed to detect the most common non-protein nitrogen contaminants, such as urea and ammonium nitrate.

In at least one segment of the food industry, the dairy industry, some countries (at least the U.S., Australia, France and Hungary), have adopted "true protein" measurement, as opposed to crude protein measurement, as the standard for payment and testing: "True protein is a measure of only the proteins in milk, whereas crude protein is a measure of all sources of nitrogen and includes nonprotein nitrogen, such as urea, which has no food value to humans. ... Current milk-testing equipment measures peptide bonds, a direct measure of true protein." Measuring peptide bonds in grains has also been put into practice in several countries including Canada, the UK, Australia, Russia and Argentina where near-infrared reflectance (NIR) technology, a type of infrared spectroscopy is used. The Food and Agriculture Organization of the United Nations (FAO) recommends that only amino acid analysis be used to determine protein in, *inter alia*, foods used as the sole source of nourishment, such as infant formula, but also provides: "When data on amino acids analyses are not available, determination of protein based on total N content by Kjeldahl (AOAC, 2000) or similar method ... is considered acceptable."

The limitations of the Kjeldahl method were at the heart of the Chinese protein export contamination in 2007 and the 2008 China milk scandal in which the industrial chemical melamine was added to the milk or glutens to increase the measured "protein".

Protein Deficiency

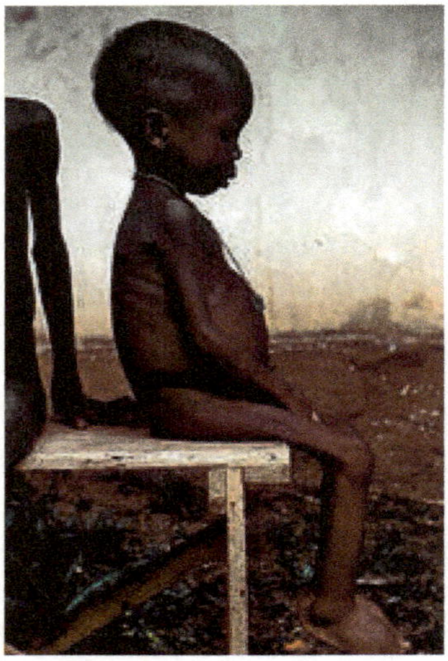

A child in Nigeria during the Biafra War suffering from kwashiorkor – one of the three protein energy malnutrition ailments afflicting over 10 million children in developing countries.

Protein deficiency and malnutrition can lead to variety of ailments including mental retardation and kwashiorkor. Symptoms of kwashiorkor include apathy, diarrhea, inactivity, failure to grow, flaky skin, fatty liver, and edema of the belly and legs. This edema is explained by the action of lipoxygenase on arachidonic acid to form leukotrienes and the normal functioning of proteins in fluid balance and lipoprotein transport.

PEM is fairly common worldwide in both children and adults and accounts for 6 million deaths annually. In the industrialized world, PEM is predominantly seen in hospitals, is associated with disease, or is often found in the elderly.

REFERENCES

1. Dietary reference intakes: macronutrients (PDF). Institute of Medicine. Retrieved 18 May 2008.
2. Food energy – methods of analysis and conversion factors. FAO. Retrieved 9 November 2007.
3. Marasmus and Kwashiorkor. Medscape Reference. May 2009.
4. Protein in diet. United States National Library of Medicine, National Institutes of Health. 2009.
5. Some individuals, especially teen boys and adult men, also need to reduce overall intake of protein foods by decreasing intakes of meats, poultry, and eggs and increasing amounts of vegetables or other underconsumed food groups.

in2015 – 2020 Dietary Guidelines for Americans: Shifts Needed To Align With Healthy Eating Patterns: A Closer Look at Current Intakes and Recommended Shifts: Protein Foods (8 ed.). U.S. Department of Health and Human Services and U.S. Department of Agriculture. December 2015. Retrieved January 9, 2016.

6. Amino acid content of foods and biological data on proteins (FAO nutritional studies number 24). Food and Agriculture Organization. 1985. ISBN 92-5-001102-4.
7. Bilsborough, Shane; Neil Mann (2006).A Review of Issues of Dietary Protein Intake in Humans. International Journal of Sport Nutrition and Exercise Metabolism (16): 129–152. Retrieved 6 December 2012.
8. Born Steve.Fueling for endurance: ten mistakes endurance athletes make and how you can avoid them. UltraCycling Magazine.
9. Boutrif, E., Food Quality and Consumer Protection Group, Food Policy and Nutrition Division, FAO, Rome:Recent Developments in Protein Quality Evaluation Food, Nutrition and Agriculture, Issue 2/3, 1991
10. D. Julian McClements.Analysis of Proteins. University of Massachusetts Amherst. Retrieved 27 April 2007.
11. Dietary Reference Intakes: The Essential Guide to Nutrient Requirements, published by the Institute of Medicine›s Food and Nutrition Board, currently available online at http://fnic.nal.usda.gov/dietary-guidance/dietary-reference-intakes/dri-reports
12. Digestion of Dietary Proteins in the Gastro-Intestinal Tract
13. Elliott P, Stamler J, Dyer AR, Appel L, Dennis B, Kesteloot H, Ueshima H, Okayama A, Chan Q, Garside DB, Zhou B (2006).Association between protein intake and blood pressure: the INTERMAP Study. Archives of Internal Medicine. 166 (1): 79–87. doi:10.1001/archinte.166.1.79. PMID 16401814. Retrieved 21 January 2013.
14. Food and Nutrition Board (2005). A Report of the Panel on Macronutrients, Subcommittees on Upper Reference Levels of Nutrients and Interpretation and Uses of Dietary Reference Intakes, and the Standing Committee on the Scientific Evaluation of Dietary Reference Intakes. Dietary Reference Intakes for Energy, Carbohydrate, Fiber, Fat, Fatty Acids, Cholesterol, Protein, and Amino Acids (Macronutrients). THE NATIONAL ACADEMIES PRESS, Washington, D.C. ISBN 0-309-08537-3.
15. Gaudichon C, Bos C, Morens C, Petzke KJ, Mariotti F, Everwand J, Benamouzig R, Dare S, Tome D, Metges CC (2002).Ileal losses of nitrogen and amino acids in humans and their importance to the assessment of amino acid requirements. Gastroenterology. 123 (1): 50–9. doi:10.1053/gast.2002.34233. PMID 12105833.
16. Genton, Laurence; Melzer, Katarina; Pichard, Claude (2010).Energy and macronutrient requirements for physical fitness in exercising subjects. Clinical Nutrition. 29 (4): 413–423. doi:10.1016/j.clnu.2010.02.002. PMID 20189694.
17. Hermann, Janice R.Protein and the Body (PDF). Oklahoma Cooperative Extension

Service, Division of Agricultural Sciences and Natural Resources • Oklahoma State University: T–3163–1 – T–3163–4.

18. http://www.cell.com/cell-metabolism/fulltext/S1550-4131%2814%2900062-X
19. Jeffery Schwartz; Bryant, Carol A.; DeWalt, Kathleen Musante; Anita Courtney (2003). The cultural feast: an introduction to food and society. Belmont, California: Thomson/Wadsworth. pp. 282, 283. ISBN 0-534-52582-2.
20. Lemon, Peter (2000).Beyond the Zone: Protein Needs of Active Individuals. Journal of the American College of Nutrition. 19 (5): 513–521. doi:10.1080/07315724.2000.10718974. PMID 11023001.
21. Lemon, PW (1995).Do athletes need more dietary protein and amino acids?. Int J Sport Nutr. 5 Suppl: S39–61. PMID 7550257.
22. Mahe S, Marteau P, Huneau JF, Thuillier F, Tome D (1994).Intestinal nitrogen and electrolyte movements following fermented milk ingestion in man. Br J Nutr. 71 (2): 169–80. doi:10.1079/BJN19940124. PMID 8142329.
23. Mahe S, Roos N, Benamouzig R, Davin L, Luengo C, Gagnon L, Gausserges N, Rautureau J, Tome D (1996).Gastrojejunal kinetics and the digestion of [15N]beta-lactoglobulin and casein in humans: the influence of the nature and quantity of the protein. Am J Clin Nutr. 63 (4): 546–52. PMID 8599318.
24. Michael C. Latham (1997).Human nutrition in the developing world. Food and Agriculture Organization of the United Nations.
25. Moore, J.C.; Devries, Jonathan W.; Lipp, Markus; Griffiths, James C.; Abernethy, Darrell R. (17 August 2010).Total Protein Methods and Their Potential Utility to Reduce the Risk of Food Protein Adulteration. Comprehensive Reviews in Food Science and Food Safety. 9 (4): 330–357. doi:10.1111/j.1541-4337.2010.00114.x.
26. Nutrition Working Group of the International Olympic Committee (2003).Nutrition for Athletes. IOC Consensus Conference on Nutrition for Sport. Lausanne.
27. P.M. VanRaden; R.L. Powell.Genetic evaluations for true protein. United States Department of Agriculture. Retrieved 27 April 2007.
28. Phillips, Stuart (2006).Dietary protein for athletes: from requirements to metabolic advantage. Appl. Physiol. Nutr. Metab. 31 (6): 647–654. doi:10.1139/H06-035. PMID 17213878.
29. Phillips, Stuart M.; Loon, Luc J. C. Van (2011-01-01).Dietary protein for athletes: From requirements to optimum adaptation. Journal of Sports Sciences. 29 (supl): S29–S38. doi:10.1080/02640414.2011.619204. ISSN 0264-0414. PMID 22150425.
30. Smith, Jack L.; Gropper, Sareen Annora Stepnick; Groff, James L. (2009). Advanced nutrition and human metabolism. Belmont, CA: Wadsworth Cengage Learning. ISBN 0-495-11657-2.
31. Snyder, Alison (August 2007).Protein Pretense: Cheating the standard protein tests is easy, but industry hesitates on alternatives. Scientific American. Retrieved 9 November 2007.

32. Steinke, Waggle; et al. (1992). New protein foods in human health: nutrition, prevention and therapy. CRC Press. pp. 91–100. ISBN 978-0-8493-6904-9.

33. Stephen Chen (18 September 2008).Melamine – an industry staple. South China Morning Post. pp. Page A2.

34. Tarnopolsky MA, Atkinson SA, MacDougall JD, Chesley A, Phillips S, Schwarcz HP (1992).Evaluation of protein requirements for trained strength athletes. Journal of Applied Physiology. 73 (5): 1986–95. PMID 1474076.

35. Ten Have, Gabriella A.M.; Engelen, Marielle P.K.J.; Luiking, Yvette C.; Deutz, Nicolaas E.P. (2007).Absorption Kinetics of Amino Acids, Peptides, and Intact Proteins. International Journal of Sport Nutrition and Exercise Metabolism. 17: S23–S36.

36. Vernon Young; Peter Pellett (1994).Plant proteins in relation to human protein and amino acid nutrition (PDF). American Journal of Clinical Nutrition. 59: 1203S-l2S.

37. Weise, Elizabeth (24 April 2007).Food tests promise tough task for FDA. USA Today. Retrieved 29 April 2007.

38. WHO, FAO, UNU (2007).Protein and amino acid requirements in human nutrition (PDF). WHO Press. Retrieved 8 July 2008.

39. Young VR (1994).Adult amino acid requirements: the case for a major revision in current recommendations (PDF). J. Nutr. 124 (8 Suppl): 1517S–1523S. PMID 8064412.

CHAPTER 9

Ketogenic Amino Acid

Chapter Contents

Ketogenesis is the release of ketones into the body when fat is broken down for energy. When carbohydrate stores are exhausted, cells turn to fat cells for fuel. These fat cells break down and release energy, and ketones are the by-product of that breakdown. Acetoacetate and acetone are usually also released.

Breaking down fat as a source of energy is generally not a normal energy production process. Carbohydrate stores in cells are replenished when carbohydrates are eaten. Eliminating carbohydrate intake for dietary or health reasons may significantly reduce these stores, leading to ketogenesis. Low carbohydrate diets and diabetic diets are two common forms of ketogenic diet.

INTRODUCTION

A **ketogenic amino acid** is an amino acid that can be degraded directly into acetyl-CoA, which is the precursor of ketone bodies. This is in contrast to the glucogenic amino acids, which are converted into glucose. Ketogenic amino acids are unable to be converted to glucose as both carbon atoms in the ketone body are ultimately degraded to carbon dioxide in the citric acid cycle.

In humans, two amino acids are exclusively ketogenic:

(remembered as all the "L" amino acids)

- Leucine
- Lysine

In humans, five amino acids are both ketogenic and glucogenic:

(remembered by the useful mnemonic "PITTT" or "FITTT", and includes all the "T" amino acids)

- Isoleucine
- Phenylalanine (abbreviated Phe or F, in contrast to Proline which is Pro or P, based on their respective pronunciations)
- Threonine
- Tryptophan
- Tyrosine

In humans, the remaining thirteen amino acids are exclusively glucogenic (i.e. are not ketogenic).

LYSINE

Lysine (abbreviated as **Lys** or **K**), encoded by the codons AAA and AAG, is an α-amino acid that is used in the biosynthesis of proteins. It contains an α-amino group (which is in the protonated $-NH_3^+$ form under biological conditions), an α-carboxylic acid group (which is in the deprotonated $-COO^-$ form under biological conditions), and a side chain lysyl ($(CH_2)_4NH_2$), classifying it as a charged (at physiological pH), aliphatic amino acid. It is essential in humans, meaning the body cannot synthesize it and thus it must be obtained from the diet.

Lysine is a base, as are arginine and histidine. The ε-amino group often participates in hydrogen bonding and as a general base in catalysis. The ε-amino group (NH_3^+) is attached to the fifth carbon from the α-carbon, which is attached to the carboxyl (C=OOH) group.

Common posttranslational modifications include methylation of the ε-amino group, giving methyl-, dimethyl-, and trimethyllysine (the latter occurring in calmodulin); also acetylation, sumoylation, ubiquitination, and hydroxylation - producing the hydroxylysine in collagen and other proteins. *O*-Glycosylation of hydroxylysine residues in the endoplasmic reticulum or Golgi apparatus is used to mark certain proteins for secretion from the cell. In opsins like rhodopsin and the visual opsins (encoded by the genes OPN1SW, OPN1MW, and OPN1LW), retinaldehyde forms a Schiff base with a conserved lysine residue, and interaction of light with the retinylidene group causes signal transduction in color vision (See visual cycle for details). Deficiencies may cause blindness, as well as many other problems due to its ubiquitous presence in proteins.

BIOSYNTHESIS

As an essential amino acid, lysine is not synthesized in animals, hence it must be ingested as lysine or lysine-containing proteins. In plants and most bacteria, it is synthesized from aspartic acid (aspartate):

- L-aspartate is first converted to L-aspartyl-4-phosphate by aspartokinase (or Aspartate kinase). ATP is needed as an energy source for this step.
- β-Aspartate semialdehyde dehydrogenase converts this into β-aspartyl-4-semialdehyde (or β-aspartate-4-semialdehyde). Energy from NADPH is used in this conversion.
- 4-hydroxy-tetrahydrodipicolinate synthase adds a pyruvate group to the β-aspartyl-4-semialdehyde, and a water molecule is removed. This causes cyclization and gives rise to (2S,4S)-4-hydroxy-2,3,4,5-tetrahydrodipicolinate.
- This product is reduced to 2,3,4,5-tetrahydrodipicolinate (or Δ^1-piperidine-2,6-dicarboxylate, in the figure: (S)-2,3,4,5-tetrahydropyridine-2,6-dicarboxylate) by 4-hydroxy-tetrahydrodipicolinate reductase. This reaction consumes an NADPH molecule and releases a second water molecule.
- Tetrahydrodipicolinate N-acetyltransferase opens this ring and gives rise to N-succinyl-L-2-amino-6-oxoheptanedionate (or N-acyl-2-amino-6-oxopimelate). Two water molecules and one acyl-CoA (succinyl-CoA) enzyme are used in this reaction.
- N-succinyl-L-2-amino-6-oxoheptanedionate is converted into N-succinyl-LL-2,6-diaminoheptanedionate (N-acyl-2,6-diaminopimelate). This reaction is catalyzed by the enzyme succinyl diaminopimelate aminotransferase. A glutamic acid molecule is used in this reaction and an oxoacid is produced as a byproduct.
- N-succinyl-LL-2,6-diaminoheptanedionate (N-acyl-2,6-diaminopimelate)is converted into LL-2,6-diaminoheptanedionate (L,L-2,6-diaminopimelate) by succinyl diaminopimelate desuccinylase (acyldiaminopimelate deacylase). A water molecule is consumed in this reaction and a succinate is produced a byproduct.
- LL-2,6-diaminoheptanedionate is converted by diaminopimelate epimerase into meso-2,6-diamino-heptanedionate (meso-2,6-diaminopimelate).
- Finally, meso-2,6-diamino-heptanedionate is converted into L-lysine by diaminopimelate decarboxylase.

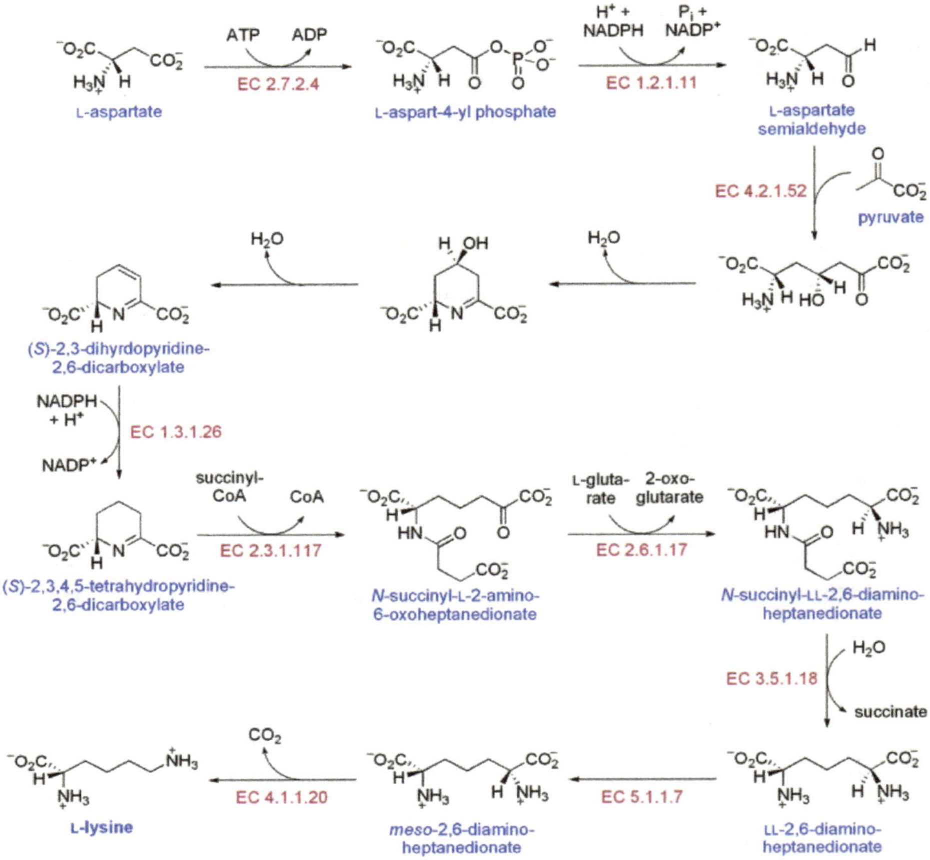

Enzymes involved in this biosynthesis include:

- Aspartokinase
- Aspartate-semialdehyde dehydrogenase
- 4-hydroxy-tetrahydrodipicolinate synthase
- 4-hydroxy-tetrahydrodipicolinate reductase
- 2,3,4,5-tetrahydropyridine-2,6-dicarboxylate N-succinyltransferase
- Succinyldiaminopimelate transaminase
- Succinyl-diaminopimelate desuccinylase
- Diaminopimelate epimerase
- Diaminopimelate decarboxylase

It is worth noting, however, that in fungi, euglenoids and some prokaryotes lysine is synthesized via the alpha-aminoadipate pathway.

Metabolism

Lysine is metabolised in mammals to give acetyl-CoA, via an initial transamination with α-ketoglutarate. The bacterial degradation of lysine yields cadaverine by decarboxylation.

Allysine is a derivative of lysine, used in the production of elastin and collagen. It is produced by the actions of the enzyme lysyl oxidase on lysine in the extracellular matrix and is essential in the crosslink formation that stabilizes collagen and elastin.

Synthesis

Synthetic, racemic lysine has long been known. A practical synthesis starts from caprolactam.Industrially, L-lysine is usually manufactured by a fermentation process using *Corynebacterium glutamicum*; production exceeds 600,000 tons a year.

L-lysine HCl is used as a dietary supplement, providing 80.03% L-lysine. As such, 1 g of L-lysine is contained in 1.25 g of L-lysine HCl.

Dietary Sources

The nutritional requirement per day, in milligrams of lysine per kilogram of body weight, is: infants (3–4 months) 103 mg/kg, children (2 years) 64 mg/kg, older children (10–12 years) 44 to 60 mg/kg, adults 12 mg/kg. For a 70 kg adult, 12 milligrams of lysine per kilogram of body weight is 0.84 grams of lysine. Recommendations for adults have been revised upwards to 30 mg/kg.

Good sources of lysine are high-protein foods such as eggs, meat (specifically red meat, lamb, pork, and poultry), soy, beans and peas, cheese (particularly Parmesan), and certain fish (such as cod and sardines).

Lysine is the limiting amino acid (the essential amino acid found in the smallest quantity in the particular foodstuff) in most cereal grains, but is plentiful in most pulses (legumes). Consequently, meals that combine cereal grains and legumes, such as the Indian dal with rice, Middle Eastern hummus, ful medames, falafel with pita bread, the Mexican beans with rice or tortilla have arisen to provide complete protein in diets that are, by choice or by necessity, vegetarian. A food is considered to have sufficient lysine if it has at least 51 mg of lysine per gram of protein (so that the protein is 5.1% lysine).

Foods containing significant proportions of lysine include:

Food	Lysine (% of protein)	Notes
Catfish, channel, farmed, raw	9.19%	Bluefish, burbot, mahi-mahi, grouper, lingcod, mackerel, pike, salmon, scup, trout, tuna, and yellowtail also have lysine content of nearly 9.2%
Beef, ground, 90% lean/10% fat, cooked	8.31%	
Chicken, roasting, meat and skin, cooked, roasted	8.11%	
Lentil, sprouts, raw	7.95%	Sprouting increases the lysine content.

Food	Lysine (% of protein)	Notes
Parmesan cheese, grated	7.75%	
Azuki bean (adzuki beans), mature seeds, raw	7.53%	
Milk, non-fat	7.48%	
Soybean, mature seeds, raw	7.42%	
Pumpkin Seed, dried	7.4%	
Egg, whole, raw	7.27%	
Pea, split, mature seeds, raw	7.22%	
Winged bean (Goa Bean or Asparagus Pea), mature seeds, raw	7.20%	
Lentil, pink, raw	6.97%	
Kidney bean, mature seeds, raw	6.87%	
Chickpea, (garbanzo beans, Bengal gram), mature seeds, raw	6.69%	
Soybean, mature seeds, sprouts	5.74%	Sprouting decreases the lysine content.
Navy bean, mature seeds, raw	5.73%	
Amaranth, grain, uncooked	5.17%	
Quinoa	5%	

Properties

L-Lysine plays a major role in calcium absorption; building muscle protein; recovering from surgery or sports injuries; and the body's production of hormones, enzymes, and antibodies.

Modifications

Lysine can be modified through acetylation (acetyllysine), methylation (methyllysine), ubiquitination, sumoylation, neddylation, biotinylation, pupylation, and carboxylation, which tends to modify the function of the protein of which the modified lysine residue(s) are a part.

Clinical Significance

A systematic Cochrane Review (investigating all clinical trials, *in vitro* studies and mechanism of action) published in 2015 showed there is no evidence that lysine supplementation is effective against herpes simplex virus and it has not been approved by the FDA for herpes simplex suppression.

Some studies have shown that lysine supplementation can decrease cold sore outbreaks and reduce healing time. Diets high in Arginine feed the herpes simplex virus and increase replication rate, while diets high in Lysine can decrease replication rate

Lysine has anxiolytic action through its effects on serotonin receptors in the intestinal tract, and is also hypothesized to reduce anxiety through serotonin regulation in the amygdala. One study on ratsshowed that overstimulation of the 5-HT4 receptors in the gut are associated with anxiety-induced intestinal pathology. Lysine, acting as a serotonin antagonist and therefore reducing the overactivity of these receptors, reduced signs of anxiety and anxiety-induced diarrhea in the sample population. Another study showed that lysine deficiency leads to a pathological increase in serotonin in the amygdala, a brain structure that is involved in emotional regulation and the stress response. Human studies have also shown correlations between reduced lysine intake and anxiety. A population-based study in Syria included 93 families whose diet is primarily grain-based and therefore likely to be deficient in lysine. Fortification of grains with lysine was shown to reduce markers of anxiety, including cortisol levels; Smiriga and colleagues hypothesized that anxiety reduction from lysine occurs through mechanism of serotonin alterations in the central amygdala; older primary research reports hypothesized lysine to reduce anxiety through the potentiation of benzodiazepine receptors (common targets of anxiolytic drugs such as Xanax and Ativan).

There are lysine conjugates that show promise in the treatment of cancer, by causing cancerous cells to destroy themselves when the drug is combined with the use of phototherapy, while leaving non-cancerous cells unharmed.

Lysine deficiency causes immunodeficiency in chickens. One cause of relative lysine deficiency is cystinuria, where there is impaired hepatic resorption of basic, or positively charged amino acids, including lysine. The accompanying urinary cysteine results because the same deficient amino acid transporter is normally present in the kidney as well.

Limited studies suggest that a high-lysine diet or L-lysine monochloride supplements may have a moderating effect on blood pressure and the incidence of stroke.

Lysine is attached to the amine of amphetamine to produce lisdexamfetamine, marketed as Vyvanse.

Use of Lysine in Animal Feed

Lysine production for animal feed is a major global industry, reaching in 2009 almost 700,000 tonnes for a market value of over €1.22 billion. Lysine is an important additive to animal feed because it is a limiting amino acid when optimizing the growth of certain animals such as pigs and chickens for the production of meat. Lysine supplementation allows for the use of lower-cost plant protein (maize, for instance, rather than soy) while maintaining high growth rates, and limiting the pollution from nitrogen excretion. In turn, however, phosphate pollution is a major environmental cost when corn is used as feed for poultry and swine.

Lysine is industrially produced by microbial fermentation, from a base mainly of sugar. Genetic engineering research is actively pursuing bacterial strains to improve the efficiency of production and allow lysine to be made from other substrates.

In Popular Culture

The 1993 film *Jurassic Park* (based on the 1990 Michael Crichton novel of the same name) features dinosaurs that were genetically altered so that they could not produce lysine. This was known as the "lysine contingency" and was supposed to prevent the cloned dinosaurs from surviving outside the park, forcing them to be dependent on lysine supplements provided by the park's veterinary staff. In reality, no animals are capable of producing lysine (it is an essential amino acid).

In 1996, lysine became the focus of a price-fixing case, the largest in United States history. The Archer Daniels Midland Company paid a fine of US$100 million, and three of its executives were convicted and served prison time. Also found guilty in the price-fixing case were two Japanese firms (Ajinomoto, Kyowa Hakko) and a South Korean firm (Sewon). Secret video recordings of the conspirators fixing lysine›s price can be found online or by requesting the video from the U.S. Department of Justice, Antitrust Division. This case served as the basis of the movie *The Informant!*, and a book of the same title.

ISOLEUCINE

Isoleucine (abbreviated as **Ile** or **I**) encoded by the codons ATT, ATC, ATA is an α-amino acid that is used in the biosynthesis of proteins. It contains an α-amino group (which is in the protonated −NH+3 form under biological conditions), an α-carboxylic acid group (which is in the deprotonated $-COO^-$ form under biological conditions), and a hydrocarbon side chain, classifying it as a non-polar, uncharged(at physiological pH), aliphatic amino acid. It is essential in humans, meaning the body cannot synthesize it, and must be ingested in our diet. Isoleucine is synthesized from pyruvate employing leucine biosynthesis enzymes in other organisms such as bacteria.

Inability to break down isoleucine, along with other amino acids, is associated with the disease called Maple Syrup Urine Disease, which results in discoloration and a sweet smell in the patient›s urine, which is where the name comes from. However, in severe cases, MSUD can lead to damage to the brain cells and ultimately death.

As an essential nutrient, it is not synthesized in the body, hence it must be ingested, usually as a component of proteins. In plants and microorganisms, it is synthesized via several steps, starting from pyruvic acid and alpha-ketoglutarate. Enzymes involved in this biosynthesis include:

- Acetolactate synthase (also known as acetohydroxy acid synthase)
- Acetohydroxy acid isomeroreductase

- Dihydroxyacid dehydratase
- Valine aminotransferase

Catabolism

Isoleucine is both a glucogenic and a ketogenic amino acid. After transamination with alpha-ketoglutarate the carbon skeleton can be converted into either Succinyl CoA, and fed into the TCA cycle for oxidation or converted into oxaloacetate for gluconeogenesis (hence glucogenic). It can also be converted into Acetyl CoA and fed into the TCA cycle by condensing with oxaloacetate to form citrate. In mammals Acetyl CoA cannot be converted back to carbohydrate but can be used in the synthesis of ketone bodies or fatty acids, hence ketogenic.

Biotin, sometimes referred to as Vitamin B7 or Vitamin H, is an absolute requirement for the full catabolism of isoleucine (as well as leucine). Without adequate biotin, the human body will be unable to fully break down isoleucine and leucine molecules.

Nutritional Sources

Even though this amino acid is not produced in animals, it is stored in high quantities. Foods that have high amounts of isoleucine include eggs, soy protein, seaweed, turkey, chicken, lamb, cheese, and fish.

Isomers of Isoleucine

Forms of Isoleucine							
Common name:	isoleucine	D-isoleucine	L-isoleucine	DL-isoleucine	allo-D-isoleucine	allo-L-isoleucine	allo-DL-isoleucine
Synonyms:		(*R*)-Isoleucine	L(+)-Isoleucine	(*R**,*R**)-isoleucine		alloisoleucine	
PubChem:	CID 791 from PubChem	CID 94206 from PubChem	CID 6306 from PubChem	CID 76551 from PubChem			
EINECS number:	207-139-8	206-269-2	200-798-2		216-143-9	216-142-3	221-464-2
CAS number:	443-79-8	319-78-8	73-32-5		1509-35-9	1509-34-8	3107-04-8

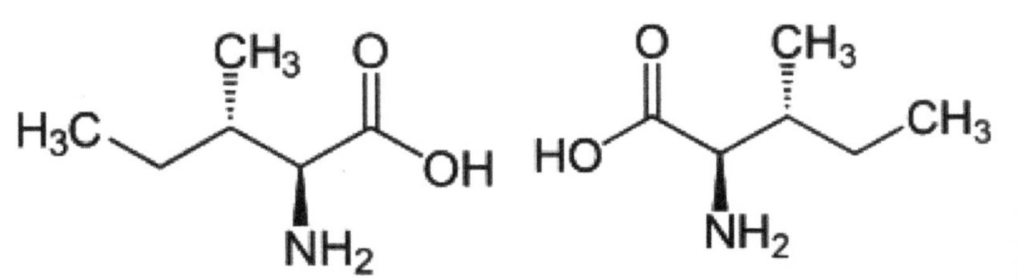

L-isoleucine (2*S*,3*S*) and D-isoleucine (2*R*,3*R*)

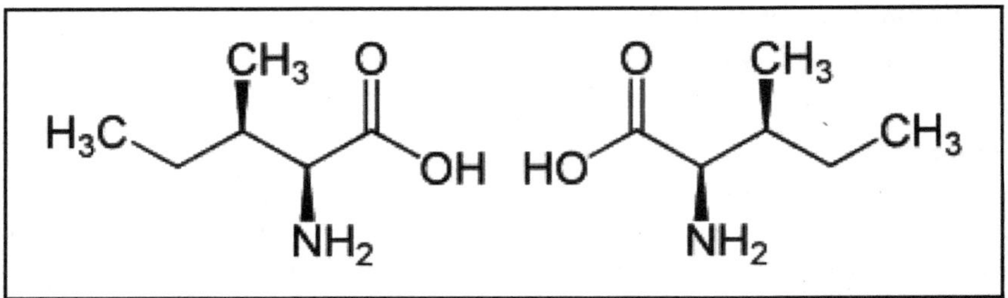

L-*allo*-isoleucine (2*S*,3*R*) and D-*allo*-isoleucine (2*R*,3*S*)

Synthesis

Isoleucine can be synthesized in a multistep procedure starting from 2-bromobutane and diethylmalonate. Synthetic isoleucine was originally reported in 1905.

German chemist Felix Ehrlich discovered isoleucine in hemoglobin in 1903.

THREONINE

Threonine (abbreviated as **Thr** or **T**) encoded by the codons ACU, ACC, ACA, and ACG is an α-amino acid that is used in the biosynthesis of proteins. It contains an α-amino group (which is in the protonated −NH+3 form under biological conditions), an α-carboxylic acid group (which is in the deprotonated $-COO^-$ form under biological conditions), and an alcohol containing side chain, classifying it as a polar, uncharged (at physiological pH) amino acid. It is essential in humans, meaning the body cannot synthesize it, and must be ingested in our diet. Threonine is synthesized from aspartate in bacteria such as *E. coli*.

Threonine sidechains are often hydrogen bonded; the commonest small motifs formed are ST turns, ST motifs (often at the beginning of alpha helices) and ST staples (usually at the middle of alpha helices).

Stereoisomerism

The threonine residue is susceptible to numerous posttranslational modifications. The hydroxyl side-chain can undergo *O*-linked glycosylation. In addition, threonine residues undergo phosphorylation through the action of a threonine kinase. In its phosphorylated form, it can be referred to as phosphothreonine.

It is a precursor of glycine, and can be used as a prodrug to reliably elevate brain glycine levels.

Threonine was discovered as the last of the 20 common proteinogenic amino acids in 1935s by William Cumming Rose, collaborating with Curtis Meyer and William Rose. The amino acid was named threonine because it was similar in structure to threose, a four-carbon monosaccharide or carbohydrate with molecular formula $C_4H_8O_4$

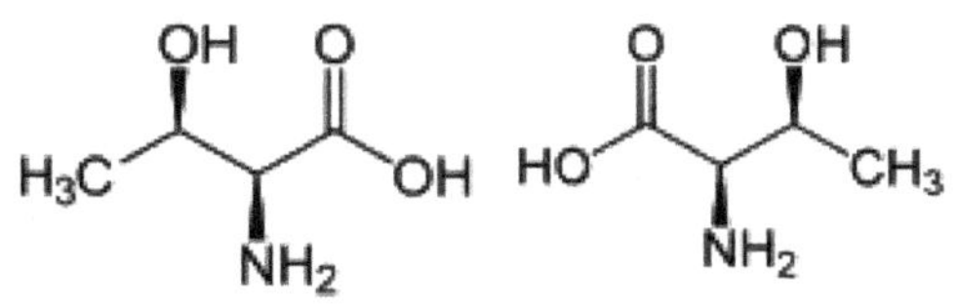

L-Threonine (2*S*,3*R*) and D-Threonine (2*R*,3*S*)

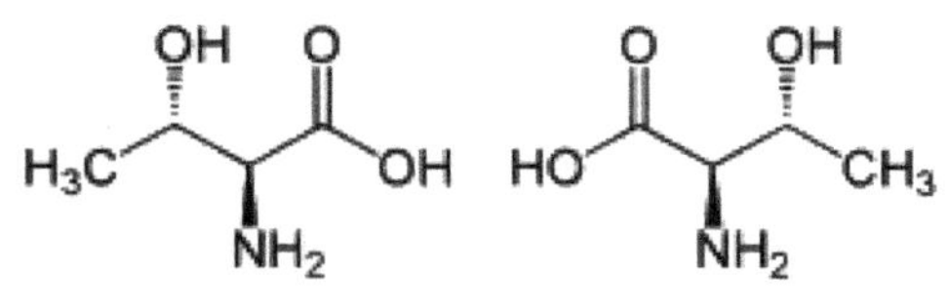

L-*allo*-Threonine (2*S*,3*S*) and D-*allo*-Threonine (2*R*,3*R*)

Threonine is one of two proteinogenic amino acids with two chiral centers. Threonine can exist in four possible stereoisomers with the following configurations: (2*S*,3*R*), (2*R*,3*S*), (2*S*,3*S*) and (2*R*,3*R*). However, the name L-threonine is used for one single diastereomer, (2*S*,3*R*)-2-amino-3-hydroxybutanoic acid. The second stereoisomer (2*S*,3*S*), which is rarely present in nature, is called L-*allo*-threonine. The two stereoisomers (2*R*,3*S*)- and (2*R*,3*R*)-2-amino-3-hydroxybutanoic acid are only of minor importance.

Biosynthesis

As an essential amino acid, threonine is not synthesized in humans, hence we must ingest threonine in the form of threonine-containing proteins. In plants and microorganisms, threonine is synthesized from aspartic acid via α-aspartyl-semialdehyde and homoserine. Homoserine undergoes *O*-phosphorylation; this phosphate ester undergoes hydrolysis concomitant with relocation of the OH group. Enzymes involved in a typical biosynthesis of threonine include:

- aspartokinase
- β-aspartate semialdehyde dehydrogenase
- homoserine dehydrogenase
- homoserine kinase
- threonine synthase.

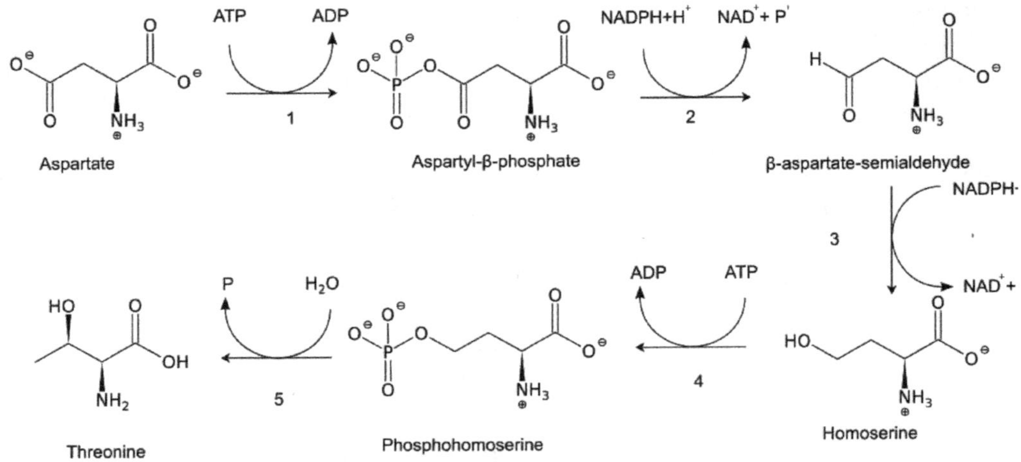

Threonine biosynthesis.

TRYPTOPHAN

Tryptophan (abbreviated as Trp or W; encoded by the codon UGG) is an α-amino acid that is used in the biosynthesis of proteins. It contains an α-amino group, an α-carboxylic acid group, and a side chain indole, classifying it as a non-polar, aromatic amino acid. It is essential in humans, meaning the body cannot synthesize it and thus it must be obtained from the diet. Tryptophan is also a precursor to the neurotransmitters serotonin and melatonin.

Like other amino acids, tryptophan is a zwitterion at physiological pH where the amino group is protonated ($-NH_3^+$; $pK_a = 9.39$) and the carboxylic acid is deprotonated ($-COO^-$; $pK_a = 2.38$).

Isolation

The isolation of tryptophan was first reported by Frederick Hopkins in 1901 through hydrolysis of casein. From 600 grams of crude casein one obtains 4-8 grams of tryptophan.

Biosynthesis and industrial production

As an essential amino acid, tryptophan is not synthesized from more basic substances in humans and other animals, who must ingest tryptophan or tryptophan-containing proteins. Plants and microorganisms commonly synthesize tryptophan from shikimic acid or anthranilate by the following process: anthranilate condenses with phosphoribosylpyrophosphate (PRPP), generating pyrophosphate as a by-product. The ring of the ribose moiety is opened and subjected to reductive decarboxylation, producing indole-3-glycerinephosphate; this, in turn, is transformed into indole. In the last step, tryptophan synthase catalyzes the formation of tryptophan from indole and the amino acid serine.

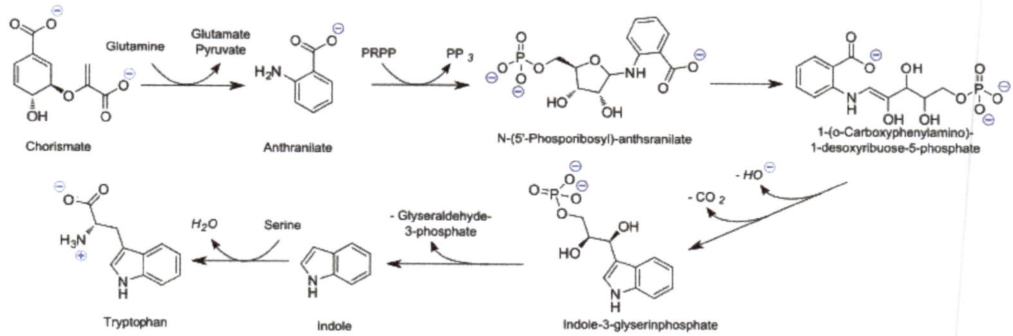

The industrial production of tryptophan is also biosynthetic and is based on the fermentation of serine and indole using either wild-type or genetically modified bacteria such as *B. amyloliquefaciens*, *B. subtilis*, *C. glutamicum* or *E. coli*. These strains carry either mutations that prevent the reuptake of aromatic amino acids or multiple/overexpressed trp operons. The conversion is catalyzed by the enzyme tryptophan synthase.

Function

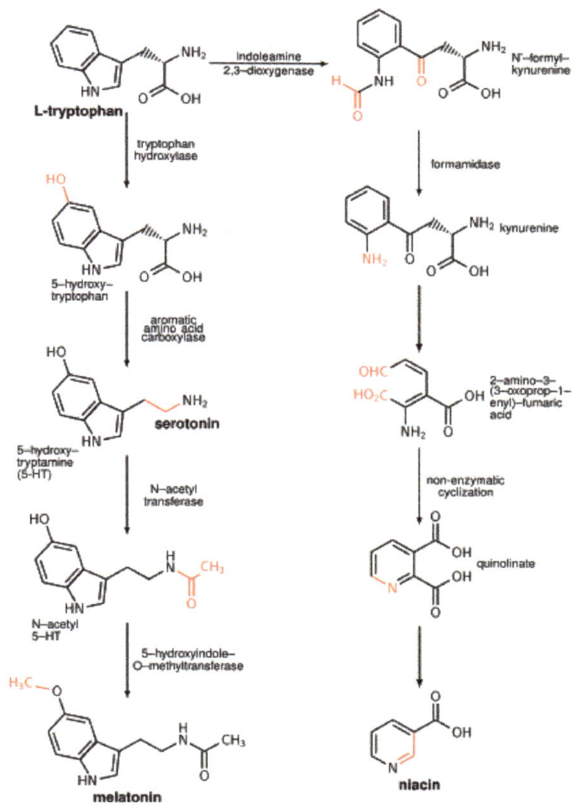

Metabolism of L-tryptophan into serotonin and melatonin (left) and niacin (right). Transformed functional groups after each chemical reaction are highlighted in red.

For many organisms (including humans), tryptophan is needed to prevent illness or death, but cannot be synthesized by the organism and must be ingested; in short, it is an essential amino acid. Amino acids, including tryptophan, act as building blocks in protein biosynthesis, and proteins are required to sustain life. In addition, tryptophan functions as a biochemical precursor for the following compounds (see also figure to the right):

- Serotonin (a neurotransmitter), synthesized via tryptophan hydroxylase. Serotonin, in turn, can be converted to melatonin (a neurohormone), via N-acetyltransferase and 5-hydroxyindole-O-methyltransferase activities.
- Niacin, also known as vitamin B_3, is synthesized from tryptophan via kynurenine and quinolinic acids as key biosynthetic intermediates.
- Auxins (a class of phytohormones) are synthesized from tryptophan.

The disorder fructose malabsorption causes improper absorption of tryptophan in the intestine, reduced levels of tryptophan in the blood, and depression. Some studies did not find reduced tryptophan in cases of lactose maldigestion.

In bacteria that synthesize tryptophan, high cellular levels of this amino acid activate a repressor protein, which binds to the trp operon. Binding of this repressor to the tryptophan operon prevents transcription of downstream DNA that codes for the enzymes involved in the biosynthesis of tryptophan. So high levels of tryptophan prevent tryptophan synthesis through a negative feedback loop and, when the cell's tryptophan levels are reduced, transcription from the trp operon resumes. The genetic organisation of the trp operon thus permits tightly regulated and rapid responses to changes in the cell›s internal and external tryptophan levels.

Tryptophan metabolism by human gastrointestinal microbiota (v · t · e)

This diagram shows the biosynthesis of bioactive compounds (indole and certain derivatives) from tryptophan by bacteria in the gut. Indole is produced from tryptophan by bacteria that express tryptophanase. *Clostridium sporogenes* metabolizes indole into 3-indolepropionic acid (IPA), a highly potent neuroprotective antioxidant that scavenges hydroxyl radicals. In the intestine, IPA binds to pregnane X receptors (PXR) in intestinal cells, thereby facilitating mucosal homeostasis and barrier function. Following absorption from the intestine and distribution to the brain, IPA confers a neuroprotective effect against cerebral ischemia and Alzheimer's disease. *Lactobacillus* species metabolize tryptophan into indole-3-aldehyde (I3A) which acts on the aryl hydrocarbon receptor (AhR) in intestinal immune cells, in turn increasing interleukin-22 (IL-22) production. Indole itself acts as a glucagon-like peptide-1 (GLP-1) secretagogue in intestinal L cells and as a ligand for AhR. Indole can also be metabolized by the liver into indoxyl sulfate, a compound that is toxic in high concentrations and associated with vascular disease and renal dysfunction. AST-120 (activated charcoal), an intestinal sorbent that is taken by mouth, adsorbs indole, in turn decreasing the concentration of indoxyl sulfate in blood plasma.

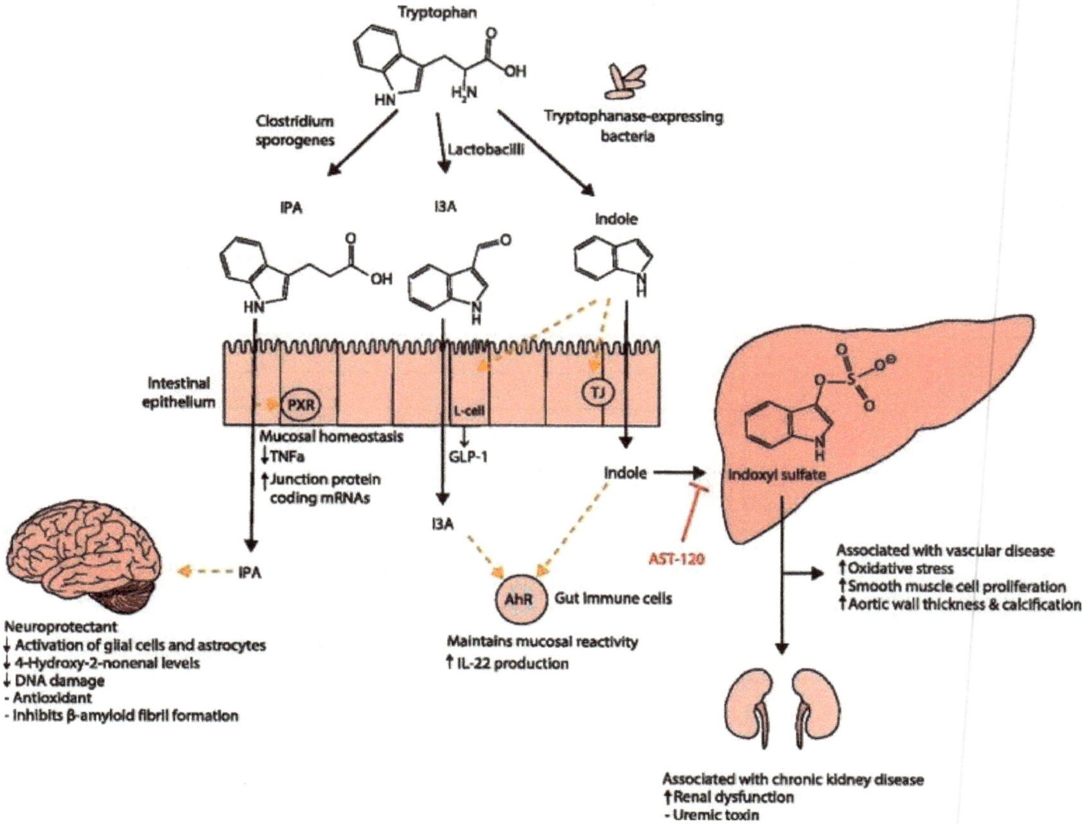

Dietary Sources

Tryptophan is a routine constituent of most protein-based foods or dietary proteins. It is particularly plentiful in chocolate, oats, dried dates, milk, yogurt, cottage cheese, red meat, eggs, fish, poultry, sesame, chickpeas, almonds, sunflower seeds, pumpkin seeds, buckwheat, spirulina, and peanuts. Contrary to the popular belief that turkey contains an abundance of tryptophan, the tryptophan content in turkey is typical of poultry.

Tryptophan (Trp) Content of Various Foods			
Food	**Tryptophan [g/100 g of food]**	**Protein [g/100 g of food]**	**Tryptophan/Protein [%]**
egg white, dried	1.00	81.10	1.23
spirulina, dried	0.93	57.47	1.62
cod, atlantic, dried	0.70	62.82	1.11
soybeans, raw	0.59	36.49	1.62
cheese, Parmesan	0.56	37.90	1.47
sesame seed	0.37	17.00	2.17
cheese, cheddar	0.32	24.90	1.29
sunflower seed	0.30	17.20	1.74

pork, chop	0.25	19.27	1.27
turkey	0.24	21.89	1.11
chicken	0.24	20.85	1.14
beef	0.23	20.13	1.12
oats	0.23	16.89	1.39
salmon	0.22	19.84	1.12
lamb, chop	0.21	18.33	1.17
perch, Atlantic	0.21	18.62	1.12
chickpeas, raw	0.19	19.30	0.96
egg	0.17	12.58	1.33
wheat flour, white	0.13	10.33	1.23
baking chocolate, unsweetened	0.13	12.9	1.23
milk	0.08	3.22	2.34
rice, white, medium-grain, cooked	0.028	2.38	1.18
quinoa, uncooked	0.167	14.12	1.2
quinoa, cooked	0.052	4.40	1.1
potatoes, russet	0.02	2.14	0.84
tamarind	0.018	2.80	0.64
banana	0.01	1.03	0.87

Turkey Meat and Drowsiness

A common assertion in the US is that heavy consumption of turkey meat results in drowsiness, due to high levels of tryptophan contained in turkey. However, the amount of tryptophan in turkey is comparable to that contained in other meats. Drowsiness after eating may be caused by other foods eaten with the turkey, particularly carbohydrates. It has been demonstrated in both animaland human tests that ingestion of a meal rich in carbohydrates triggers release of insulin. Insulin in turn stimulates the uptake of large neutral branched-chain amino acids (BCAA), but not tryptophan into muscle, increasing the ratio of tryptophan to BCAA in the blood stream. The resulting increased tryptophan ratio reduces competition at the large neutral amino acid transporter (which transports both BCAA and aromatic amino acids), resulting in more uptake of tryptophan across the blood–brain barrier into the cerebrospinal fluid (CSF). Once in the CSF, tryptophan is converted into serotonin in the raphe nuclei by the normal enzymatic pathway. The resultant serotonin is further metabolised into melatonin by the pineal gland. Hence, this data suggests that "feast-induced drowsiness"—or postprandial somnolence—may be the result of a heavy meal rich in carbohydrates, which indirectly increases the production of sleep-promoting melatonin in the brain.

Use as a Dietary Supplement

Tryptophan is sold over the counter in the United States, Canada, and the United Kingdom as a dietary supplement for use as an antidepressant, anxiolytic, and sleep aid. It is also marketed as a prescription drug in some European countries for the indication of major depression under various trade names.

Since tryptophan is converted into 5-hydroxytryptophan (5-HTP) which is subsequently converted into the neurotransmitter serotonin, it has been proposed that consumption of tryptophan or 5-HTP may therefore improve depression symptoms by increasing the level of serotonin in the brain. In 2001 a Cochrane Review of the effect of 5-HTP and tryptophan on depression was published. The authors included only studies of a high rigor and included both 5-HTP and tryptophan in their review because of the limited data on either. Of 108 studies of 5-HTP and tryptophan on depression published between 1966 and 2000, only two met the authors' quality standards for inclusion, totaling 64 study participants. The substances were more effective than placebo in the two studies included but the authors state that, "the evidence was of insufficient quality to be conclusive," and note, "because alternative antidepressants exist which have been proven to be effective and safe, the clinical usefulness of 5-HTP and tryptophan is limited at present." The use of tryptophan as an adjunctive therapy in addition to standard treatment for mood and anxiety disorders is not supported by the scientific evidence. Due to the lack of high quality studies and preliminary nature of studies showing effectiveness and the lack of adequate study on their safety, the use of tryptophan and 5-HTP is not highly recommended or thought to be clinically useful.

There is evidence that blood tryptophan levels are unlikely to be altered by changing the diet, but tryptophan is available in health food stores as a dietary supplement. Consuming purified tryptophan increases brain serotonin whereas eating foods containing tryptophan does not. This is because the transport system which brings tryptophan across the blood-brain barrier is also selective for the other amino acids which are contained in protein food sources. High blood plasma levels of other large neutral amino acids prevent the plasma concentration of tryptophan from increasing brain concentration levels.

Side effects

Potential side effects of tryptophan include nausea, diarrhea, drowsiness, lightheadedness, headache, dry mouth, blurred vision, sedation, euphoria, and nystagmus (involuntary eye movements).Because tryptophan has not been thoroughly studied in a clinical setting, possible side effects and interactions with other drugs are not well known.

Interactions

Tryptophan taken as a dietary supplement (such as in tablet form) has the potential to cause serotonin syndrome when combined with antidepressants of the MAOI or SSRI class or other strongly serotonergic drugs.

RESEARCH

In 1912 Felix Ehrlich demonstrated that yeast attacks the natural amino acids essentially by splitting off carbon dioxide and replacing the amino group with hydroxyl. By this reaction, tryptophan gives rise to tryptophol.

Tryptophan affects brain serotonin synthesis when given orally in a purified form and is used to modify serotonin levels for research in psychology. Low brain serotonin is induced by administration of tryptophan-poor protein in a technique called ‹acute tryptophan depletion›. Studies using this method have evaluated the effect of serotonin on mood and social behavior, finding that serotonin reduces aggression and increases agreeableness.

Fluorescence

Tryptophan is an important intrinsic fluorescent probe (amino acid), which can be used to estimate the nature of microenvironment of the tryptophan. Most of the intrinsic fluorescence emissions of a folded protein are due to excitation of tryptophan residues.

Safety

Eosinophilia–myalgia Syndrome

There was a large outbreak of eosinophilia-myalgia syndrome (EMS) in the U.S. in 1989, with more than 1,500 cases reported to the CDC and at least 37 deaths. After preliminary investigation revealed that the outbreak was linked to intake of tryptophan, the U.S. Food and Drug Administration (FDA) banned most tryptophan from sale in the US in 1991, and other countries followed suit.

Subsequent epidemiological studies suggested that EMS was linked to specific batches of L-tryptophan supplied by a single large Japanese manufacturer, Showa Denko. It eventually became clear that recent batches of Showa Denko›s L-tryptophan were contaminated by trace impurities, which were subsequently thought to be responsible for the 1989 EMS outbreak. However, other evidence suggests that tryptophan itself may be a potentially major contributory factor in EMS.

The FDA loosened its restrictions on sales and marketing of tryptophan in February 2001, but continued to limit the importation of tryptophan not intended for an exempted use until 2005.

The fact that the Showa Denko facility used genetically engineered bacteria to produce the contaminated batches of L-tryptophan later found to have caused the outbreak of eosinophilia-myalgia syndrome has been cited as evidence of a need for "close monitoring of the chemical purity of biotechnology-derived products." Those calling for purity monitoring have, in turn, been criticized as anti-GMO activists who overlook possible non-GMO causes of contamination and threaten the development of biotech.

LEUCINE

Leucine (abbreviated as **Leu** or **L**; encoded by the six codons UUA, UUG, CUU, CUC, CUA, and CUG) is an α-amino acid used in the biosynthesis of proteins. It contains an α-amino group (which is in the protonated −NH+3 form under biological conditions), an α-carboxylic acid group (which is in the deprotonated $-COO^-$ form under biological conditions), and an isobutyl side chain, classifying it as a nonpolar (at physiological pH) amino acid. It is essential in humans—meaning the body cannot synthesize it and thus must obtain from the diet.

Leucine is a major component of the subunits in ferritin, astacin, and other "buffer" proteins.

Biology

Leucine is used in the liver, adipose tissue, and muscle tissue. Adipose and muscle tissue use leucine in the formation of sterols. Combined leucine use in these two tissues is seven times greater than in the liver.

Biosynthesis in Plants

Valine is an essential amino acid in the diet of animals because they lack the complete enzyme pathway to synthesize it *de novo* from potential precursor compounds. Consequently, they must ingest it, usually as a component of proteins. Plants and microorganisms synthesize leucine from pyruvic acid with a series of enzymes:

- Acetolactate synthase
- Acetohydroxy acid isomeroreductase
- Dihydroxyacid dehydratase
- α-Isopropylmalate synthase
- α-Isopropylmalate isomerase
- Leucine aminotransferase

Synthesis of the small, hydrophobic amino acid valine also includes the initial part of this pathway.

Metabolism in Humans

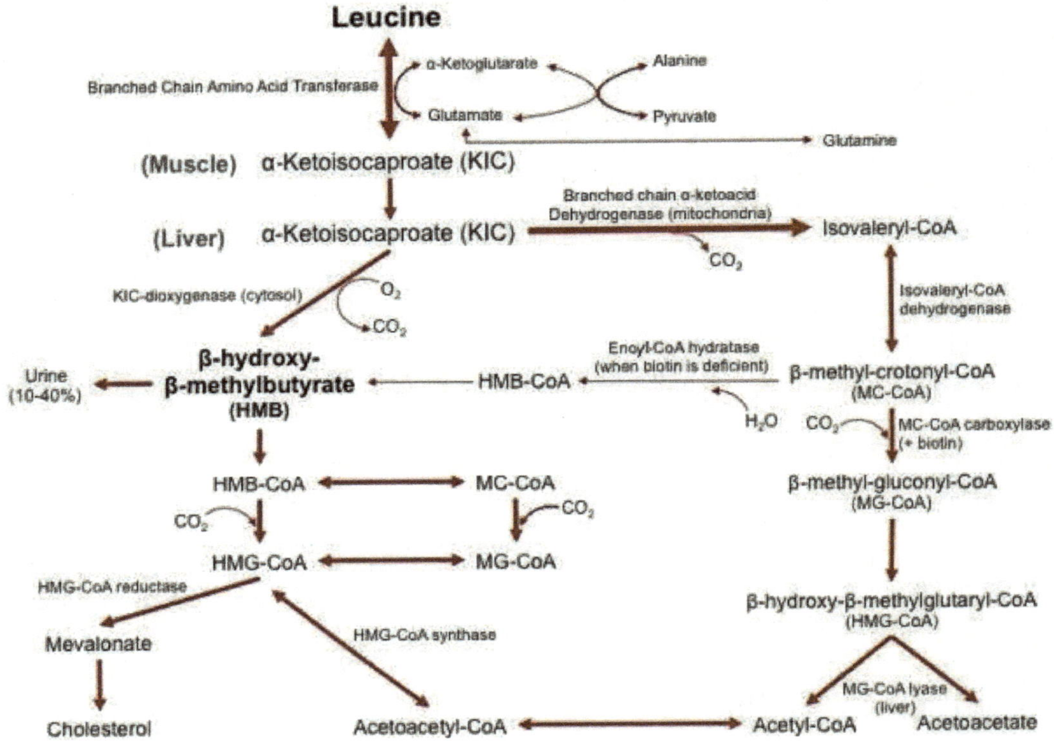

Human metabolic pathway for β-hydroxy β-methylbutyric acid (HMB) and isovaleryl-CoA, relative to l-leucine. Of the two major pathways, leucine is mostly metabolized into isovaleryl-CoA, while only about 5% is metabolized into HMB.

In healthy individuals, approximately 60% of dietary l-leucine is metabolized after several hours, with roughly 5% (2–10% range) of dietary l-leucine being converted to β-hydroxy β-methylbutyric acid (HMB). Around 40% of dietary l-leucine is converted to acetyl-CoA, which is subsequently used in the synthesis of other compounds.

The vast majority of l-leucine metabolism is initially catalyzed by the branched-chain amino acid aminotransferase enzyme, producing α-ketoisocaproate (α-KIC). α-Ketoisocaproate is mostly metabolized by the mitochondrial enzyme branched-chain α-ketoacid dehydrogenase, which converts it to isovaleryl-CoA. Isovaleryl-CoA is subsequently metabolized by isovaleryl-CoA dehydrogenase and converted to β-methylcrotonoyl-CoA (MC-CoA), which is used in the synthesis of acetyl-CoA and other compounds. During biotin deficiency, HMB can be synthesized from MC-CoA via enoyl-CoA hydratase and an unknown thioesterase enzyme, which convert MC-CoA into β-hydroxy β-methylbutyryl-CoA (HMB-CoA) and HMB-CoA into HMB respectively. A relatively small amount of α-KIC is metabolized in the liver by the cytosolic enzyme 4-hydroxyphenylpyruvate dioxygenase (*KIC dioxygenase*), which converts α-KIC to HMB.

In healthy individuals, this minor pathway – which involves the conversion of l-leucine to α-KIC and then HMB – is the predominant route of HMB synthesis.

A small fraction of l-leucine metabolism – less than 5% in all tissues except the testes where it accounts for about 33% – is initially catalyzed by leucine aminomutase, producing β-leucine, which is subsequently metabolized into β-ketoisocaproate (β-KIC), β-ketoisocaproyl-CoA, and then acetyl-CoA by a series of uncharacterized enzymes. HMB could be produced via certain metabolites that are generated along this pathway, but as of 2015 the associated enzymes and reactions involved are not known.

The metabolism of HMB is initially catalyzed by an uncharacterized enzyme which converts it to HMB-CoA. HMB-CoA is metabolized by either enoyl-CoA hydratase or another uncharacterized enzyme, producing MC-CoA or hydroxymethylglutaryl-CoA (HMG-CoA) respectively. MC-CoA is then converted by the enzyme methylcrotonyl-CoA carboxylase to methylglutaconyl-CoA (MG-CoA), which is subsequently converted to HMG-CoA by methylglutaconyl-CoA hydratase. HMG-CoA is then cleaved into to acetyl-CoA and acetoacetate by HMG-CoA lyase or used in the production of cholesterol via the mevalonate pathway.

Effects

Leucine is an mTOR activator. It is a dietary amino acid with the capacity to directly stimulate muscle protein synthesis. As a dietary supplement, leucine has been found to slow the degradation of muscle tissue by increasing the synthesis of muscle proteins in aged rats. However, results of comparative studies are conflicted. Long-term leucine supplementation does not increase muscle mass or strength in healthy elderly men. More studies are needed, preferably ones based on an objective, random sample of society. Factors such as lifestyle choices, age, gender, diet, exercise, etc. must be factored into the analyses to isolate the effects of supplemental leucine as a standalone, or if taken with other branched chain amino acids (BCAAs). Until then, dietary supplemental leucine cannot be associated as the prime reason for muscular growth or optimal maintenance for the entire population.

Leucine potently activates the mammalian target of rapamycin kinase that regulates cell growth. Infusion of leucine into the rat brain has been shown to decrease food intake and body weight via activation of the mTOR pathway. Several sensing mechanisms have been proposed; most recently, it has been demonstrated that sestrin 2 can directly bind to leucine and activate mTORC1 activity by promoting its localization to the lysosome.

Both L-leucine and D-leucine protect mice against seizures. D-leucine also terminates seizures in mice after the onset of seizure activity, at least as effectively as diazepam and without sedative effects. Decreased dietary intake of L-leucine promotes adiposity in mice. High blood levels of leucine are associated with insulin resistance in humans, mice, and rodents.

Safety

Leucine toxicity, as seen in decompensated maple syrup urine disease (MSUD), causes delirium and neurologic compromise, and can be life-threatening.

Excess leucine may be a cause of pellagra, whose main symptoms are "the four D›s": diarrhea, dermatitis, dementia and death, though the relationship is unclear.

Leucine at a dose exceeding 500 mg/kg/d was observed with hyperammonemia. As such, the UL for leucine in healthy adult men can be suggested at 500 mg/kg/d or 35 g/d under acute dietary conditions.

Dietary Sources

Food sources of leucine	
Food	**g/100g**
Soybeans, mature seeds, roasted, salted	2.868
Hemp seed, hulled	2.163
Beef, round, top round, separable lean and fat, trimmed to 3 mm ($\frac{1}{8}$ in) fat, select, raw	1.76
Peanuts	1.672
Salami, pork	1.63
Fish, salmon, pink, raw	1.62
Wheat germ	1.571
Almonds	1.488
Chicken, broilers or fryers, thigh, meat only, raw	1.48
Chicken egg, yolk, raw, fresh	1.40
Oat	1.284
soybeans, Edamame, green, raw	0.926
Beans, pinto, cooked	0.765
Lentils, cooked	0.654
Chickpea, cooked	0.631
Corn, yellow	0.348
Cow milk, whole, 3.25% milk fat	0.27
Rice, brown, medium-grain, cooked	0.191
Milk, human, mature, fluid	0.10

Chemical Properties

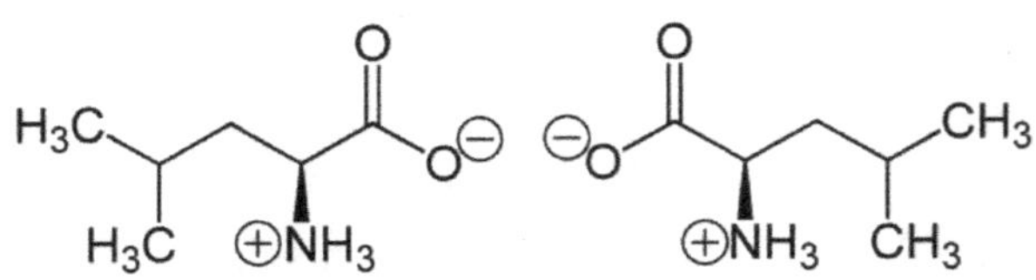

(*S*)-Leucine (or L-leucine), left; (*R*)-leucine (or D-leucine), right, in zwitterionic form at neutral pH.

Leucine is a branched-chain amino acid (BCAA) since it possesses an aliphatic side-chain that is non-linear.

Racemic leucine had been subjected to circularly polarized synchrotron radiation to better understand the origin of biomolecular asymmetry. An enantiomeric enhancement of 2.6% had been induced, indicating a possible photochemical origin of biomolecules' homochirality.

REFERENCES

1. "Dietary Supplement Database: Blend Information (DSBI)". L-LYSINE HCL 10000820 80.03% lysine
2. "Erowid Cacti Vault : Cactus Growers Guide". Erowid.org. 2008-03-08. Retrieved 2013-04-16.
3. "Homo sapiens: 4-hydroxyphenylpyruvate dioxygenase reaction". MetaCyc. SRI International. 20 August 2012. Retrieved 6 June 2016.
4. "KEGG Reaction: R04137". Kyoto Encyclopedia of Genes and Genomes. Kanehisa Laboratories. Retrieved 24 June 2016.
5. "KEGG Reaction: R10759". Kyoto Encyclopedia of Genes and Genomes. Kanehisa Laboratories. Retrieved 24 June 2016.
6. "Leucine metabolism". BRENDA. Technische Universität Braunschweig. Retrieved 8 June 2016.
7. "MetaCyc: L-lysine biosynthesis I".
8. "Norwegian granted for improving lysine production process"
9. "Subjective response to lysine in the therapy of herpes simplex". Journal of Antimicrobial Chemotherapy. 12.
10. "Tyrosine". The Columbia Electronic Encyclopedia, 6th ed. Infoplease.com — Columbia University Press. 2007. Retrieved 2008-04-20.
11. "Tyrosine". University of Maryland Medical Center. Retrieved 2011-03-17.
12. Abelson, Philip (March 1999). "A Potential Phosphate Crisis". Science. 283 (5410): 2015. doi:10.1126/science.283.5410.2015. PMID 10206902.
13. Bapurao S, Krishnaswamy K (1978). "Vitamin B6 nutritional status of pellagrins and their leucine tolerance". Am J Clin Nutr. 31 (5): 819–24. PMID 206127.
14. Booth, A N; Masri, M S; Robbins, D J; Emerson, O H; Jones, F T; Deeds, F (1960). "Urinary phenolic acid metabolities of tyrosine". Journal of Biological Chemistry. 235 (9): 2649–2652.
15. Braun, J. V. (1909). "Synthese des inaktiven Lysins aus Piperidin". Berichte der deutschen chemischen Gesellschaft. 42: 839–846. doi:10.1002/cber.190904201134.
16. Brioche T, Pagano AF, Py G, Chopard A (April 2016). "Muscle wasting and aging: Experimental models, fatty infiltrations, and prevention". Mol. Aspects Med. doi:10.1016/j.mam.2016.04.006. PMID 27106402.
17. Broadley KJ (March 2010). "The vascular effects of trace amines and amphetamines". Pharmacol. Ther. 125 (3): 363–375. doi:10.1016/j.pharmthera.2009.11.005. PMID 19948186.
18. Chantranupong, Lynne; Wolfson, Rachel L.; Orozco, Jose M.; Saxton, Robert

A.; Scaria, Sonia M.; Bar-Peled, Liron; Spooner, Eric; Isasa, Marta; Gygi, Steven P. (9 October 2014). "The Sestrins interact with GATOR2 to negatively regulate the amino-acid-sensing pathway upstream of mTORC1". Cell Reports. 9 (1): 1–8. doi:10.1016/j.celrep.2014.09.014. ISSN 2211-1247. PMC 4223866 . PMID 25263562.

19. Chavez-Bejar, M., J. Baez-Viveros, A. Martinez, F. Bolivar, G. Gosset. (2012) Biotechnological production of L-tyrosine and derived compounds. Process Biochemistry. 47: 1017-1026
20. Chavez-Bejar, M., J. Baez-Viveros, A. Martinez, F. Bolivar, G. Gosset. (2012) Biotechnological production of L-tyrosine and derived compounds. Process Biochemistry. 47: 1017-1026
21. Chen C, Sander JE, Dale NM (2003). "The effect of dietary lysine deficiency on the immune response to Newcastle disease vaccination in chickens". Avian Dis. 47 (4): 1346–51. doi:10.1637/7008. PMID 14708981.
22. Chinevere TD, Sawyer RD, Creer AR, Conlee RK, Parcell AC (2002). "Effects of L-tyrosine and carbohydrate ingestion on endurance exercise performance". J. Appl. Physiol. 93 (5): 1590–7. doi:10.1152/japplphysiol.00625.2001 (inactive 2015-01-09). PMID 12381742.
23. Ching-Chi Chi1, Shu-Hui Wang, Finola M Delamere, Fenella Wojnarowska, Mathilde C Peters, Preetha P Kanjirath (2015). "Interventions for prevention of herpes simplex labialis (cold sores on the lips)". Cochrane Database of Systematic Reviews (8). doi:10.1002/14651858.CD010095.pub2. CD010095.
24. Connor, J.M.; "Global Price Fixing" 2nd Ed. Springer-Verlag: Heidelberg, 2008. ISBN 978-3-540-78669-6.
25. Cota D, Proulx K, Smith KA, Kozma SC, Thomas G, Woods SC, Seeley RJ (2006). "Hypothalamic mTOR signaling regulates food intake". Science. 312 (5775): 927–930. doi:10.1126/science.1124147. PMID 16690869.
26. Coyne, Jerry A. (October 10, 1999). "The Truth Is Way Out There". The New York Times. Retrieved 2008-04-06.
27. Dawson, R.M.C., et al., Data for Biochemical Research, Oxford, Clarendon Press, 1959.
28. Deijen JB, Orlebeke JF (1994). "Effect of tyrosine on cognitive function and blood pressure under stress". Brain Res. Bull. 33 (3): 319–23. doi:10.1016/0361-9230(94)90200-3. PMID 8293316.
29. Deijen JB, Wientjes CJ, Vullinghs HF, Cloin PA, Langefeld JJ (1999). "Tyrosine improves cognitive performance and reduces blood pressure in cadets after one week of a combat training course". Brain Res. Bull. 48 (2): 203–9. doi:10.1016/S0361-9230(98)00163-4. PMID 10230711.
30. Douglas Harper (2001). "Tyrosine". Online Etymology Dictionary. Retrieved 2008-04-20.
31. Drugs.com. "Herpes Simplex, Suppression Medications". Retrieved 2014-05-19.
32. Eck, J. C.; Marvel, C. S. (1943). "dl-Lysine Hydrochlorides" (PDF). Organic

Syntheses, Collected. 2: 374.

33. Eichenwald, Kurt.; "The Informant: a true story" Broadway Books: New York, 2000. ISBN 0-7679-0326-9.
34. Elango R, Chapman K, Rafii M, Ball RO, Pencharz PB (2012). "Determination of the tolerable upper intake level of leucine in acute dietary studies in young men".
35. Etzel MR (2004). "Manufacture and use of dairy protein fractions". The Journal of Nutrition. 134 (4): 996S–1002S. PMID 15051860.
36. FAO/WHO/UNU (2007). "PROTEIN AND AMINO ACID REQUIREMENTS IN HUMAN NUTRITION" (PDF). WHO Press., page 150-152
37. Flodin 1997[clarification needed]
38. Fontana, Luigi; Cummings, Nicole E.; Arriola Apelo, Sebastian I.; Neuman, Joshua C.; Kasza, Ildiko; Schmidt, Brian A.; Cava, Edda; Spelta, Francesco; Tosti, Valeria (21 June 2016). "Decreased Consumption of Branched-Chain Amino Acids Improves Metabolic Health". Cell Reports. 16: 520–30. doi:10.1016/j.celrep.2016.05.092. ISSN 2211-1247. PMC 4947548 . PMID 27346343.
39. Hao S, Avraham Y, Bonne O, Berry EM (2001). "Separation-induced body weight loss, impairment in alternation behavior, and autonomic tone: effects of tyrosine". Pharmacol. Biochem. Behav. 68 (2): 273–81. doi:10.1016/S0091-3057(00)00448-2. PMID 11267632.
40. Hartman AL, Santos P, O'Riordan KJ, Stafstrom CE, Marie Hardwick J (2015). "Potent anti-seizure effects of D-leucine". Neurobiology of Disease. 82: 46–53. doi:10.1016/j.nbd.2015.05.013. PMID 26054437. Retrieved 26 November 2015.
41. Hegyi J, Schwartz R, Hegyi V (2004). "Pellagra: dermatitis, dementia, and diarrhea". Int J Dermatol. 43 (1): 1–5. doi:10.1111/j.1365-4632.2004.01959.x. PMID 14693013.
42. Helena Kloosterman; USDA National Nutrient Database for Standard Reference. "Essential Amino Acids Search, catfish farmed". Retrieved 2010-10-10.
43. Helena Kloosterman; USDA National Nutrient Database for Standard Reference. "Essential Amino Acids Search, beef ground 90 10 cooked". Retrieved 2010-10-10.
44. Helena Kloosterman; USDA National Nutrient Database for Standard Reference. "Essential Amino Acids Search, chicken roasting meat skin". Retrieved 2010-10-10.
45. Helena Kloosterman; USDA National Nutrient Database for Standard Reference. "Essential Amino Acids Search, lentils sprouted". Retrieved 2010-10-10.
46. Helena Kloosterman; USDA National Nutrient Database for Standard Reference. "Essential Amino Acids Search, parmesan cheese". Retrieved 2010-10-10.
47. Helena Kloosterman; USDA National Nutrient Database for Standard Reference. "Essential Amino Acids Search, adzuki bean". Retrieved 2010-10-10.

48. Helena Kloosterman; USDA National Nutrient Database for Standard Reference. "Essential Amino Acids Search, milk nonfat". Retrieved 2010-10-10.

49. Helena Kloosterman; USDA National Nutrient Database for Standard Reference. "Essential Amino Acids Search, soybean seeds". Retrieved 2010-10-10.

50. Helena Kloosterman; USDA National Nutrient Database for Standard Reference. "Essential Amino Acids Search, egg whole". Retrieved 2010-10-10.

51. Helena Kloosterman; USDA National Nutrient Database for Standard Reference. "Essential Amino Acids Search, pea split". Retrieved 2010-10-10.

52. Helena Kloosterman; USDA National Nutrient Database for Standard Reference. "Essential Amino Acids Search, winged bean seeds". Retrieved 2010-10-10.

53. Helena Kloosterman; USDA National Nutrient Database for Standard Reference. "Essential Amino Acids Search, lentils". Retrieved 2010-10-10.

54. Helena Kloosterman; USDA National Nutrient Database for Standard Reference. "Essential Amino Acids Search, kidney bean". Retrieved 2010-10-10.

55. Helena Kloosterman; USDA National Nutrient Database for Standard Reference. "Essential Amino Acids Search, chickpea". Retrieved 2010-10-10.

56. Helena Kloosterman; USDA National Nutrient Database for Standard Reference. "Essential Amino Acids Search, soybeans sprouted". Retrieved 2010-10-10.

57. Helena Kloosterman; USDA National Nutrient Database for Standard Reference. "Essential Amino Acids Search, navy bean". Retrieved 2010-10-10.

58. Helena Kloosterman; USDA National Nutrient Database for Standard Reference. "Essential Amino Acids Search, amaranth". Retrieved 2010-10-10.

59. Hoffhines AJ, Damoc E, Bridges KG, Leary JA, Moore KL (2006). "Detection and purification of tyrosine-sulfated proteins using a novel anti-sulfotyrosine monoclonal antibody". J. Biol. Chem. 281 (49): 37877–87. doi:10.1074/jbc.M609398200. PMC 1764208 . PMID 17046811.

60. http://ndb.nal.usda.gov/ndb/nutrients/report/nutrientsfrm?max=25&offset=0&totCount=0&nutrient1=505&nutrient2=203&nutrient3=&subset=1&fg=&sort=c&measureby=g

61. Humphrey, Cara E.; Furegati, Markus; Laumen, Kurt; La Vecchia, Luigi; Leutert, Thomas; Müller-Hartwieg, J. Constanze D.; Vögtle, Markus (2007). "Optimized Synthesis of L-m-Tyrosine Suitable for Chemical Scale-Up". Organic Process Research & Development. 11: 1069–1075. doi:10.1021/op700093y.

62. Institute of Medicine of the National Academies. "Dietary Reference Intakes for Macronutrients". Retrieved 2010-10-10.

63. IUPAC-IUBMB Joint Commission on Biochemical Nomenclature (1983). "Nomenclature and Symbolism for Amino Acids and Peptides". Recommendations on Organic & Biochemical Nomenclature, Symbols & Terminology. Retrieved 2007-05-17.

64. IUPAC-IUBMB Joint Commission on Biochemical Nomenclature. "Nomenclature and Symbolism for Amino Acids and Peptides". Recommendations on Organic &

Biochemical Nomenclature, Symbols & Terminology etc. Retrieved 2007-05-17.

65. J. Rosenthal, et al. Department of Medicine, University of Toronto, Toronto, Canada. "Metabolic fate of leucine: A significant sterol precursor in adipose tissue and muscle". American Journal of Physiology Vol. 226, No. 2, p. 411-418. Retrieved 25 March 2008.
66. Kohlmeier M (2015). "Leucine". Nutrient Metabolism: Structures, Functions, and Genes (2nd ed.). Academic Press. pp. 385–388. ISBN 9780123877840. Retrieved 6 June 2016. Figure 8.57: Metabolism of L-leucine
67. L. Combaret, et al. Human Nutrition Research Centre of Clermont-Ferrand. "A leucine-supplemented diet restores the defective postprandial inhibition of proteasome-dependent proteolysis in aged rat skeletal muscle". Journal of Physiology Volume 569, issue 2, p. 489-499. Retrieved 25 March 2008.
68. Leathwood PD, Pollet P (1982). "Diet-induced mood changes in normal populations". Journal of Psychiatric Research. 17 (2): 147–54. doi:10.1016/0022-3956(82)90016-4. PMID 6764931.
69. Lieberman HR, Corkin S, Spring BJ, Wurtman RJ, Growdon JH (1985). "The effects of dietary neurotransmitter precursors on human behavior". Am J Clin Nutr. 42 (2): 366–370. PMID 4025206.
70. Lindemann L, Hoener MC (May 2005). "A renaissance in trace amines inspired by a novel GPCR family". Trends Pharmacol. Sci. 26 (5): 274–281. doi:10.1016/j.tips.2005.03.007. PMID 15860375.
71. Lutke-Eversloh, T., Santos, C.N.S. (2007) Perspectives of biotechnological production of L-tyrosine and its applications. Appl. Microbiol. Biotechnol. 77: 751-762. PMID 17968539
72. Lutke-Eversloh, T., Santos, C.N.S. (2007) Perspectives of biotechnological production of L-tyrosine and its applications. Appl. Microbiol. Biotechnol. 77: 751-762
73. Lynch, Christopher J.; Adams, Sean H. (1 December 2014). "Branched-chain amino acids in metabolic signalling and insulin resistance". Nature Reviews. Endocrinology. 10 (12): 723–736. doi:10.1038/nrendo.2014.171. ISSN 1759-5037. PMC 4424797 . PMID 25287287.
74. Lysine. The Biology Project, Department of Biochemistry and Molecular Biophysics, University of Arizona.
75. Magill RA, Waters WF, Bray GA, Volaufova J, Smith SR, Lieberman HR, McNevin N, Ryan DH (2003). "Effects of tyrosine, phentermine, caffeine D-amphetamine, and placebo on cognitive and motor performance deficits during sleep deprivation". Nutritional Neuroscience. 6 (4): 237–46. doi:10.1080/10284 15031000120552. PMID 12887140.
76. Mahoney CR, Castellani J, Kramer FM, Young A, Lieberman HR (2007). "Tyrosine supplementation mitigates working memory decrements during cold exposure". Physiology and Behavior. IN PRESS (4): 575–82. doi:10.1016/j.physbeh.2007.05.003. PMID 17585971.

77. Meierhenrich: Amino acids and the asymmetry of life, Springer-Verlag, 2008, ISBN 978-3-540-76885-2.

78. Mock DM, Stratton SL, Horvath TD, Bogusiewicz A, Matthews NI, Henrich CL, Dawson AM, Spencer HJ, Owen SN, Boysen G, Moran JH (November 2011).

79. Molnár GA, Nemes V, Biró Z, Ludány A, Wagner Z, Wittmann I (2005). "Accumulation of the hydroxyl free radical markers meta-, ortho-tyrosine and DOPA in cataractous lenses is accompanied by a lower protein and phenylalanine content of the water-soluble phase". Free Radic. Res. 39 (12): 1359–66. doi:10.1080/10715760500307107. PMID 16298866.

80. Molnár GA, Wagner Z, Markó L, Kó Szegi T, Mohás M, Kocsis B, Matus Z, Wagner L, Tamaskó M, Mazák I, Laczy B, Nagy J, Wittmann I (2005). "Urinary ortho-tyrosine excretion in diabetes mellitus and renal failure: evidence for hydroxyl radical production". Kidney Int. 68 (5): 2281–7. doi:10.1111/j.1523-1755.2005.00687.x. PMID 16221230.

81. National Nutrient Database for Standard Reference. U.S. Department of Agriculture. Retrieved 16 September 2009.

82. Nelson, D. L.; Cox, M. M. "Lehninger, Principles of Biochemistry" 3rd Ed. Worth Publishing: New York, 2000. ISBN 1-57259-153-6.

83. Neri DF, Wiegmann D, Stanny RR, Shappell SA, McCardie A, McKay DL (1995). "The effects of tyrosine on cognitive performance during extended wakefulness". Aviation, space, and environmental medicine. 66 (4): 313–9. PMID 7794222.

84. Oelke, E.A.; Putnam, D.H.; Teynor, T.M.; Oplinger, E.S. "Quinoa". Alternative Field Crops Manual. University of Wisconsin Cooperative Extension. Retrieved 11 September 2012.

85. Pfefferle, W.; Möckel, B.; Bathe, B.; Marx, A. (2003). "Biotechnological manufacture of lysine". Advances in Biochemical Engineering/Biotechnology. Advances in Biochemical Engineering/Biotechnology. 79: 59–112. doi:10.1007/3-540-45989-8_3. ISBN 978-3-540-43383-5. PMID 12523389.

86. Rasmussen B, Gilbert E, Turki A, Madden K, Elango R (2016). "Determination of the safety of leucine supplementation in healthy elderly men". Amino Acids. 48: 1707–16. doi:10.1007/s00726-016-2241-0. PMID 27138628. Retrieved 6 May 2016. the upper limit for leucine intake in healthy elderly could be set similar to young men at 500 mg kg-1 day-1 or ~35 g/day for an individual weighing 70 kg

87. Rasmussen DD, Ishizuka B, Quigley ME, Yen SS (1983). "Effects of tyrosine and tryptophan ingestion on plasma catecholamine and 3,4-dihydroxyphenylacetic acid concentrations". J. Clin. Endocrinol. Metab. 57 (4): 760–3. doi:10.1210/jcem-57-4-760. PMID 6885965.

88. Reinstein DK, Lehnert H, Wurtman RJ (1985). "Dietary tyrosine suppresses the rise in plasma corticosterone following acute stress in rats". Life Sci. 37 (23): 2157–63. doi:10.1016/0024-3205(85)90566-1. PMID 4068899.

89. Sadoul K, Boyault C, Pabion M, Khochbin S (February 2008). "Regulation of protein turnover by acetyltransferases and deacetylases". Biochimie. 90 (2):

306–12. doi:10.1016/j.biochi.2007.06.009. PMID 17681659.

90. Saxton, Robert A.; Knockenhauer, Kevin E.; Wolfson, Rachel L.; Chantranupong, Lynne; Pacold, Michael E.; Wang, Tim; Schwartz, Thomas U.; Sabatini, David M. (1 January 2016). "Structural basis for leucine sensing by the Sestrin2-mTORC1 pathway". Science. 351 (6268): 53–58. doi:10.1126/science.aad2087. ISSN 1095-9203. PMC 4698039 . PMID 26586190.
91. ScienceDaily. "Chemists Kill Cancer Cells With Light-activated Molecules". Retrieved 2008-01-24.
92. Sebastiaan Boll and Evelien M. Bunnik (November 2015). "Lysine supplementation is not effective for the prevention or treatment of feline herpesvirus 1 infection in cats: a systematic review". BMC Veterinary Research. 11 (1): 284. doi:10.1186/s12917-015-0594-3. PMC 4647294 . PMID 26573523.
93. Smriga and Torii; Torii, K (2003). "l-Lysine acts like a partial serotonin receptor 4 antagonist and inhibits serotonin-mediated intestinal pathologies and anxiety in rats". PNAS. 100 (26): 15370–5. doi:10.1073/pnas.2436556100. PMC 307574 . PMID 14676321.
94. Smriga, Ghosh, Mouneimne, Pellett, and Scrimshaw (May 2004). "Lysine fortification reduces anxiety and lessens stress in family members in economically weak communities in Northwest Syria". Proceedings of the National Academy of Sciences. 101 (22): 8285–8288. doi:10.1073/pnas.0402550101.
95. Smriga, Kameishi, Uneyama, and Torii (December 2002). "Dietary L-Lysine Deficiency Increases Stress-Induced Anxiety and Fecal Excretion in Rats". The Journal of Nutrition. 132 (12): 3744–6. PMID 12468617.
96. Strüder HK, Hollmann W, Platen P, Donike M, Gotzmann A, Weber K (1998). "Influence of paroxetine, branched-chain amino acids and tyrosine on neuroendocrine system responses and fatigue in humans". Horm. Metab. Res. 30 (4): 188–94. doi:10.1055/s-2007-978864. PMID 9623632.
97. Thomas JR, Lockwood PA, Singh A, Deuster PA (1999). "Tyrosine improves working memory in a multitasking environment". Pharmacol. Biochem. Behav. 64 (3): 495–500. doi:10.1016/S0091-3057(99)00094-5. PMID 10548261.
98. title=Nutrition Data url=http://nutritiondata.self.com/facts/nut-and-seed-products/3066/2
99. Toride Y. "Lysine and other amino acids for feed: production and contribution to protein utilization in animal feeding". Retrieved 2011-01-25.
100. United Nations Food & Agriculture Organization : Agriculture and Consumer Protection. "Energy and protein requirements: 5.6 Requirements for essential amino acids". Retrieved 2010-10-10.
101. University of Maryland Medical Center. "Lysine". Retrieved 2009-12-30.
102. Verhoeven, Suzanne; Vanschoonbeek, Kristof; Verdijk, Lex B.; Koopman, René; Wodzig, Will K.W.H.; Dendale, Paul; van Loon, Luc JC (May 2009). "Long-term leucine supplementation does not increase muscle mass or strength in healthy elderly men". Am J Clin Nutr. 89 (5): 1468–75. doi:10.3945/ajcn.2008.26668.

PMID 19321567.

103. Wang X, Li J, Dong G, Yue J (February 2014). "The endogenous substrates of brain CYP2D". Eur. J. Pharmacol. 724: 211–218. doi:10.1016/j.ejphar.2013.12.025. PMID 24374199. CYP2D4 (433 μm) > CYP2D2 ≈ CYP2D6 > CYP2D18 (688 μm) for p-tyramine

104. Wilson JM, Fitschen PJ, Campbell B, Wilson GJ, Zanchi N, Taylor L, Wilborn C, Kalman DS, Stout JR, Hoffman JR, Ziegenfuss TN, Lopez HL, Kreider RB, Smith-Ryan AE, Antonio J (February 2013). "International Society of Sports Nutrition Position Stand: beta-hydroxy-beta-methylbutyrate (HMB)". J. Int. Soc. Sports. Nutr. 10 (1): 6. doi:10.1186/1550-2783-10-6. PMC 3568064 . PMID 23374455.

105. Winter, Ruth (2009). A consumer's dictionary of food additives (7th ed.). New York: Three Rivers Press. ISBN 0307408922.

106. Wolfson, Rachel L.; Chantranupong, Lynne; Saxton, Robert A.; Shen, Kuang; Scaria, Sonia M.; Cantor, Jason R.; Sabatini, David M. (1 January 2016). "Sestrin2 is a leucine sensor for the mTORC1 pathway". Science. 351 (6268): 43–48. doi:10.1126/science.aab2674. ISSN 1095-9203. PMC 4698017 . PMID 26449471.

107. Wu, G (2009). "Amino acids: Metabolism, functions, and nutrition". Amino Acids. 37 (1): 1–17. doi:10.1007/s00726-009-0269-0. PMID 19301095.

108. Young VR, Pellett PL (1994). "Plant proteins in relation to human protein and amino acid nutrition" (PDF). American Journal of Clinical Nutrition. 59 (5 Suppl): 1203S–1212S. PMID 8172124.

109. Zanchi NE, Gerlinger-Romero F, Guimarães-Ferreira L, de Siqueira Filho MA, Felitti V, Lira FS, Seelaender M, Lancha AH (April 2011). "HMB supplementation: clinical and athletic performance-related effects and mechanisms of action". Amino Acids. 40 (4): 1015–1025. doi:10.1007/s00726-010-0678-0. PMID 20607321. HMB is a metabolite of the amino acid leucine (Van Koverin and Nissen 1992), an essential amino acid.

Index

S

T

V